Ethics in Psychiatry: A Review

Guest Editors

LAURA WEISS ROBERTS, MD, MA
JINGER G. HOOP, MD, MFA

PSYCHIATRIC CLINICS OF NORTH AMERICA

www.psych.theclinics.com

June 2009 • Volume 32 • Number 2

SAUNDERS an imprint of ELSEVIER, Inc.

W.B. SAUNDERS COMPANY
A Division of Elsevier Inc.

1600 John F. Kennedy Boulevard • Suite 1800 • Philadelphia, PA 19103-2899

http://www.theclinics.com

PSYCHIATRIC CLINICS OF NORTH AMERICA Volume 32, Number 2
June 2009 ISSN 0193-953X, ISBN-13: 978-1-4377-0535-5, ISBN-10: 1-4377-0535-9

Editor: Sarah E. Barth
Developmental Editor: Donald Mumford

Psychiatric Clinics of North America (ISSN 0193-953X) is published quarterly by Elsevier Inc., 360 Park Avenue South, New York, NY 10010-1710. Months of issue are March, June, September, and December. Business and Editorial Offices: 1600 John F. Kennedy Blvd., Suite 1800, Philadelphia, PA 19103-2899. Periodicals postage paid at New York, NY and additional mailing offices. Subscription prices are $230.00 per year (US individuals), $398.00 per year (US institutions), $116.00 per year (US students/residents), $275.00 per year (Canadian individuals), $495.00 per year (Canadian Institutions), $342.00 per year (foreign individuals), $495.00 per year (foreign institutions), and $171.00 per year (international & Canadian students/residents). Foreign air speed delivery is included in all *Clinics'* subscription prices. All prices are subject to change without notice. **POSTMASTER:** Send address changes to *Psychiatric Clinics of North America*, Elsevier Periodicals Customer Service, 11830 Westline Industrial Drive, St. Louis, MO 63146. Customer Service: 1-800-654-2452 (US). From outside the United States, call 1-314-453-7041. Fax: 1-314-453-5170. E-mail: JournalsCustomer Service-usa@elsevier.com (for print support) and JournalsOnlineSupport-usa@elsevier.com (for online support).

Reprints. For copies of 100 or more, of articles in this publication, please contact the Commercial Reprints Department, Elsevier Inc., 360 Park Avenue South, New York, New York 10010-1710. Tel.: (212) 633-3813, Fax: (212) 462-1935, E-mail: reprints@elsevier.com.

Psychiatric Clinics of North America is covered in *MEDLINE/PubMed (Index Medicus)*, *Current Contents/Social and Behavioral Sciences*, *Social Science Citation Index*, *Embase/Excerpta Medica*, and PsycINFO.

Printed and bound by CPI Group (UK) Ltd, Croydon, CR0 4YY
Transferred to Digital Print 2011

Contributors

GUEST EDITORS

LAURA WEISS ROBERTS, MD, MA
Charles E. Kubly Professor and Chairman, Department of Psychiatry and Behavioral Medicine, Medical College of Wisconsin; and Professor of Bioethics, Department of Population Health, Medical College of Wisconsin, Milwaukee, Wisconsin

JINGER G. HOOP, MD, MFA
Assistant Professor, Department of Psychiatry and Behavioral Medicine, Medical College of Wisconsin, Milwaukee, Wisconsin

AUTHORS

GEORGE N. APPENZELLER, MD, LTC, MC, USA
Medical Chief of Staff, Winn Army Community Hospital, Fort Stewart, Georgia

ROBERT A. BAILEY, MD
Professor, Department of Psychiatry, and Associate Dean for Clinical Affairs, University of New Mexico School of Medicine, Albuquerque, New Mexico

LILIANA KALOGJERA BARRY, JD
Assistant Clinical Professor, Department of Psychiatry and Behavioral Medicine, Medical College of Wisconsin; and Staff Attorney, United States Department of Veterans Affairs, Office of Regional Counsel, Milwaukee, Wisconsin

JERALD BELITZ, PhD
Associate Professor and Chief Psychologist, Department of Psychiatry, University of New Mexico School of Medicine, Albuquerque, New Mexico

DAVID M. BENEDEK, MD, COL, MC, USA
Professor, Department of Psychiatry, Uniformed Services University of the Health Sciences, Bethesda, Maryland

MICHAEL P. BOGENSCHUTZ, MD
Professor and Vice-Chair for Addictions, Department of Psychiatry, University of New Mexico School of Medicine, Albuquerque, New Mexico

PHILIP J. CANDILIS, MD
Associate Professor of Psychiatry, Law and Psychiatry Program, University of Massachusetts Medical School, Worcester, Massachusetts

DONNA T. CHEN, MD, MPH
Assistant Professor of Biomedical Ethics, Psychiatry, and Public Health Sciences, Center for Biomedical Ethics and Humanities, University of Virginia Health System; Department of Public Health Sciences, University of Virginia School of Medicine; and Department of Psychiatry and Neurobehavioral Sciences, University of Virginia School of Medicine, Charlottesville, Virginia

JOHN COVERDALE, MD, MEd, FRANZCP
Professor of Psychiatry and Behavioral Sciences and of Medical Ethics, Menninger
Department of Psychiatry and Behavioral Sciences, and Center for Medical Ethics and
Health Policy, Baylor College of Medicine, Houston, Texas

LAURA B. DUNN, MD
Associate Professor and Director of Psycho-oncology, Department of Psychiatry,
University of California, San Francisco, California

ANITA EVERETT, MD, DFAPA
Section Director, Community and General Psychiatry, Johns Hopkins School of Medicine,
Bayview Campus, Baltimore, Maryland

CYNTHIA M.A. GEPPERT, MD, PhD, MPH
Chief Consultation, Psychiatry and Ethics, New Mexico Veterans Affairs Health Care
System; and Associate Professor of Psychiatry and Director of Ethics Education,
Department of Psychiatry, University of New Mexico School of Medicine, Albuquerque,
New Mexico

THOMAS A. GRIEGER, MD, DFAPA, CAPT, MC, USN (Ret)
Department of Psychiatry, Uniformed Services University of the Health Sciences,
Bethesda, Maryland

JINGER G. HOOP, MD, MFA
Assistant Professor, Department of Psychiatry and Behavioral Medicine, Medical College
of Wisconsin, Milwaukee, Wisconsin

CHARLES HUFFINE, MD
Assistant Medical Director, Child and Adolescent Programs, King County Mental Health,
Chemical Abuse and Dependency Service, Seattle, Washington

SHAILI JAIN, MD
General Adult Psychiatrist, Aurora Psychiatric Hospital, Wauwatosa; and Clinical
Assistant Professor of Psychiatry, Department of Psychiatry and Behavioral Medicine,
Medical College of Wisconsin, Milwaukee, Wisconsin

LAURENCE B. McCULLOUGH, PhD
Dalton Tomlin Chair in Medical Ethics and Health Policy, Baylor College of Medicine,
Houston, Texas

LAURA J. MILLER, MD
Professor and Director, Women's Mental Health Program, Department of Psychiatry,
University of Illinois at Chicago, Chicago, Illinois

SAHANA MISRA, MD
Staff Psychiatrist and Assistant Professor, Mental Health Division, Portland VA Medical
Center; Department of Psychiatry, Oregon Health & Science University, Portland, Oregon

LAURA WEISS ROBERTS, MD, MA
Charles E. Kubly Professor and Chairman, Department of Psychiatry and Behavioral
Medicine, Medical College of Wisconsin; and Professor of Bioethics, Department of
Population Health, Medical College of Wisconsin, Milwaukee, Wisconsin

LOIS L. SHEPHERD, JD
Associate Professor of Biomedical Ethics and Public Health Sciences, and Professor of Law, Center for Biomedical Ethics and Humanities, University of Virginia Health System; Department of Public Health Sciences, University of Virginia School of Medicine; School of Law, University of Virginia, Charlottesville, Virginia

RYAN SPELLECY, PhD
Assistant Professor, Center for the Study of Bioethics, Medical College of Wisconsin; and Assistant Professor, Department of Psychiatry and Behavioral Medicine, Medical College of Wisconsin, Milwaukee, Wisconsin

ART WALASZEK, MD
Associate Professor of Psychiatry and Residency Training Director, Department of Psychiatry, University of Wisconsin School of Medicine and Public Health, Madison, Wisconsin

CHRISTOPHER H. WARNER, MD, MAJ, MC, USA
Department of Behavioral Medicine, Winn Army Community Hospital, Fort Stewart, Georgia

MARK T. WRIGHT, MD
Associate Professor, Department of Psychiatry and Behavioral Medicine, Medical College of Wisconsin; and Associate Professor, Department of Neurology, Medical College of Wisconsin, Milwaukee, Wisconsin

Contents

Preface   xiii

Laura Weiss Roberts and Jinger G. Hoop

Clinical Ethics for the Treatment of Children and Adolescents:
A Guide for General Psychiatrists   243

Jerald Belitz and Robert A. Bailey

> This article is written for the general psychiatrist whose practice does not customarily include children and adolescents but has occasion to work with youths who present with neurobiological disorders or serious emotional disorders that fall under the rubric of childhood psychiatric diagnoses. It discusses the unique ethical considerations that general psychiatrists may not routinely encounter. It reviews ethical concerns related to such themes as informed consent, confidentiality, documentation about other family members, familial and cultural practices, professional competence, mandatory treatment, evidence-based practices, boundary issues, and research practices. The intent is to provide psychiatrists with an enhanced awareness of those ethical considerations, a broad framework for comprehending and addressing those issues, and additional resources for further development. The goal is to help the reader achieve competency, rather than expertise.

Ethical Issues in Perinatal Mental Health   259

Laura J. Miller

> The principles of medical ethics can guide clinicians toward solutions to dilemmas involving the mental health treatment of women who are pregnant, postpartum, or trying to conceive. In situations that seem to pit the needs of a perinatal woman against the needs of her fetus or baby, clinicians can reframe the problem to find a solution that most benefits the mother–baby dyad. A woman's ability to make informed decisions about medical care includes her ability to decide on behalf of her fetus. Explanations of the risks of psychiatric treatments must be balanced with explanations of the risks of the untreated symptoms. Using these guidelines helps ensure that women are not stigmatized by having psychiatric disorders or by being pregnant.

Ethical Considerations in Military Psychiatry   271

Christopher H. Warner, George N. Appenzeller, Thomas A. Grieger,
David M. Benedek, and Laura Weiss Roberts

> Military psychiatrists face multiple unique issues in combat and at home. At the root of many of these issues is the question "For whom does the psychiatrist work—the service member-patient or the military?" We review several of the key issues faced by a military psychiatrist, including confidentiality, informed consent, dual agency, boundaries, dealing with

detainees, determining fitness for deployments, treatment in combat, and separation from the military.

Ethics in Substance Use Disorder Treatment   283

Cynthia M.A. Geppert and Michael P. Bogenschutz

Substance use disorders are a significant public health problem in the United States and because of their prevalence almost every clinician encounters ethical dilemmas in this area. Although substance abuse treatment is grounded in the principles and values of clinical ethics, the increased stigma, diminished autonomy, and lack of social justice in substance abuse treatment represent distinct contextual features. Three salient features of that distinctiveness frame this review of ethics in substance use disorders treatment. The first is social stigma and the way it has influenced confidentiality protections in substance use treatment and research. The second is the role of autonomy and personal responsibility as it relates to informed consent and decisional capacity. The third is social justice as manifested in the struggle for parity.

Ethics in Psychotherapy: A Focus on Professional Boundaries and Confidentiality Practices   299

Shaili Jain and Laura Weiss Roberts

This article examines two key ethics topics in psychotherapy: professional boundaries and confidentiality. These topics pertain to all therapeutic modalities, encompassing supportive and cognitive-behavioral therapy, psychoanalysis, psychodynamic and combined medication management, and related psychotherapy approaches undertaken by psychiatrists. The discussion demonstrates a continued relevance to the contemporary therapist. The nature of the dilemmas may have changed (eg, how to use e-mail communication in therapy), but the need for the therapist to display ethical competence remains vital. In light of the issues of the medical profession in relation to the public trust, the ethics of psychotherapy may be more critical than ever before.

A Basic Decision-Making Approach to Common Ethical Issues in Consultation-Liaison Psychiatry   315

Mark T. Wright and Laura Weiss Roberts

Ethical dilemmas abound in psychosomatic medicine, and for many reasons, consultation-liaison psychiatrists are called on to help resolve complex ethical issues in clinical care settings. Unfortunately, most psychiatrists have had little training in clinical ethics to prepare them for this important professional responsibility. Consultation-liaison psychiatrists do not need to become clinical ethicists, but these subspecialty physicians may find it valuable to have increased expertise when handling the ethical issues commonly seen in diverse clinical settings. Here, we offer a method of ethical analysis and decision making (the Four Topics Method) and four illustrations drawn from real and complicated medical-psychiatric cases that may be useful to consultation-liaison psychiatrists.

Ethics in Contemporary Community Psychiatry   **329**

Anita Everett and Charles Huffine

This article builds on the existing values and ethical foundations of medical ethics and develops them such that they are applicable to community psychiatry. The authors address ethical foundations that apply to clinical settings and administrative and advocacy roles. This article has two central goals: (1) to provide community psychiatrists a framework in which to approach a novel ethical situation and (2) to provide general psychiatrists with a broadened understanding of applied ethics in the many novel situations encountered in contemporary community psychiatry practice.

Clinical Ethics Issues in Geriatric Psychiatry   **343**

Art Walaszek

Psychiatrists treating older adults must address a rich mixture of medical, psychiatric, and psychosocial issues that may lead to ethical dilemmas involving autonomy, patient welfare, and social justice. Because of the potentially disabling effects of neuropsychiatric conditions disproportionately affecting older adults, their autonomy may become compromised. Psychiatrists thus become involved in assessing decisional and other types of capacity and in treating conditions that may affect capacity. The balance of risks and benefits of medical interventions must be weighed carefully in older adults, especially in the settings of dementia and end-of-life care. Finally, the care of older adults raises difficult questions about the allocation of scarce medical resources.

When, Why, and How to Conduct Research in Child and Adolescent Psychiatry: Practical and Ethical Considerations   **361**

Donna T. Chen and Lois L. Shepherd

Several excellent overviews of the ethical issues that arise in child and adolescent psychiatric research have been published in recent years and serve to focus attention on the many ethical and practical challenges inherent in this work. This article extends these discussions by focusing on some important decision points through case discussions.

Ethical Issues in Psychiatric Research   **381**

Liliana Kalogjera Barry

The psychiatric research imperative remains strong, as investigators strive for greater understanding of mental illness, which affects millions of people in the United States alone. With the need for research, however, comes an obligation to conduct such research in a manner that protects and respects participants. Accordingly, the field of psychiatric research ethics continues to grow in depth and breadth. Initial debates, which focused on the ethical permissibility of research involving participants who have mental illness, have evolved into more nuanced inquiries, both theoretical and empirical. These inquiries can provide a greater understanding of the imperatives and boundaries for psychiatric research.

Research Ethics Issues in Geriatric Psychiatry   395

Laura B. Dunn and Sahana Misra

With an aging population and with the prevalence of psychiatric illness in the older population expected to rise dramatically in coming decades, advances in geriatric psychiatry research are urgently needed. Ethical issues in the design, conduct, and monitoring of research involving older adults parallel the same issues as related to human subjects research generally. However, a number of special issues relevant to geriatric psychiatry research merit further discussion. These special issues include: the assessment of capacity in populations where cognitive disorders are more prevalent; the role of surrogate decision makers; the legal status of surrogate consent; the use of advanced directives for research participation; and research involving suicidal individuals.

The Ethics of Psychiatric Education   413

John Coverdale, Laurence B. McCullough, and Laura Weiss Roberts

This article discusses the central elements of the ethics of psychiatric education. This discussion is framed in light of the work of John Gregory, whose medical ethics helped shape medicine as a profession. References to John Gregory's medical ethics are used here to inform the ethics of psychiatric education in three selected areas of importance to the profession: the management of suicidal patients, managing sexual boundaries between psychiatrists and patients, and avoiding conflicts of interest.

The Revolution in Forensic Ethics: Narrative, Compassion, and a Robust
Professionalism   423

Philip J. Candilis

For 5 decades modern forensic psychiatry has struggled with the seminal question of which master it serves: is it a field that answers chiefly to the law or to psychiatry? It is the law, after all, that privileges forensic experts in the courtroom, but it is psychiatry that grounds them in the medical ethics of care and cure. In reviewing the historical narrative of modern forensic ethics, this article explores whether the field has developed to the point that it is insufficient to apply legal or medical ethics alone. Rather, a more robust professionalism of broader perspectives, mixed theories, and basic ethical habits and skills may foster better understanding of the complex intersection of psychiatry and the law.

Philosophical and Ethical Issues at the Forefront of Neuroscience and Genetics: An Overview for Psychiatrists   **437**

Jinger G. Hoop and Ryan Spellecy

The rapid pace of research advances in neuroscience and genetics has given rise to a new field of study, neuroethics, which seeks to explore the moral questions that arise from the use of new brain-based therapies and from our growing understanding of the biology of human behavior, cognition, and emotion. The authors present an overview of selected topics in neuroethics that may be of special interest to psychiatrists, including a discussion of how genetics and functional neuroimaging have added nuance and complexity to mind/body dualism, the concept of free will, and the proper role of emotion in morality. Other topics include the use of brain-based therapies such as neuromodulation, psychopharmacology, and genetic technologies as enhancements to normal mental functioning.

Index   **451**

FORTHCOMING ISSUES

September 2009
Anxiety
Hans-Ulrich Wittchen, MD and
Andrew T. Gloster, PhD, *Guest Editors*

December 2009
Schizophrenia Comorbidities
Michael Hwang, MD and
Henry Nasrallah, MD, *Guest Editors*

March 2010
Genetics
James B. Potash, MD,
Guest Editor

RECENT ISSUES

March 2009
Child and Adolescent Psychiatry
for the General Psychiatrist
Malia McCarthy, MD and
Robert L. Hendren, DO,
Guest Editors

December 2008
Sexually Compulsive Behavior:
Hypersexuality
Mark F. Schwartz, ScD and
Fred S. Berlin, MD, PhD, *Guest Editors*

September 2008
Recent Research in Personality Disorders
Joel Paris, MD, *Guest Editor*

RELATED INTEREST

Child and Adolescent Psychiatry Clinics of North America, January 2008
(Vol. 17, No. 1)
Ethics
Mary Lynn Dell, MD, MTS, ThM, *Guest Editor*

THE CLINICS ARE NOW AVAILABLE ONLINE!

Access your subscription at:
www.theclinics.com

Preface

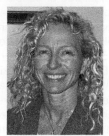 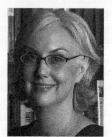

Laura Weiss Roberts, MD, MA   Jinger G. Hoop, MD, MFA
Guest Editors

All good psychiatrists are ethicists. Sound ethical reasoning and moral judgment are essential to the work of a physician. Psychiatrists make ethically complex decisions on a daily basis: Which details about a patient's care should be disclosed to an insurer? Where should the therapeutic frame boundaries be set? How should suspicions of impairment in a colleague be handled? When is it best to visit—and revisit—informed consent discussions in providing care for diseases that may be relentless in their effects on cognition and volition? When should the privilege of confidentiality be set aside in obeying the law? And when is it appropriate to intervene with a patient in grave danger due to severe neuropsychiatric illnesses? For this reason, psychiatrists develop specialized expertise in certain kinds of ethics issues just as they develop specialized expertise in certain aspects of clinical medicine. Over time, the thoughtful, self-reflective practice of psychiatry can strengthen one's ethics skills of identifying, approaching, and resolving moral dilemmas that arise in professional work (eg, clinical care, consultation, research, and training) with people living with mental illness. Over time, good psychiatrists may also develop wisdom as they repeatedly enact their commitment to the virtues of compassion, empathy, fidelity, veracity, self-effacement, and integrity.

In assembling this collection of articles, we viewed the current landscape of psychiatric ethics through two converging lenses: One focused on ethical issues arising in relation to mental illness prior to birth until old age and the other focused on the diverse roles that psychiatrists assume in the course of their professional work. This issue thus begins with eight articles on the ethical practice of clinical psychiatry. In the first article, "Clinical Ethics for the Treatment of Children and Adolescents: A Guide for General Psychiatrists," Belitz and Bailey provide general psychiatrists with a succinct overview of the ethical issues of distinct importance in mental health care involving children and adolescents. Next, Miller's review, "Ethical Issues in Perinatal Mental Health," uses case examples to explore several concepts that are key to the mental health treatment of women during the perinatal period, including relational ethics, preventive ethics, and principles of informed consent.

"Ethical Considerations in Military Psychiatry," by Warner, Appenzeller, Grieger, Benedek, and Roberts, presents the key ethical dilemma facing military psychiatrists

Psychiatr Clin N Am 32 (2009) xiii–xv
doi:10.1016/j.psc.2009.04.001
0193-953X/09/$ – see front matter © 2009 Elsevier Inc. All rights reserved.

as one of dual agency: "For whom does the psychiatrist work—the service member–patient or the military?" The article by Geppert and Bogenschutz, "Ethics in Substance Abuse Treatment," describes how the contextual features of substance abuse treatment—stigma, diminished autonomy, and lack of parity—add a deep moral complexity to the care of patients struggling with addiction. "Ethics in Psychotherapy," by Jain and Roberts, demonstrates the continued relevance of discussions of professional boundaries and confidentiality practices for all contemporary psychotherapeutic modalities. In the article by Wright and Roberts, "A Basic Decision-Making Approach to Common Ethical Issues in Consultation-Liaison Psychiatry," a useful method for analyzing dilemmas in complex medical-psychiatric cases is offered, based on Jonsen and Siegler's[1,2] "four topics" model of ethical analysis and decision-making. Everett and Huffine's article, "Ethics in Contemporary Community Psychiatry," describes the ethical issues particular to clinical care in the context of public funding, nontraditional settings, and multidisciplinary teams. Rounding out the set of eight clinical articles is Walaszek's "Clinical Ethical Issues in Geriatric Psychiatry," which emphasizes the importance of respect for autonomy, patient welfare, and social justice in the care of older adults.

The next three articles provide a developmental perspective on psychiatric research ethics. First is Chen and Shepherd's "When, Why, and How to Conduct Research in Child and Adolescent Psychiatry," which uses case discussions to highlight key ethical considerations for clinical psychiatrists contemplating involvement in research. Next, "Ethical Issues in Psychiatric Research," by Barry, is a concise overview of the major topics in psychiatric research involving adults. After touching upon the initial debates over the ethical permissibility of research involving participants with mental illness, the article delves into more nuanced inquiries involving informed consent, placebo trials, and emerging research methods. Finally, "Research Ethics Issues in Geriatric Psychiatry," by Dunn and Misra, highlights special ethical issues in research on older patients—including assessment of decisional capacity, use of alternative decision-makers and advanced directives, and research involving suicidal individuals.

The final three articles demonstrate the importance of ethics to psychiatric endeavors beyond the treatment of patients and the conduct of research. These articles have a deeper grounding in history and moral philosophy, and they offer perspectives of importance to the future. Coverdale, McCullough, and Roberts' "The Ethics of Psychiatric Education" uses the seminal work of the eighteenth-century physician John Gregory as a touchstone for discussing psychiatric education regarding suicidal patients, boundaries, and conflicts of interest. Candilis' "Perspectives on the Revolution in Forensic Ethics" presents a historical narrative of the field of forensic psychiatry in terms of what the author identifies as its central ethical tension: "Is it a field that answers chiefly to the law or to psychiatry?" The issue concludes with a look at emerging issues in psychiatric ethics. Hoop and Spellecy survey the burgeoning field of neuroethics, which studies the ethical implications arising from research advances in the biology of brain functioning.

This collection is the first on the topic of psychiatric ethics to appear in *Psychiatric Clinics of North America* since 2002, when an issue on the same topic was published under the esteemed guest editorship of Glen O. Gabbard, MD.[3] A comparison of the content of the 2002 issue to the current one shows how the connection between psychiatry and ethics has evolved over the past 7 years. The psychiatric community's thinking about many fundamental clinical ethics issues—such as the clinical management of boundaries and confidentiality—appears to have changed little. However, our understanding of issues related to decisional capacity, especially for research participation, has clearly become more nuanced, thanks in part to a concerted effort by the National Institutes of Health to fund the work of dedicated psychiatric ethics researchers in this area. The 2002 issue included an article by terrorism expert Jerrold M. Post[4] regarding psychiatric profiling of political figures. The sweep of history since the terrorist attacks on the United States in 2001 now leads us to focus on the role of the psychiatrist in caring for the more than 100,000 actively deployed United States service personnel.

Finally, some ethics topics in 2009 appear to have become more salient in the past several years: the involvement of children, suicidal individuals, and other "vulnerable" persons in mental health research; social justice issues surrounding access to mental health care and substance abuse treatment; psychiatric care of veterans and soldiers; real and apparent conflicts of interest among psychiatrists with ties to industry; and profound moral questions raised by advances in cognitive neuroscience and molecular genetics. We look forward to robust discussion and debate among our psychiatrist colleagues on these and other ethical issues in the years to come.

Ethics is integral to contemporary psychiatry, and it has been our honor to edit this issue, which demonstrates this connection so clearly. We wish to express our sincere appreciation to our authors and to our editorial colleagues—Sarah Barth at Elsevier Publishing and Ann Tennier at the Medical College of Wisconsin.

Laura Weiss Roberts, MD, MA
Jinger G. Hoop, MD, MFA

Department of Psychiatry and Behavioral Medicine
Medical College of Wisconsin
8701 Watertown Plank Road
Milwaukee, WI 53226

E-mail addresses:
RobertsL@mcw.edu
jhoop@mcw.edu

REFERENCES

1. Siegler M. Decision-making strategy for clinical-ethical problems in medicine. Arch Intern Med 1982;142:2178–9.
2. Jonsen AR, Siegler M, Winslade WJ. Clinical ethics: a practical approach to ethical decisions in clinical medicine. 6th edition. New York: McGraw Hill, Medical Pub. Division; 2006.
3. Gabbard GO, editor. Ethics in psychiatry. Psychiatric Clin North Am 2002;25: 509–684.
4. Post JM. Ethical considerations in psychiatric profiling of political figures. Psychiatric Clin North Am 2002;25:635–46.

Box 1

Caring for children—core ethical issues

1. Children are inherently more vulnerable than adults.

2. Children's abilities are more variable and change over time.

3. Children are more reliant upon others and upon their environment.

4. Ethical principles and practices in the treatment of adults must be modified in response to the child's current developmental abilities and legal status.

5. Boundary and role issues are often more prevalent and more complex when caring for children than for adults.

6. Adult psychiatric practices, and the adult psychiatric knowledge base, do not transfer reliably to the care of children.

7. Practitioners must develop skills to work with families, agencies, and systems.

8. It is key to monitor one's own actions and motivations.

9. Seeking consultation and advice is helpful in difficult situations.

10. It is essential to maintain an absolute commitment to the safety and well-being of the patient.

---

present with neurobiological disorders or serious emotional disorders that fall under the rubric of childhood psychiatric diagnoses. It discusses the unique ethical considerations that general psychiatrists may not routinely encounter. It reviews ethical concerns related to such themes as informed consent, confidentiality, documentation about other family members, familial and cultural practices, professional competence, mandatory treatment, evidence-based practices, boundary issues, and research practices. The intent is to provide psychiatrists with an enhanced awareness of those ethical considerations, a broad framework for comprehending and addressing those issues, and additional resources for further development. The goal is to help the reader achieve competency, rather than expertise.

CHILDREN ARE DIFFERENT

Children are smaller than adults. This fact is obvious, but the practical and ethical implications are substantial. Being smaller, children are more readily intimidated by adults, even if unintentionally. Adults unavoidably look down at children, and children unavoidably look up at adults. The world is largely designed for adults; so although adults sit down, children must climb up. These simple physical facts both establish and illustrate the relative imbalance of power, influence, and authority between children and adults.

Children are inherently more vulnerable than most adults. The responsibility for assuring ethical action therefore resides more with the psychiatrist than is common with adult patients. Also, psychiatrists may simply acknowledge that adult patients are responsible for the consequences of their actions; however, adults have a responsibility to protect or buffer child patients from more substantial and unintended negative consequences. For example, if a responsible adult patient decides to quit his or her job, that decision may be respected as the patient's autonomous choice. In contrast, if a young adolescent decides to quit school, questions arise as to how informed a young adolescent is about the consequences of such an act, how competent the adolescent is to make such a choice, and the degree to which the psychiatrist (as well as parents) may be obliged to question or confront such action.

Children also differ from one another. In a very real way, there is no such category as "children." Infants differ from toddlers, who differ from preschoolers, who differ from school-aged children, and so on. Furthermore, within any one group of children there is wide variability in size, ability, and maturity. Many children experience significant variability among their own maturational abilities—physical, cognitive, emotional, social, and moral. Finally, the individual child may progress and regress in the face of various challenges or traumas, being "childish" one day and a "young man" or "young lady" the next. Essentially, although adulthood certainly has particular developmental stages, children manifest much broader developmental and individual variability than do adults. As a consequence, the psychiatrist must attend much more closely to the state and abilities of the child patient, at times even from moment to moment. The child's ability to engage in particular aspects of care, including its ethical aspects, or to move toward particular goals of treatment may vary with the child's immediate developmental abilities, themes, challenges, and tasks.

Another consequence of the relatively rapid development of children is that small actions may have much greater consequences. A small nudge toward health may, over time, be of great benefit; on the other hand, a small negative deviation in the developmental course early on may be of great consequence by adulthood. As a result, the child's psychiatrist must be especially attentive to the possible negative developmental implications of each intervention. Although there may be less tolerance for error in treating children, this risk is balanced positively by the fact that children often are more forgiving of adults and may reward relatively small investments of resources with disproportionate positive outcomes.

Children also are more reliant upon their environment, especially their social environment. Children are less able to shape their environment to meet their needs and consequently must accommodate themselves to their external world. Indeed, the child who is especially assertive in attempting to alter the environment may be perceived as presumptuous, willful, or oppositional. Young children depend upon adults for the basics of life—food, clothing, shelter—and, fundamentally, their very survival. The emotional implications of such dependency and vulnerability cannot be overestimated. Additionally, children are psychologically and emotionally dependent on their parents, teachers, and other significant adults. Children are more receptive to adult support and sustenance; however, they also are more susceptible to experiencing adults as negating and invalidating. Because of this dependence, unthinkingly treating a youth as an autonomous ethical agent may be well intentioned but may require more than the child can deliver and therefore may go against the child's best interests. As Winnicott[1] perceptively noted, even the adolescent who is seemingly striving for autonomy may at times very much need the freedom to be immature that is made possible only by a firm and reassuring parental presence. This consideration in no way diminishes the importance of respecting each child's integrity and right to assent voluntarily to treatment.

As a rule, children have many more expectations and mandates placed on them by society, have a more limited set of adaptive abilities, and are granted fewer behavioral options than adults. For example, adults have a relatively broad range of vocational options available, each with its own set of advantages and demands; children, however, must go to school. Adults may avoid certain behavioral or ethical demands simply by avoiding the circumstances in which they arise; children often are unable to avail themselves of such environmental and behavioral flexibility.

PROFESSIONAL COMPETENCY

This section addresses the competency of the treating psychiatrist, rather than the child's decision-making competency (discussed elsewhere in this article). A fundamental principle of medical ethics is that, outside of extenuating circumstances, physicians provide only care that they are competent to deliver. Clinical competency is especially important when working with children, given the greater potential impact on their developing brains and selves and their greater vulnerability.

In areas of abundant resources, upholding this principle is relatively straightforward. In many communities, however, child mental health resources are uncommon to nonexistent, thus creating an "extenuating circumstance." In communities with scare resources, the general psychiatric practitioner often is pressed into providing clinical care for children who have psychiatric needs. In addition to being clinically challenging, such requests produce ethical challenges.[2-4] Similarly, the general psychiatrist practicing family therapy may be implored by a family to provide individual treatment to a specific child. In such circumstances, the general psychiatrist often is practicing at the ambiguous edge of competency and must monitor whether he or she is straying across that edge.

In particular, general psychiatrists need to be aware that many interventions that have been validated empirically for adult populations have not been researched in child populations and have no evidenced benefit for youth. For example, the efficacy of tricyclic antidepressants is much less well established in the treatment of child and adolescent affective disorders than in adults.[5,6] Thus, reliance on adult-based evidence and experience may lead to care that lacks beneficence or is even dangerous.[7]

Enhancing one's competency requires more than a literature review. General psychiatrists are encouraged to engage in all forms of learning opportunities, including workshops, distance learning, and a careful reading of the literature. Because local consultation is likely to be limited, psychiatrists can access resources such as Internet consultation groups (eg, the Physician Access Line at the University of New Mexico Health Sciences Center, http://hsc.unm.edu/som/telehealth/pals.shtml, or the Hopkins Access Line at The Johns Hopkins Hospital, http://www.hopkinshospital.org/hospital/referring.html#hal, telemedicine conferences, or telephone consultation with an academic medical center).

As well as being mindful of one's own competency, the general psychiatrist must be mindful of the availability and competency of collaborators. In the current health care environment, it is increasingly common for pediatricians to have significant experience in providing psychopharmacological care for their child and adolescent patients, and they may provide useful consultation or collaboration. Similarly, schools are long-experienced in addressing their students' behavioral issues and can function as important, reliable, and experienced treatment allies. In contrast, the psychiatrist's professional colleagues cannot be assumed to have the necessary competency to work with children.

Despite the potential difficulty of arranging for a consultation or even for a transfer of care outside the local community, general psychiatrists are asked to consider these measures in situations where their expertise may be especially challenged:

- Acute suicidality, particularly in a young child who may not be cognitively able to understand death
- Multiple psychiatric comorbidities, particularly those that may interact negatively (eg, bipolar affective disorder, conduct disorder and substance abuse)

- Polypharmacy or multiple short-term medication trials
- Significant lack of response to treatment, particularly with life-threatening disorders such as anorexia nervosa
- Mixed psychiatric disorder(s) and neurodevelopmental disorder(s)
- Atypical presentation or symptomatology (raising the possibility of a missed psychiatric or somatic diagnosis)
- Rare childhood psychiatric disorder(s) (eg, schizophrenia before the age of 9 years)
- A primary diagnosis uncommon in an adult practice (eg, childhood disintegrative disorder, separation anxiety disorder)
- A child patient who has little or no reliable family or social support
- Unremitting anxiety on the part of the treating psychiatrist

The capacity to access consultation when one is uncertain or unclear about the appropriate course of action is the hallmark of a competent and ethical psychiatrist.[8]

PSYCHOPHARMACOLOGY

Several ethical aspects of child and adolescent psychopharmacology warrant specific mention.[9,10] As noted earlier, competency in general psychopharmacology does not guarantee competency in child psychopharmacology. The brain continues to develop through adolescence.[11] Neurotransmitter and neuromodulator systems develop at varying rates and change functions.[12] Medications with proven efficacy in adults may not demonstrate such efficacy in children.[13]

Also, many medications that are approved by the Food and Drug Administration for use in adults do not have such approval for children or even for adolescents.[14] Child and adolescent psychiatrists frequently find themselves having to practice off-label if they are to care for their patients adequately. As a cautionary note, some data suggest that children have a high placebo response rate[15,16] that can complicate both assessment of efficacy for the individual patient and assessment of data from clinical trials, especially for clinicians less familiar with children. In addition to raising complex questions about the ethics of off-label or less well-substantiated use of medications, such practice also may incur increased legal liability. On the other hand, depriving children of potentially valuable treatments raises another set of ethical issues.[17]

As with many such ethical dilemmas, the psychiatrist's best recourse is to assess consciously and conscientiously the needs and risks for each particular patient, including the certainty of the diagnosis, the risks of prescribing and not prescribing, one's own level of competence, and the availability of more expert treatment resources. Such specific and thoughtful deliberation avoids the dangers of overgeneralization and poorly considered care and increases the likelihood of providing the best possible individualized care to the particular patient.

As discussed elsewhere in this article, consent to pharmacologic treatment also varies with the cognitive abilities of the child or adolescent.

INFORMED CONSENT

Informed consent is identified as the foundation of ethical health care.[18] Before a patient's consent can be considered informed, the individual must possess decisional capacity, understand the risks and benefits of accepting or declining the treatment and the potential outcomes of alternative treatments, and provide a voluntary and non-coerced decision. Psychiatrists are obliged to recognize the individual patient's dignity, autonomy, and capacity for self-determination.

Because minors are determined to lack decisional capacity, parents or legal guardians are assigned the responsibility of furnishing informed consent for health care interventions. In respecting children's dignity, physicians are expected to include them in the consent process and ask the youths to assent to treatment participation. Doing so requires communicating the treatment goals and interventions to the child in a format appropriate to the child's developmental capacity in the cognitive, emotional, and social domains. Essentially, the youth is accepting the physician's invitation to participate in the therapeutic process. It is important to replicate this discussion as the child's functionality improves with age and developmental maturation.

In recent years, legislators and clinicians have recognized the rights of a mature minor, an adolescent who possesses the necessary cognitive and emotional aptitude to provide his or her own informed consent. Empirical research[18] demonstrates that by age 14 years, adolescents manifest emotional maturity, cognitive capabilities, and decisional competence comparable to adults. They exhibit the ability to understand factual issues, potential outcomes, the consequences of each alternative, and the meaning of the decision within the framework of their personal values. Consequently, all 50 states have legislation that grants mature minors the authority to consent to health care decisions related to contraceptives, pregnancy, sexually transmitted diseases, mental health, or substance abuse.[19] Importantly, these statutes do not mandate parental notification. In states that do not explicitly grant mature minors confidential access to mental health care, physicians regularly treat adolescents they appraise to be mature, especially if their state has laws allowing minors to access similar services. Psychiatrists are advised to document evidence of the adolescent's maturity and the reasoning for their decision to treat the patient absent parental consent.

The Society for Adolescent Medicine emphasizes the merit of allowing adolescents to access confidential services for sensitive health concerns.[20] The Society asserts that many adolescents, especially those who engage in high-risk or dangerous activities, will abstain from health care or refrain from honest communication with their physician. When adolescents are permitted to consent to confidential treatment, the ethical standards of patient autonomy, beneficence, nonmaleficence, and justice are preserved.

Psychiatrists, however, are compelled to use clinical judgment, knowledge of state laws, and professional guidelines with respect to confidential treatment of adolescents. There is contrasting research that questions the capacity of adolescents to provide informed consent independently.[18] Age is an arbitrary delineation of maturity, because not all adolescents achieve developmental milestones at the same rate or sequence. Each specific patient's capacity to provide voluntary consent should be assessed within the context of the complexity of the decision and the youth's psychosocial level of development and current mental and emotional status. As an example, substance abuse has been associated with cognitive impairments in the areas of attention, concentration, processing of information, motivation, and perception, and, consequently, damages decisional capacity.[21] Additionally, much of the research demonstrating adolescents' decisional capabilities has occurred in laboratory settings and may not always generalize to real-world settings, especially when the youth lacks all the relevant information provided in a research environment.[18]

CONFIDENTIALITY

With children, the privilege of releasing confidential information resides with the guardian who initially consented to the treatment. Many states also require adolescents over the age of 14 years to consent to the release of information. Typically, mature minors who have confidentially consented to their mental health treatment can independently allow or deny the release their records. Virtually every state allows exceptions to the principles of confidentiality. Physicians may disclose protected health information with other providers free of any release in situations that are considered medically necessary for the continuity of care or necessary to protect the minor, others, or the public against imminent harm.[22]

Determining when to share information with parents is, perhaps, the most problematical challenge for a psychiatrist. Several states that sanction confidential treatment for mature minors also allow physicians to communicate with parents when such an intervention clearly is in the best interest of the youth. Conversely, many states permit physicians to deny guardians access to the medical record or protected information if the disclosure is likely to cause harm to the minor. The privacy guidelines of the Health Insurance Portability and Accountability Act[22,23] authorize health care professionals, when acting in the best interest of the minor, to determine if or when guardians can have access to protected information. Although these regulations direct practice, they require clinical judgment to serve as the pilot.

Successful resolution of this dilemma begins at the initiation of treatment when psychiatrists establish whether the patient is the minor or the family and the psychiatrist's relationship with each family member. The psychiatrist then elucidates the limits of confidentiality in a manner that is congruent with the youth's developmental level. This discussion includes clarification of terms such as the best interest of the child and behaviors that may entail parental notification, including personal neglect, imminent harm, self-injury, and high-risk behavior. It is respectful to explore with older youth the clinical process by which sensitive material will be shared with parents. More specifically, doing so involves deciding who conveys the information and the context in which the material is shared. This understanding enables the youth to make an independent decision about what and when to disclose information to the psychiatrist.

Children who lack the legal status of a mature minor can be assured a measure of confidentiality when the guardians understand the importance of the therapeutic relationship between doctor and patient and agree to respect the confidentiality that is inherent in that relationship. This understanding is not an enforceable agreement and does not release the psychiatrist from the obligation of acting in the best interest of the child.

COMMUNICATION WITH THIRD PARTIES

Unintended disclosures to third parties represent a significant threat to confidentiality.[24,25] Potential problems associated with documentation and record-keeping should be discussed openly at the onset of treatment. Records often contain personal information about family members and can be shared inadvertently even when a release of information is signed. This problem can be avoided by restricting documentation to relevant details about the identified minor, deleting sensitive material about family members from the medical record before releasing it to another provider, obtaining separate releases of information from each participant, or maintaining discrete records for each participant.

Communications with third parties who mandate treatment for the minor or reimburse the provider for those services can produce violations to confidentially. Frequently, insurance carriers request clinical details and treatment plans before authorizing payment for services and frequently assume that with payment comes the right to dictate treatment. Psychiatrists are encouraged to negotiate this potential conflict early in the treatment while preserving collaborative communication and therapeutic alliances with payors. General psychiatrists who work with managed care entities may be familiar with this dynamic. When information is disclosed, physicians are counseled to minimize these reports, including only the information necessary to secure authorization.

Likewise, courts, juvenile justice systems, social services agencies, and schools that mandate treatment for minors may request protected information as evidence of the youth's compliance or as justification of remuneration for the services. It is essential for the treating psychiatrist to help the payor understand that it is paying for the psychiatrist's best efforts, which may or may not be completely synchronous with the payor's agenda. The optimal resolution is an agreement among the child and family, the referring agency, and the psychiatrist that restricts communication to attendance and general information about progress toward the identified goals. Again, the objective is to share the least amount of protected information to sustain medically necessary treatment. If the referring agency demands more protected information than is ethically required, the psychiatrist has the option to refuse services and refer the minor to other providers.

ASSESSMENT AND DIAGNOSIS

Because younger children typically have less experience, knowledge, and verbal fluency than adults, psychiatric assessment of children requires increased reliance on supplemental sources of information, including recurrent observation of the child, nonverbal interactions such as play, garnering information from parents, teachers, and other significant adults, and medical histories and other historical sources. It is important for psychiatrists to adjust their language and cognitive level to match the child's abilities. A comprehensive child psychiatric assessment requires more time than is characteristic of an adult assessment. It also is important to discuss the results of the assessment with the child in a way that is congruent with the child's cognitive and emotional level of functioning.

As with all psychiatric care, psychiatric diagnosis is fundamental for children. A good diagnosis provides valuable treatment guidance; a poor diagnosis rapidly leads one astray. Children often come to a practitioner with a pre-existing diagnosis, or at least with a hypothesized diagnosis. Obviously, it is important to determine objectively whether that diagnosis is accurate. Also, psychiatric disorders may manifest differently in children than in adults; for example, the broad phenotype of pediatric bipolar disorder may manifest fewer discrete manic or depressed episodes than seen with adult bipolar disorder.[26] As noted earlier, psychiatrists must evaluate their level of competency when assessing and diagnosing children and seek consultation when needed.

As with adult patients, psychiatric assessments of children may be put to uses beyond clinical care. Schools may ask for assessments to determine whether a child qualifies for special education. Lawyers or courts may ask for an assessment to determine whether a child's or adolescent's actions were willful or were caused by a psychiatric disorder—put differently, and with different implications, whether or not the child is responsible and accountable for those actions. Adoption agencies may request psychiatric screening before adoption. Divorcing parents, their lawyers, or the divorce court may request a psychiatric assessment to determine who should have custody of a child. Managed care entities may wish to know whether they are obliged, under the terms of their contract, to pay for a child's care. The assessing psychiatrist always considers whether the child's best interests are being protected and whether one's professional competency boundaries are being overly tested.

Considering the difficulties of assessment, a diagnosis should not be ascertained by the youth's initial response to a specific intervention. Although it often is tempting to make such a diagnosis, doing so is no more reliable or justified than it is with adults. For example, a positive response to stimulant medication does not confirm a diagnosis of attention-deficit/hyperactivity disorder, because most individuals would respond to stimulant medication with increased attention and enhanced cognitive performance.

ROLES AND BOUNDARY ISSUES

Clinical work with children can present uncertainties associated with potential boundary violations such as accepting hugs from patients, escorting children to the bathroom or assisting a preschooler with toileting, giving food as a reward; buying fund-raising items, accepting invitations to significant events, giving gifts to patients, and restraining out-of-control patients.[27] Clinicians tend to be more flexible with their interventions when working with younger children. Understanding one's professional perspective on boundaries and childhood developmental issues is vital to maintain a consistently therapeutic relationship with the youth.

Children commonly ask psychiatrists about their personal life and experiences or their personal views on controversial subjects.[25,28] These inquiries may be innocent questions regarding the physician's age or more sensitive, and less comfortable, questions about the provider's religion, views on adolescent sexuality, or history of substance use. The wisest course of action is to maintain focus on the meaning of the question within the context of the patient's phenomenological world and to provide a response that is congruent with the child's intent behind the question, therapeutic needs, and emotional and cognitive developmental level. Of course, each psychiatrist establishes and reevaluates his or her professional boundaries concerning self-disclosure before initiating treatment.

Competing world views between the child and parents present unique practice dilemmas.[25] This problem often is manifested at the initiation of treatment when the youth disagrees with the parents' formulation of the problem behaviors and treatment goals. It may surface later on when the youth divulges beliefs or practices that are not necessarily dangerous or illegal but violate the parents' moral, religious, or cultural values. A therapeutic alliance may not develop if the youth perceives the psychiatrist as an extension of the parental system. Alternately, the parents may terminate treatment if they perceive the clinician as overly identified with the child. The clinical and ethical task includes facilitating discussion between the child and parent. As indicated earlier, this task incorporates delineating who is the patient and facilitating communication that is contingent on the age and developmental level of the child, the therapeutic needs of the child, and the a priori agreement concerning what and how information will be shared with parents. Similarly, psychiatrists are cautioned to be aware of their own world views about families, discipline practices, and acceptable or unacceptable child and adolescent behaviors so that these standards are not imposed on the patient. When the child or parents are from a culture different from that of the psychiatrist, care should be not taken to assume a shared understanding of roles within the family.[29] Ethical treatment occurs when the provider understands and respects the child's and the family's values.

Psychiatrists assume many roles while interacting with children.[30] Psychiatrists frequently are asked by schools, lawyers, courts, adoption agencies, insurance companies, and others to provide an objective expert opinion about a child. In such circumstances it is important for the psychiatrist to understand clearly whose agent they are and what role they are assuming. In situations in which the psychiatrist's opinion may have an adverse outcome for the child, such as when a psychiatrist is asked by a court to render an opinion about a child's mental competency, clarity about role and agency is especially important and should be explained carefully to the child and family. In particular, the psychiatrist should inform the child explicitly when an assessment is done other than for treatment reasons or when the usual standards of patient confidentiality do not apply. Such explanations should be made with consideration for the child's cognitive and linguistic abilities. Similarly, a research psychiatrist should be clear with the child subject about the differences between research and clinical encounters.

A unique set of boundary issues exists in rural or small communities.[2,3,31] Because of a scarcity of resources in rural environments, a psychiatrist may be the sole provider for youths who otherwise would be referred to another clinician. In small communities, families may solicit care from a trusted member of their defined group so that they will feel understood and valued. Most salient is the complexity of managing overlapping relationships with patients with whom psychiatrists regularly interact in the daily routine of community life. It is the psychiatrist's responsibility to define the therapeutic relationship and the principles of confidentiality and to clarify that clinical discussion cannot transpire with the child or parent in any environment outside the designated clinical time. This explanation requires an open dialogue that acknowledges that the nonprofessional relationship may be affected. Additionally, the physician's spouse or children may have personal or professional relationships with the minor patient or minor's family at school, church, recreational, or other community activities. The psychiatrist must practice confidentiality rigorously.

PROTECTING CHILDREN AND CHILD ABUSE REPORTS

Psychiatrists who work with children have a special obligation to protect youth from harm. These responsibilities encompass the clinically ethical treatment of youths who may be neglected or abused by their parents or other designated care providers.

Ethical conflicts frequently are associated with disclosures of physical or sexual abuse of a child and the state requirements designating psychiatrists as mandatory reporters. Every state has a statute mandating mental health professionals to report suspected child abuse to an identified state agency. States impose penalties for failure to report and provide immunity from liability against good-faith reports.[25] These reports, however, challenge the principles of confidentiality and threaten the therapeutic relationship. Often, children and parents feel betrayed when a report is made, especially if the limits of confidentiality were not discussed at the beginning of treatment.

Conflicts revolve around the questions of when and how to report. Most states do not define abuse explicitly or establish the norm for suspicion. Providers are encouraged to consult with state officials and trusted colleagues about the community's paradigms of reportable abuse, particularly concerning physical and emotional abuse. Psychiatrists are encouraged to explore further their own values regarding corporal punishment, shouting, shaming, and other discipline styles before determining whether a child is being abused. Of course, all clinicians are responsible for acting in the best interest of the youth and must report any behavior that crosses their threshold of suspected abuse.

Additionally, the guiding principles are to maintain ethical and legal conduct while using every clinical effort to maintain the therapeutic relationship with the child and family. The decision of how to report depends on the imminent risk to the child. If the youth has endured serious harm or is at risk of serious harm, a report must be made immediately, regardless of the psychological impact on the child or family. Physicians, however, are expected to use their clinical skills to prepare the child for the likely consequences of such a report. In situations of minimal risk, providers need to assess the psychological status of the child and family and the probable effects of the report. One possibility is to help the child and/or parent make the report during the treatment session so that it is incorporated into the therapeutic work. Likewise, the psychiatrist may report in the presence of the child and/or family for the same therapeutic reasons. Or, a report may be made without informing the youth or family.

These obligations also direct treatment practices in a hospital or other setting in which the psychiatrist is clinically responsible for the care provided by allied mental health professionals and paraprofessionals. The psychiatrist has the ethical charge of comprehending the prevailing guidelines related to least restrictive treatment and the working definitions of seclusion, restraint, punishment, and aversive interventions and to ensure that the patients are receiving clinically appropriate and beneficial treatment. This responsibility translates to the preclusion of coercive, punitive, painful, or developmentally inappropriate interventions and the unnecessary use of physical, mechanical, or chemical restraints.

Although nurses and other providers may not report directly to the physician, the psychiatrist has the responsibility of assuring that each patient receives individualized care that is clinically appropriate. Ethical dilemmas may emerge if the physician observes the institution or a particular staff member engaging in harmful practices or failing to employ beneficial practices. To avoid these problems, the psychiatrist may need to provide psychosocial education and consultation to the staff regarding such issues as cognitive, emotional, and moral development, symptomatology of specific diagnoses, and boundary violations; to the administrators regarding such issues as clinical standards of care; and to parents regarding their child's right to safe and helpful treatment. As in situations discussed previously, a report to a Child Protective Services agency may be warranted.

RESEARCH ISSUES

Inherent to psychiatric research with minors is the conflict between gaining essential scientific data about childhood disorders and the need to protect the rights and integrity of the participants.[6] The insufficiency of empirically validated treatments, particularly in the domain of psychopharmacological therapies, denies youth the benefit of evidence-based care. Consequently, untested care can be construed as experimental and unethical in that the interventions may lack beneficence or may cause unintended harm.[32] This situation was recognized by the National Institutes of Health[33] when it established the goal of increasing the participation of minors in research that investigates the treatment of disorders that affect children. This research is intended to benefit children and adolescents who are diagnosed as having specific disorders and to improve the public health status of minors. Children, however, are identified as a vulnerable population that requires specific safeguards to protect them against exploitation and any undue harm.[34] These youths are additionally vulnerable because they have medical, psychiatric, or developmental disorders.[35]

Legal precedent assumes that minors lack the capacity to consent to their inclusion in research. Because consent can be imparted only by the individual partaking in the research, the minor's participation requires permission by the parents or guardians. The Department of Health and Human Services (DHHS)[34] guidelines, however, require minors to assent or affirmatively to agree to their participation. The absence of an objection does not translate to an assent. Significantly, children can veto their participation and withdraw from the project at any time during the research protocol. This ability to withdraw essentially protects their right to volunteerism.

Information about the research must be presented to the minor at a level proportionate to the child's age and developmental level. A child's capacity to assent is determined by the child's age, developmental maturity, and psychological state at the time of recruitment. Although children usually are not considered capable of giving assent until age 7 years, younger children have the right to learn about the research and to assent to their involvement.[6,32,34]

As discussed earlier, the concept of a "mature minor" has emerged recently in the psychiatric, ethical, and legal literature.[19,36] This concept has been expanded to allow mature minors the opportunity to consent independently to their involvement in a research project. The Institutional Review Board (IRB) that sanctions a specific research trial has the authority to waive the requirement for parental permission, thus permitting mature minors to consent to confidential participation in that specific investigation. Recent Federal regulations[37] established three criteria that IRBs must follow before granting mature minors this right: that the research involves no more than minimal risk; that the waiver of parental permission will not affect the welfare of the research participant adversely; and that the research project could not be performed practically without the waiver of parental permission.

Research with adolescents who are homeless or who engage in high-risk or illegal behaviors would not transpire if the construct of mature minor did not exist. The Society for Adolescent Medicine[38] argues that adolescents who engage in substance abuse and other sensitive behaviors will not participate in research unless they are assured of confidentiality. Without the participation of these youths, important data about effective prevention and treatment interventions will not be obtained.

The DHHS systematizes the safeguards necessary to protect minors from the potential harm associated with the research. Risk is determined by appraising the risk to the participant, the benefit to the participant, the benefit to similar children or children in general, and the minor's capacity to assent. Minimal risk is defined as a situation with risks no greater than those experienced in children's daily lives, assuming that a daily life represents a safe and caring environment.[6,32,34] If the study exposes the child to no more than minimal risk, the minor's participation is acceptable with one parent's permission and the child's assent.

When the study presents more than minimal risk, minors can participate if the benefits are greater than the risks. In this circumstance, permission of both parents, when applicable, and the assent of the minor is required. The benefit to the specific participant must be at least equal to that of the other treatments available to children who have the same disorder. Participation can proceed if one parent grants permission, and the child assents. Research that exposes children to more than minimal risk and offers no direct benefit to the participant can proceed only if the study is likely to generate useful data that will benefit other children who have the same disorder. Importantly, the minor must not incur any unpleasant experiences that exceed those routinely sustained in a medical, dental, psychological, social, or educational encounter.[6,23,34]

SUMMARY

Clinical work—psychotherapy, assessment, consultation, or research—with emotionally ill children and adolescents is challenging, complex, and exceedingly rewarding. Psychiatrists must remain mindful of children's vulnerabilities but also remain respectful of their rights, regardless of any legal barriers or developmental limitations that exist. To varying degrees, youths are afforded the rights of integrity, autonomy, informed consent or assent, protection of health care information, and participation in research. All physicians who work with children and adolescents are obliged to possess the requisite skills necessary for the provision of beneficial assessments, psychotherapy and psychopharmacology, the protection and advocacy that vulnerable children may require, and the ability to collaborate with families, schools, and other systems in which children regularly function. This work requires self-examination and awareness of one's values and attitudes about children and families and self-monitoring of one's motivations and intents during therapeutic interactions. Additionally, psychiatrists are reminded to seek consultation from valued colleagues whenever an ethical quandary presents itself. Finally, while negotiating the multiple requirements of children, families, communities, legal statutes, and professional ethics and standards, psychiatrists must maintain an ardent commitment to the safety and well-being of their young patients.

APPENDIX 1: ADDITIONAL RESOURCES

Readers who wish to pursue this topic further or who wish to consult additional resources may find the following items of use:

1. American Academy of Child and Adolescent Psychiatry Code of Ethics. Available at: http://www.aacap.org/galleries/AboutUs/CodeOfEthics.PDF.
2. Schetky DH, editor. Ethics. *Child and Adolescent Psychiatric Clinics of North America* 1995;4(4).
3. Dell ML, Trivedi HK, editors. Ethics. *Child and Adolescent Psychiatric Clinics of North America* 2008;17(1).
4. Schetky DH. Ethics in the practice of child and adolescent psychiatry. In: Lewis M, editor. Child and adolescent psychiatry: a comprehensive textbook. 3rd edition. Philadelphia: Lippincott, Williams, and Wilkins; 2002. p. 1442–6.
5. American Association of Child and Adolescent Psychiatry Practice Parameters. Available at: http://www.aacap.org/cs/root/member_information/practice_information/practice_parameters/practice_parameters.
6. American Academy of Pediatrics Committee on Bioethics policy statements. Available at: http://www.aacap.org/galleries/AboutUs/CodeOfEthics.PDF.
7. Dulcan MK, Martini DR. Concise guide to child & adolescent psychiatry. 2nd edition. Washington DC: American Psychiatric Publishing, Inc.; 1999.
8. The *Journal of the American Academy of Child & Adolescent Psychiatry* regularly publishes 10-year reviews of a variety of topics on child psychiatry.

REFERENCES

1. Winnicott DW. Adolescent immaturity. In: Winnicott DW, editor. Home is where we start from: essays by a psychoanalyst. New York: WW Norton & Company; 1986. p. 150–66.
2. Roberts LW, Dyer AL. Concise guide to ethics in mental health. Washington, DC: American Psychiatric Publishing; 2004.

3. Roberts LW, Battaglia J, Epstein RS. Frontier ethics: mental health care needs and ethical dilemmas in rural communities. Psychiatr Serv 1999;50(4):497–503.

4. Roberts LW, Battaglia J, Smithpeter M, et al. An office on Main Street. Health care dilemmas in small communities. Hastings Cent Rep 1999;29(4):28–37.

5. Ambrosini PJ, Bianchi MD, Rabinovich H, et al. Antidepressant treatments in children and adolescents. I. Affective disorders. J Am Acad Child Adolesc Psychiatry 1993;32(1):1–6.

6. Tsapakis EM, Soldani F, Tondo L, et al. Efficacy of antidepressants in juvenile depression: meta-analysis. Br J Psychiatry 2008;193:10–7.

7. Hoop JG, Smyth AC, Roberts LW. Ethical issues in psychiatric research on children and adolescents. Child Adolesc Psychiatr Clin N Am 2008;17:127–48.

8. Roberts LW, McCarty T, Roberts BB, et al. Clinical ethics teaching in psychiatric supervision. Acad Psychiatry 1996;20:176–88.

9. Spetie L, Arnold LE. Ethical issues in child psychopharmacology research and practice: emphasis on preschoolers. Psychopharmacology 2007;191(1):15–26.

10. Koelch M, Schnoor K, Fegert JM. Ethical issues in psychopharmacology of children and adolescents. Curr Opin Psychiatry 2008;21:598–605.

11. Lenroot RK, Giedd JN. Brain development in children and adolescents: insights from anatomical magnetic resonance imaging. Neurosci Biobehav Rev 2006; 30(6):718–29.

12. Herlenius E, Lagercrantz H. Neurotransmitters and neuromodulators during early human development. Early Hum Dev 2001;65(1):21–37.

13. Keller MB, Ryan ND, Strober M, et al. Efficacy of paroxetine in the treatment of adolescent major depression: a randomized, controlled trial. J Am Acad Child Adolesc Psychiatry 2001;40(7):762–72.

14. Dell ML, Vaughan BS, Kratochvil CJ. Ethics and the prescription pad. Child Adolesc Psychiatr Clin N Am 2008;17(1):93–111.

15. Rheims S, Cucherat M, Arzimanoglou A, et al. Greater response to placebo in children than in adults: a system review and meta-analysis in drug-resistant partial epilepsy. PLoS Med 2008;5(8):1223–37.

16. Birmaher B, Ryan ND, Williamson DE, et al. Childhood and adolescent depression: a review of the past 10 years. Part 1. J Am Acad Child Adolesc Psychiatry 1996;35:1427–39.

17. Ringold S. Antidepressant warning focuses attention on unmet need for child psychiatrists. JAMA 2005;293(5):537–8.

18. Kuther TZ. Medical decision-making and minors: issues of consent and assent. Adolescence 2003;38:343–58.

19. Boonstra H, Nash E. Minors and the right to consent to health care. Guttmacher Rep Public Policy 2000;2:1–6.

20. Ford C, English A, Sigman G. Confidential Health Care for Adolescents: position paper of the society for adolescent medicine. J Adolesc Health 2004;35:160–7.

21. Brody JL, Waldron HB. Ethical issues in research n the treatment of alcohol substance abuse. Addict Behav 2000;35:160–7.

22. English A, Ford CA. The HIPPA privacy rule and adolescents: legal questions and clinical challenges. Perspect Sex Reprod Health 2004;36:80–6.

23. U.S. Department of Health and Human Services: Office for Civil Rights—HIPAA. Medical privacy—national standards to protect the privacy of personal health information. Available at: http://www.hhs.gov/ocr/hipaa/finalreg.html. 2002; Accessed December 17, 2008.

24. Recupero PR. Ethics of medical records and professional communication. Child Adolesc Psychiatr Clin N Am 2008;17:37–51.

25. Belitz J. Caring for children. In: Roberts LW, Dyer AR, editors. Concise guide to ethics in mental health care. Washington, DC: American Psychiatric Publishing; 2004. p. 119–35.
26. Pavuluri MN, Birmaher B, Naylor MW. Pediatric bipolar disorder: a review of the past 10 years. J Am Acad Child Adolesc Psychiatry 2005;44(9):846–71.
27. Mannheim CI, Sancilio M, Phipps-Yonas S, et al. Ethical ambiguities in the practice of child clinical psychology. Research and Practice 2002;35:24–9.
28. Ascherman LI, Rubin S. Current ethical issues in child and adolescent psychotherapy. Child Adolesc Psychiatr Clin N Am 2008;17:21–35.
29. Banu az-Zubair MK. Who is a parent? Parenthood in Islamic ethics. J Med Ethics 2008;33:605–9.
30. Black D, Subotsky F. Medical ethics and child psychiatry. J Med Ethics 1982; 8:5–8.
31. Stockman AF. Dual relationships in rural mental health practice: an ethical dilemma. J Rural Community Psychol 1990;11:31–45.
32. Rosato J. The ethics of clinical trials: a child's view. J Law Med Ethics 2000;28: 362–78.
33. National Institutes of Health. NIH policy and guidelines on the inclusion of children as participants in research involving human subjects. Bethesda (MD): U.S. Department of Health and Human Services; 1998.
34. U.S. Department of Health and Human Services: code of federal regulations, Title 45: public welfare. Part 46: protection of human subjects regulations governing protection afforded children in research (Subpart D). Washington, DC: U.S. Department of Health and Human Services; 1983.
35. Koocher GP, Keith-Spiegel PC. Children, ethics and the law. Lincoln (NE): University of Nebraska Press; 2000.
36. Dailard C. New medical records privacy rule: the interface with teen access to confidential care. Guttmacher Rep Public Policy 2003;6:6–7.
37. Diviak KR, Curry SJ, Emery SL, et al. Human participants challenges in youth tobacco cessation research: researcher's perspective. Ethics Behav 2004;14: 321–34.
38. Santelli JS, Rogers AS, Rosenfeld WD, et al. Guidelines for adolescent health research: a position paper of the Society for Adolescent Medicine. J Adolesc Health 2003;33:396–409.

Ethical Issues in Perinatal Mental Health

Laura J. Miller, MD

KEYWORDS

• Ethics • Perinatal • Depression • Schizophrenia
• Bipolar disorder • Schizoaffective disorder

Balancing ethical tenets in psychiatric practice is often challenging. These challenges increase in complexity when clinicians must consider simultaneously the needs of a pregnant woman and her fetus, a postpartum woman and her baby, or a woman planning a pregnancy and her not-yet-conceived child.

Legal opinions regarding psychiatric interventions for perinatal women sometimes complicate ethical dilemmas more than they clarify them. This situation exists, in part, because many judgments have been governed by perspectives on two extremes. From one such perspective, a mother and her fetus or baby are considered adversaries, with child-protection statutes invoked and guardians appointed to protect the fetus or baby from the mother and/or the mother's clinician.[1] The other extreme is that a fetus is not considered a person and therefore has no rights.[2] From this standpoint, the health and well-being of a fetus does not have to be considered at all in making decisions about a woman's psychiatric treatment.

Neither of these stances is consistent with the clinical reality that the health and well-being of women and their babies are intimately intertwined. Untreated perinatal psychiatric symptoms can increase the risk of preterm delivery, abnormal stress responses, growth problems, and emotional and behavioral disturbances in offspring.[3–7] Conversely, health complications in neonates lead to a high risk of psychiatric symptoms in their mothers.[8]

This article reviews ethical principles that can help clinicians simultaneously consider the needs of perinatal mentally ill women and their offspring. The principles of beneficence, nonmaleficence, respect for autonomy, and justice are widely regarded as the cornerstones of medical ethics and have been validated empirically as governing physicians' clinical decision-making.[9] The application of these principles to ethical dilemmas during preconception, during pregnancy, and postpartum is described using case examples, along with concepts that have proven useful in helping to balance these

Women's Mental Health Program, Department of Psychiatry, University of Illinois at Chicago, 912 South Wood Street, M/C 913, Chicago, IL 60612, USA
E-mail address: ljm@psych.uic.edu

Psychiatr Clin N Am 32 (2009) 259–270
doi:10.1016/j.psc.2009.02.002
0193-953X/09/$ – see front matter © 2009 Elsevier Inc. All rights reserved.

psych.theclinics.com

principles. These concepts include relational ethics, substituted judgment, preventive ethics, directive counseling, and avoiding omission bias.

AUTONOMY, BENEFICENCE, AND RELATIONAL ETHICS

Case 1: When a woman whose bipolar disorder had been well controlled for years learned she was pregnant, she discontinued lithium to avoid harmful effects to her fetus. In her third trimester, she developed a manic episode with psychotic features. Acting on a delusional belief that the fetus was an evil spirit, she entered an alley and attempted to puncture her amniotic sac with a knitting needle, with the intent of pulling the fetus out. She had boiled the needle to sterilize it and was taking care not to injure herself in the process. Police officers brought her to an emergency room. There she refused psychiatric treatment because she thought treatment would interfere with her efforts to rid herself of the evil spirit. She declared her intent to continue trying to destroy the fetus until she succeeded but was adamant that she would take care not to harm herself in the process. She appeared well nourished, and there was no evidence of other high-risk behaviors.

Clinicians have an ethical obligation to respect patient autonomy. In general, patients are the ones who decide whether to accept medical treatments, based on their values, beliefs, and priorities. Clinicians also have an ethical obligation to act with beneficence—that is, to promote a patient's best interest by taking the course of action that most benefits the patient. Ethical dilemmas arise when these two obligations collide, for example, when a patient refuses treatment that a clinician believes is essential.[10] In this case, the dilemma is more complicated. Here there is no evidence that the untreated symptoms are directly placing the patient herself at risk. Although it is possible the patient will harm herself inadvertently while attempting to rid herself of her fetus, she has demonstrated meticulous efforts to protect herself from doing so. There is more compelling reason to believe that her fetus is at risk of harm. Does a clinician's ethical obligation of beneficence extend to a patient's fetus, and, if so, does that obligation outweigh the obligation for patient autonomy?

Long-standing ethical and legal precedents support the notion that clinicians caring for pregnant women have an obligation to promote a baby's right to be born alive and healthy.[11] That obligation includes treating maternal conditions that pose risks to the fetus, as in this case. History, however, is replete with instances of excessively forcing pregnant women to accept medical intervention they disagree with for the sake of their fetuses.[12] An ethical standard that protects fetal well-being while steering clear of coercion or paternalism is to respect a woman's refusal of treatment except when the proposed treatment leads to "clear and overwhelming" benefit to her fetus.[10,13] This standard is widely, although not universally, accepted.

Another principle that can guide clinical decision-making in cases of apparent conflict between maternal and fetal interests is that of relational ethics. Relational ethics emphasizes the perspective that the patient's well-being and her baby's well-being are intertwined, rather than at odds.[14] For example, most women who kill their babies because of delusions suffer profoundly later.[15] In the case example here, if the patient remained untreated and succeeded in harming her fetus, it is likely that her own subsequent mental health would deteriorate. From this vantage point, treating the patient despite her current lack of consent is done as much for her own well-being as for the well-being of her fetus.

A further consideration is whether the patient's ability to make authentic, autonomous decisions is compromised by the symptoms of her illness.[16] In this case, before her mania recurred, this patient tried to protect her fetus from harm by discontinuing lithium. Her subsequent decision to refuse treatment, thereby endangering her fetus, is based on a delusional belief and is not congruent with her baseline values. When psychiatric symptoms grossly impair a patient's capacity to make authentic decisions about treatment, a surrogate decision-maker can weigh the risks and benefits of proposed treatment based on two standards: substituted judgment and/or best interests. Substituted judgment decisions are based on what the patient probably would have chosen if she were not psychotic. Although not universally accepted, this standard typically is used in court cases involving refusal of psychotropic medication[17] and is recommended for pregnant women who have psychotic disorders who need surrogate decision-making about psychiatric care.[18] When it is difficult to discern what decision the patient would have made if competent, decisions can be based on community standards of what would be in the patient's best interest. In this case example, a substituted judgment standard can be applied: the patient's long track record of taking lithium consistently suggests that when not psychotic she desires treatment, and her previously protective behavior toward her fetus suggests that when not psychotic she strongly values the well-being of her fetus.

JUSTICE AND DIRECTIVE COUNSELING

Case 2: A 27-year-old woman has a 10-year history of chronic paranoid schizophrenia and is in her thirty-second week of pregnancy. She has had no prenatal care but has been taking quetiapine regularly as prescribed, before and throughout her pregnancy. She is brought to the emergency room by her mother, who saw blood on the bathroom floor at home. The patient does not seem to be in acute physical or emotional distress. She acknowledges she had a "small amount" of bleeding from her vagina earlier that day, but she refuses vital signs, physical examination, or other intervention. She fully understands the physician's explanation of the purpose and nature of the examination and the risks to herself and her fetus of unchecked bleeding. Although she has had delusions in the past, she has none now. She says she is refusing because she is a loner, does not like to be examined, and feels this is her private business. She states that if the baby was meant to be okay, it will be okay on its own. She agrees, however, to return to the emergency room if she later develops more copious bleeding.

As in the first case, this woman has a psychotic disorder and is refusing intervention, thus placing herself and/or her fetus at risk. In this case, however, there is no evidence that the patient's psychiatric disorder is interfering with her decision-making. She is not acutely psychotic, and by a substituted judgment standard she consistently would make the same decision she is making now, as evidenced by her past history of consistent acceptance of psychotropic medication but lack of acceptance of prenatal care or any other type of physical examination.

A key ethical principle to consider in this case is that of justice. In medical ethics, justice generally refers to the concept that both the benefits and the burdens of health care should be shared equitably in society.[19] This concept includes the implication that patients who have psychiatric disorders should not be treated differently from non–mentally ill patients. In this case, if a woman without schizophrenia has the autonomy to refuse examination, justice requires the same level of autonomy for this woman who does have schizophrenia. The concept of justice also applies to her pregnancy status. In situations in which a nonpregnant woman would have the autonomy to refuse examination, justice requires that a pregnant woman be afforded the same choice, unless overriding her decision affords clear and overwhelming benefit to her fetus.

The American Medical Association Code of Ethics typifies most ethical standards in upholding a woman's right to make an informed decision to refuse medical interventions designed to benefit her fetus, except in rare circumstances of grave danger to the fetus and minimal invasiveness to the pregnant woman.[20] Legal opinions generally have upheld that pregnant women's privacy rights prevail over fetal rights, with rare exceptions based on the level of risk to the fetus, the viability of the fetus, and the invasiveness of the proposed medical intervention.[21]

That being said, it is possible to probe further into the patient's reasons for refusal and even to try to influence her decision, without violating her autonomy. This process is known as "directive counseling."[13] Unlike nondirective counseling, the clinician doing directive counseling holds a definite opinion that the patient should accept the proffered medical intervention, expresses that opinion clearly, and attempts to persuade the patient to accept the intervention. Unlike coercion, however, directive counseling assumes that the patient's decision will be respected, even if it continues to differ from that of the clinician.[22] Unlike paternalism, directive counseling does not assume that physicians' decisions are inherently superior or that patients should accept physicians' recommendations unquestioningly.[23]

In this case, empathic inquiry might uncover historical reasons for the patient's dislike of physical examinations, such as sexual trauma and/or prior insensitive, stressful physical examinations. The clinician then could negotiate with the patient acceptable terms of examination (eg, scrupulous attention to privacy, explicit permission to touch, and presence of a supportive significant other).

SUBSTITUTE DECISION MAKERS AND PREVENTIVE ETHICS

Case 3: A woman who had schizoaffective disorder had had a good therapeutic response to valproate and aripiprazole but then discontinued both medications because she felt she no longer needed them. Three months later, she developed manic symptoms, including hypersexuality and impaired judgment. She was hospitalized and had a positive pregnancy test on admission. Ultrasound examination confirmed an early intrauterine pregnancy. The patient maintained the delusional belief that she was not pregnant. She wished to resume her prior medications. Her physician was aware that valproate could increase the risk of neural tube defects and developmental delay in her fetus[24] and that aripiprazole had not been studied systematically in human pregnancy. He tried to discuss these risks with the patient and to raise alternative treatment strategies, but the patient remained steadfast in her insistence that she was not pregnant and had no intention of becoming pregnant.

In this case, the patient is capable of weighing the general risks and benefits of medication and of making an informed treatment decision on her own behalf, but her delusional denial of pregnancy interferes with her ability to weigh the risks and benefits of medication for her fetus.[25] Her clinician is faced with the need to balance beneficence toward the patient (alleviating her symptoms by resuming her medications, as she wishes) with nonmaleficence (the ethical imperative not to do harm) toward her fetus. The concept of relational ethics amplifies the dilemma, because harm to the fetus might prove ultimately harmful to the mother's mental health if she regrets the risks of fetal medication exposure once she regains her baseline mental state.

For these reasons, informed consent to treatment during pregnancy encompasses a woman's ability to make autonomous decisions on behalf of her fetus as well as herself. A substitute decision-maker is indicated if psychotic symptoms interfere with her ability to make such decisions. In some jurisdictions, courts approach this situation by appointing a guardian ad litem for the fetus. Unfortunately, this practice stems from an adversarial framework in which the interests of the mother and of the fetus are considered separate and opposed.[26] The role of the guardian ad litem for the fetus is to consider fetal well-being in isolation from maternal well-being, as if the mother were an inert container. Generally in such cases the mother has a separate guardian ad litem, and the two substitute decision-makers argue their separate (usually opposing) positions before a judge. In such circumstances, a clinician can educate all parties about the ways in which maternal and fetal well-being are linked and advocate for a balanced solution that will treat the patient's symptoms effectively while reducing risks to the fetus. For example, this approach might involve advocating for a medication regimen that treats the patient's symptoms effectively while posing fewer risks to her fetus.

This case also illustrates the value of preventive ethics—anticipating and preventing ethical dilemmas in clinical practice. A preventive ethical approach suggests that clinicians should discuss family planning proactively with women of reproductive age when prescribing medications that could pose risks in pregnancy and should include pregnancy-related risks in informed consent discussions about new medications.[27] In this case, it could have been predicted that the patient was at high risk for unintended pregnancy while manic, because of a history of hypersexuality and impaired judgment in prior episodes. Had she been informed of the pregnancy-related risks of her medications at the time of her initial prescriptions, she might have chosen a different medication regimen. Alternately, she still might have chosen that regimen, and then it would have been clear that the choice reflected her authentic, informed decision. Knowing the effect of her manic episodes on her risk of unplanned pregnancy, she also might have considered long-acting contraception that would protect her even during bouts of hypersexuality and impaired judgment.[28]

Some states honor psychiatric advance directives, which are contracts that facilitate preventive ethics. These directives are legal documents drafted and signed by a person who has a recurrent psychiatric disorder while he or she is not delusional about treatment, stating what sort of treatment he or she wants to authorize in advance during future episodes.[29] During those future episodes, if psychotic symptoms interfere with the patient's judgment, the patient's nonpsychotic baseline decisions are honored. When women of reproductive age use psychiatric advance directives, it is helpful to include their preferences for treatment continuation or modification should they be pregnant during an episode of illness.

PERINATAL MEDICATION DECISIONS AND OMISSION BIAS

Case 4: A woman who has recurrent major depression discontinued her antidepressant medication while attempting to become pregnant because she wanted to reduce medication risks to a fetus. She was thrilled when she became pregnant, but during her second trimester she developed a major depressive episode and began to believe that she would not be an adequate mother. She told her physician that she planned to give up her baby for adoption at the time of the baby's birth and then to kill herself. She refused to resume antidepressant medication because her physician had explained to her that some newborns exposed to antidepressants in utero develop medication withdrawal effects at birth. She had experienced antidepressant withdrawal in the past and found it highly distressing to imagine her baby going through that experience. She was convinced that the best outcome for the baby was to remain free of medication and to be raised by a non–mentally ill mother and that her own well-being was irrelevant.

In this case, the patient is not psychotic and accurately understands the risks of medication for her baby. She also understands the risks to herself of remaining off medication, but she does not believe those risks are relevant. What is the prevailing ethical consideration—autonomy (respecting her right to value her baby's needs over her own) or beneficence (forcing medication against her will because the risk of untreated illness far outweighs the risk of medication for the baby)?

Untangling this dilemma begins with a clinical assessment of the influence of depression on the patient's ability to make decisions. On the one hand, it is the norm for new mothers to value their babies' well-being over their own. In a study of nondepressed postpartum women, for example, 64% endorsed the belief that their lives should be centered wholly on their infants.[30] On the other hand, major depression can color a woman's perceptions in the direction of devaluing herself and emotionally overestimating the significance of risks to her fetus, even when reality testing and cognition are intact.[13] This situation compromises decision-making ability, increasing the relative importance of a beneficence-based approach. When this depressive bias becomes extreme, a substitute decision-maker may be needed.

Before it is concluded that a substitute decision-maker is essential, however, other approaches can be considered. One problem that may have amplified the ethical dilemma in this case is omission bias. The physician's explanation of the risks of anti-depressant medication for the newborn was detailed, clear, and specific. Was the physician equally detailed, clear, and specific in describing the risks to the baby that could result from untreated maternal depression? Studies of medical decision-making show that in most cases, the answer is no, because of omission bias. In general, physicians worry more about the risks of commission (eg, medications they prescribe, or procedures they perform) than about the risks of omission (eg, of not prescribing medication or performing a procedure).[31] This situation seems to be caused by a difference in perceived causality: physicians feel more responsible for causing harm if the harm results from something they do than if it results from something they do not do. Eliminating omission bias, thus giving the pregnant patient a balanced assessment of the risks to both her and her baby of untreated symptoms versus medications, allows a patient to make accurately informed decisions.

A relational ethics approach also might help in this case. The physician could acknowledge the patient's desire to value her baby's well-being first and foremost and modify recommended treatment accordingly. For example, instead of recommending that the patient take a full dose of antidepressant medication throughout pregnancy, even if the physician considers that dosage optimal, the physician could suggest a partial dose taper during the last few weeks of pregnancy. Although this approach would pose some risk of maternal symptom relapse, it would be far less risky for the patient than going without her medication altogether, and it might reduce the risk of neonatal withdrawal from abrupt medication discontinuation.[32] Combined with therapeutic interventions to help the patient regain a sense that her own life and health have value, this effort to find an acceptable compromise between the patient's values and the clinician's judgment might preclude the need for coercion.

ETHICAL ASSESSMENT OF PARENTING RISKS

Case 5: A 35-year-old woman who has schizophrenia comes to a mental health clinic for a preconception planning consultation, accompanied by her husband. The couple would like to start a family and seek consultation about whether the patient should maintain, discontinue, or change her medication regimen while trying to conceive or during pregnancy. The evaluating physician feels that, because of her diagnosis, the patient should not try to become pregnant or parent a child. The physician wonders about her ethical obligations to the patient and to the potential unborn child.

In this case, the physician feels a sense of responsibility toward a potential life, a child not yet conceived. If the physician assumes that the patient's parenting capability will be compromised solely because of the patient's having schizophrenia, the physician's thinking is influenced by bias and stigma. Studies demonstrate that insight into mental illness, a working knowledge of child development, and social support influence parenting behavior and risk, whereas diagnosis per se does not.[33–35] In this case, the patient's proactive planning suggests excellent insight, and her husband's presence suggests some social support. The ethical principle of justice implies that physicians cannot hold women who have mental illness to a different standard of parenting than other women. If a physician would not question the decision to conceive a child by a woman who has well-controlled diabetes, the physician cannot ethically question the same decision by a woman who has well-controlled schizophrenia.

The principle of nonmaleficence also underscores the ethical mandate for physicians to remain free of bias against women who have psychiatric disorders who want to bear children. In *An Unquiet Mind*, her account of her struggle with bipolar disorder, Dr. Kay Redfield Jamison recounts the long-lasting emotional pain that can result from such bias, as she describes a session with a new physician:

I told him that I very much wanted to have children, which immediately led to his asking me what I planned to do about taking lithium during pregnancy. I started to tell him that it seemed obvious to me that the dangers of my illness far outweighed any potential problems that lithium might cause a developing fetus, and that I therefore would choose to stay on lithium. Before I finished, however, he broke in to ask me if I knew that manic-depressive illness was a genetic disease. Stifling for the moment an urge to remind him that I had spent my entire professional life studying manic-depressive illness and that, in any event, I wasn't entirely stupid, I said, "Yes, of course." At that point, in an icy and imperious voice that I can hear to this day, he stated, as though it were God's truth, which he no doubt felt that it was—"You shouldn't have children. You have manic-depressive illness."[36]

But what about situations in which a physician believes a woman would be at high risk for maltreating a future child, not because of bias but for specific clinical reasons, such as a history of maltreating other children, poor insight, or nonadherence to treatment? Does the physician have an ethical obligation toward her patient's not-yet-conceived child?

This obligation is an area of controversy, with some ethicists contending there is no such obligation. The relational ethics construct, however, suggests that if a physician steers clear of bias, it is not only ethically justified but ethically important to counsel women about known risks posed by their disorders to themselves and to their offspring should they become pregnant. This counseling constitutes preventive ethics, in that women who anticipate potential risks can put preventive interventions in place. For example, if the physician informs a patient who has schizophrenia that the postpartum period is a high-risk time for exacerbation of that disorder, the patient can arrange additional social support in advance. When indicated, a physician can recommend psychosocial rehabilitation, parenting classes, or other measures to reduce risks and bolster parenting capability before a woman becomes pregnant or gives birth.

ETHICAL CONSIDERATIONS IN SCREENING FOR MATERNAL MENTAL ILLNESS

Case 6: A woman brought her 4-week-old son to his first well-baby visit with a pediatrician. On a maternal mental health screening tool, she disclosed that she has bipolar disorder. In answer to the pediatrician's follow-up questions, she explained that her illness had been diagnosed 7years ago and that she has taken medication regularly ever since with only one recurrent mood episode 4 years ago, managed on an outpatient basis with a medication change. The baby appears healthy and well cared for, and the mother appears attentive to the baby. The pediatrician is uneasy about the risks to the baby from the mother's mental illness. Because he is unable to conduct a comprehensive evaluation of the mother, he wonders if he should report her to the child welfare agency for them to evaluate, "just in case."

A compelling body of data demonstrates that a mother's postpartum mental health has profound short- and long-term effects on the physical and mental health of her offspring.[37–39] This is why pediatricians increasingly are called upon to include maternal mental health screens as a routine part of well-baby checkups.[40] Unfortunately, surveys of pediatricians find that most have not been trained adequately to address maternal mental health problems once such problems are identified.[41] Thus, screening for maternal mental health problems poses ethical conundrums for pediatricians. The baby's mother is not the pediatrician's patient. Even if trained, pediatricians are not in a position to diagnose and treat illnesses in mothers of their patients. So having identified a potential mental health problem in a patient's mother, does a pediatrician have ethical obligations toward that mother? Do pediatricians' ethical responsibilities to their patients, the babies, imply that they should err on the side of caution and notify child welfare agencies about suspected maternal major mental illness?

Some ethicists underscore the ethical costs of postpartum depression screening, including the risks of misclassification, and conclude that the benefits of screening do not warrant these costs.[42] It is possible, however, to find approaches that reduce the ethical costs of screening while amplifying the benefits. For example, a meta-analysis shows that depression screening alone, in the absence of adequate follow-up systems, does not improve patient entry into mental health treatment and does not lead to improvement in symptoms.[43] This finding suggests that the ethical costs indeed outweigh the benefits in clinics that screen mothers with no system in place for addressing "positive" screens (screens with scores suggestive of psychiatric problems). A clinic that has guidelines for addressing positive screens, trains its clinicians, uses relevant clinical tools and referral resources, and has back-up mental health consultation available, however, is positioned to improve outcomes for mothers and their offspring substantially.[44]

Physicians are legally mandated to report risk of child maltreatment to child welfare agencies. The principle of justice is a useful guide to physicians wondering whether to report maternal mental illness. Ethical practice is to approach a mother who has a psychiatric disorder in the same way the physician would approach a mother with any other disorder that could affect a baby. For example, a pediatrician might have no qualms about a mother who has a well-controlled seizure disorder caring for a baby but might have grave concerns about a mother who has poorly controlled, frequent generalized tonic-clonic seizures who lives alone, does not take her anticonvulsant medication, drinks alcohol, and already has injured her baby once by dropping the baby during a seizure. Similarly, there is no indication that well-controlled bipolar disorder compromises safe and effective parenting, but symptomatic bipolar disorder, especially in the context of additive risk factors, can affect parenting and outcome for offspring adversely.[45,46]

A pediatrician with ethical obligations to a baby of necessity has ethical obligations to the baby's caregivers, because the baby's well-being is so dependent on the well-being of those caregivers. Pediatricians are well positioned to practice preventive ethics. If they note maternal psychiatric symptoms that do not lead to child maltreatment but nevertheless interfere with optimal bonding and parenting, pediatricians can recommend maternal psychiatric evaluation and treatment, parenting classes, parenting coaching, and/or co-parenting arrangements with significant others.[47] For more extreme cases in which parenting capacity might be compromised episodically by acute symptoms, physicians can recommend standby guardianship where available. These legal documents, supported by legislation in some states, are used by patients who have recurring illnesses (medical or psychiatric) to designate proactively someone as a temporary guardian for their children during episodes of illness.[48] Their use reduces the risk of permanent loss of custody.

SUMMARY

The principles of autonomy, beneficence, nonmaleficence, and justice can guide clinicians in finding ethical approaches to the treatment of women who have psychiatric disorders during preconception, pregnancy, and postpartum. **Table 1** summarizes some clinical dilemmas in perinatal mental health care, the ethical conundrums posed by these situations, and guiding principles or tools that can help clinicians resolve ethical conflicts.

Table 1
Approaches to ethical dilemmas in perinatal mental health care

Clinical Situation	Ethical Dilemma	Helpful Approaches
Mother tries to harm her fetus because of delusions	Maternal autonomy versus beneficence to fetus	Relational ethics Substituted judgment
Nondelusional refusal of obstetric care	Maternal autonomy versus beneficence to mother and fetus	Justice Directive counseling
Denial of pregnancy affecting mother's decisions about treatment	Maternal autonomy versus nonmaleficence to fetus	Substitute decision maker Preventive ethics Psychiatric advance directives
Depression and concern for fetus affecting mother's decisions about treatment	Maternal autonomy versus beneficence to mother	Avoid omission bias Relational ethics
Woman who has major mental illness wants to conceive	Beneficence toward potential life versus nonmaleficence toward mother	Justice Relational ethics Preventive ethics
Maternal major mental illness found by pediatrician doing maternal mental health screening	Ethical costs versus benefits of screening	Justice Adequate follow-up system for screening Standby guardianship

The concept of relational ethics helps resolve apparent mother–offspring ethical conflicts, and the practice of preventive ethics helps anticipate and reduce the risk of ethical dilemmas and adverse clinical outcomes. These central principles suggest the following guidelines in caring for perinatal women:

- In situations that seem to pit the needs of a pregnant or postpartum woman against the needs of her fetus or baby, reframe the problem to find a solution that most benefits the mother–baby dyad while posing the least risk to the dyad.
- In evaluating a pregnant woman's ability to make autonomous, informed decisions about medical care, assess her ability to decide on behalf of both herself and her fetus.
- When explaining the risks of treatments such as psychotropic medication during pregnancy, avoid errors of omission by also explaining the risks of withholding the treatments.
- Apply the principle of justice to ensure that women are not stigmatized by having psychiatric disorders or by being pregnant.
- When screening for maternal psychiatric symptoms, ensure that the benefits of screening outweigh the ethical costs by designing effective follow-up systems for helping women who have positive screens.
- When treating women of reproductive age for psychiatric disorders, proactively discuss family planning and, when appropriate, the anticipated risks of the illness and the treatment during future pregnancies. Offer preventive interventions to reduce these risks.

REFERENCES

1. Johnsen D. A new threat to pregnant women's autonomy. Hastings Cent Rep 1987;August:33–40.
2. Curran WJ. An historical perspective on the law of personality and status with special regard to the human fetus and the rights of women. Milbank Mem Fund Q Health Soc 1983;61(1):58–75.
3. Dayan J, Creveuil C, Marks MN, et al. Prenatal depression, prenatal anxiety, and spontaneous preterm birth: a prospective cohort study among women with early and regular care. Psychosom Med 2006;68(6):938–46.
4. Davis EP, Glynn LM, Schetter CD, et al. Prenatal exposure to maternal depression and cortisol influences infant temperament. J Am Acad Child Adolesc Psychiatry 2007;46(6):737–46.
5. Poobalan AS, Aucott LS, Ross L, et al. Effects of treating postnatal depression on mother-infant interaction and child development: systematic review. Br J Psychiatry 2007;191:378–86.
6. Rahman A, Bunn J, Lovel H, et al. Association between antenatal depression and low birthweight in a developing country. Acta Psychiatr Scand 2007;115(6):481–6.
7. Li D, Liu L, Odouli R. Presence of depressive symptoms during early pregnancy and the risk of preterm delivery: a prospective cohort study. Hum Reprod 2009;24(1):146–53.
8. Shaw RJ, Deblois T, Ikuta L, et al. Acute stress disorder among parents of infants in the neonatal intensive care nursery. Psychosom 2006;47(3):206–12.
9. Ebbesen M, Pedersen BD. Empirical investigation of the ethical reasoning of physicians and molecular biologist—the importance of the four principles of biomedical ethics. Philos Ethics Humanit Med 2007;2:23–38.

10. Chervenak FA, Mccullough LB. A practical method of analysis of the physician's ethical obligations to the fetus and pregnant woman in obstetric care. Resid Staff Physician 1989;January:79–87.

11. Ament M. The right to be well-born. J Leg Med 1974;2(6):24–30.

12. Kolder VEB, Gallagher J, Parsons MT. Court-ordered obstetrical interventions. N Engl J Med 1987;316(19):1192–6.

13. Coverdale JH, McCullough LB, Chervenak FA, et al. Clinical implications of respect for autonomy in the psychiatric treatment of pregnant patients with depression. Psychiatr Serv 1997;48(2):209–12.

14. Seeman MV. Relational ethics: when mothers suffer from psychosis. Arch Womens Ment Health 2004;7(3):201–10.

15. Holden CE, Burland AS, Lemmen CA. Insanity and filicide: women who murder their children. New Dir Ment Health Serv 1996;69:25–34.

16. Roberts LW, Dunn LB. Obstet Gynecol Clin North Am 2003;30(3):559–82.

17. Ciccone JR, Tokoli JF, Clements CD, et al. Right to refuse treatment: impact of Rivers v Katz. Bull Am Acad Psychiatry Law 1990;18(2):203–15.

18. Coverdale JH, McCullough LB, Chervenak FA. Assisted and surrogate decision making for pregnant patients who have schizophrenia. Schizophr Bull 2004; 30(3):659–64.

19. Roberts LW, Geppert CM. Ethical use of long-acting medications in the treatment of severe and persistent mental illness. Compr Psychiatry 2004;45(3):161–7.

20. American Medical Association Code of Medical Ethics. Available at: www.ama-assn.org. Accessed March 31, 2009.

21. Mohaupt SM, Sharma KK. Forensic implications and medical-legal dilemmas of maternal versus fetal rights. J Forensic Sci 1998;43(5):985–92.

22. Sjostrand M, Helgesson G. Coercive treatment and autonomy in psychiatry. Bioethics 2008;22(2):113–20.

23. McCoy M. Autonomy, consent, and medical paternalism: legal issues in medical intervention. J Altern Complement Med 2008;14(6):785–92.

24. Yonkers KA, Wisner KL, Stowe Z, et al. Management of bipolar disorder during pregnancy and the postpartum period. Am J Psychiatry 2004;161(4): 608–20.

25. Miller LJ. Denial of pregnancy. In: Spinelli M, editor. Infanticide: psychosocial and legal perspectives on mothers who kill. Washington, DC: American Psychiatric Press; 2003. p. 81–104.

26. French CM. Protecting the "right" to choose of women who are incompetent: ethical, doctrinal, and practical arguments against fetal representation. Case West Reserve Law Rev 2005;56(2):511–46.

27. McCullough LB, Coverdale J, Bayer T, et al. Ethically justified guidelines for family planning interventions to prevent pregnancy in female patients with chronic mental illness. Am J Obstet Gynecol 1992;167(1):19–25.

28. Miller LJ, Finnerty M. Family planning knowledge, attitudes and practices in women with schizophrenia spectrum disorders. J Psychosom Obstet Gynaecol 1998;19(4):210–7.

29. Swanson J, Swartz M, Ferron J, et al. Psychiatric advance directives among public mental health consumers in five U.S. cities: prevalence, demand, and correlates. J Am Acad Psychiatry Law 2006;34(1):43–57.

30. Hall PL, Wittkowski A. An exploration of negative thoughts as a normal phenomenon after childbirth. J Midwifery Womens Health 2006;51(5):315–94.

31. Kordes-de Vaal JH. Intention and the omission bias: omission perceived as non-decision. Acta Psychol (Amst) 1996;93(1–3):161–72.

32. Miller LJ, Bishop J, Fischer J, et al. Balancing risks: dosing strategies for antidepressants near the end of pregnancy. J Clin Psychiatry 2008;69(2):323–4.
33. Mullick M, Miller LJ, Jacobsen T. Insight into mental illness and child maltreatment risk among mothers with major psychiatric disorders. Psychiatr Serv 2001;52(4): 488–92.
34. Leventhal A, Jacobsen T, Miller L, et al. Caregiving attitudes and at-risk maternal behavior among mothers with major mental illness. Psychiatr Serv 2004;55(12): 1431–3.
35. Jacobsen T, Miller LJ. Attachment quality in young children of mentally ill mothers: contribution of maternal caregiving abilities and foster care context. In: Solomon J, George CC, editors. Attachment disorganization. New York: Guilford Press; 1999. p. 347–78.
36. Jamison KR. An unquiet mind. New York: Knopf; 1995. p.191.
37. Murray L, Sinclair D, Cooper P, et al. The socioemotional development of 5-year-old children of postnatally depressed mothers. J Child Psychol Psychiatry 1999; 40(8):1259–71.
38. O'Brien LM, Cardner Heycock E, Hanna M, et al. Postnatal depression and faltering growth: a community study. Pediatrics 2004;113(5):1242–7.
39. Galler JR, Ramsey FC, Harrison RH, et al. Postpartum maternal moods and infant size predict performance on a national high school entrance examination. J Child Psychol Psychiatry 2004;45(6):1064–75.
40. Chaudron LH, Sziliagyi PG, Kitzman HJ, et al. Detection of postpartum depressive symptoms by screening at well-child visits. Pediatrics 2004;113(3):551–8.
41. Heneghan AM, Johnson Silver E, Bauman LJ, et al. Do pediatricians recognize mothers with depressive symptoms? Pediatrics 2000;106(6):1367–73.
42. Krantz I, Eriksson B, Lundquist-Persson C, et al. Screening for postpartum depression with the Edinburgh Postnatal Depression Scale (EPDS): an ethical analysis. Scand J Public Health 2008;36(2):211–6.
43. Gilbody S, Sheldon T, House A. Screening and case-finding instruments for depression: a meta-analysis. CMAJ 2008;18(8):997–1003.
44. Chaudron LH, Szilagyi PG, Campbell AT, et al. Legal and ethical considerations: risks and benefits of postpartum depression screening at well-child visits. Pediatrics 2007;19(1):123–8.
45. Mowbray CT, Bybee D, Oyserman D, et al. Psychosocial outcomes for adult children of parents with severe mental illnesses: demographic and clinical history predictors. Health Soc Work 2006;31(2):99–108.
46. Vance YH, Huntley Jones S, Espie J, et al. Parental communication style and family relationships in children of bipolar parents. Br J Clin Psychol 2008; 47(Pt. 3):355–9.
47. Nicholson J, Miller LJ. Parenting and schizophrenia. In: Mueser KT, Jeste DV, editors. Clinical handbook of schizophrenia. New York: Guilford; 2008. p. 471–80.
48. Geballe SD. Guardianship as a therapeutic option. Child Adolesc Psychiatr Clin N Am 2000;9(2):407–24.

Ethical Considerations in Military Psychiatry

Christopher H. Warner, MD, MAJ, MC, USA[a],*,
George N. Appenzeller, MD, LTC, MC, USA[b],
Thomas A. Grieger, MD, CAPT, MC, USN (Ret)[c],
David M. Benedek, MD, DFAPA, COL, MC, USA[c],
Laura Weiss Roberts, MD, MA[d]

KEYWORDS

- Military psychiatry • Ethics • Confidentiality
- Dual agency • Deployment health

Psychiatrists have been serving in uniform since World War I and caring for service members in times of war and peace. In the early years, military psychiatrists perceived that the rationale for the military's activities sufficiently satisfied the criteria for a "just" war and saw little role conflict or moral dilemma associated with encouraging the service member-patient to return to combat.[1] During the Vietnam War, however, the psychiatric community began to debate the appropriate role for psychiatrists during time of war, especially for those serving in the military.[1] At the root of this issue was the question "For whom does the psychiatrist work—the individual service member-patient or the military organization?"

A military psychiatrist is guided as a physician by the Hippocratic Oath and the American Psychiatric Association's code of ethics. As a military officer, psychiatrists are also guided by the Uniformed Code of Military Justice and the mission of the military medical officer to "maintain the fighting force." Currently, there are more than 540,000 individuals in military service, with more than 250 military and civilian psychiatrists providing direct care and offering expertise to the military related to key mental

Financial and Proprietary Disclosure: This article was not supported by pharmaceutical companies. The work herein was part of our employment with the federal government and is therefore in the public domain. The stated views are those of the authors and do not represent the views or the policy of the Department of Defense. No industry grants or financial support were used in this project.

[a] Department of Behavioral Medicine, Winn Army Community Hospital, 1061 Harmon Avenue, Fort Stewart, GA 31314, USA

[b] Winn Army Community Hospital, 1061 Harmon Avenue, Fort Stewart, GA 31314, USA

[c] Department of Psychiatry, Uniformed Services University of the Health Sciences, Bethesda, MD 20814, USA

[d] Department of Psychiatry and Behavioral Medicine, Medical College of Wisconsin, Milwaukee, WI 53226, USA

* Corresponding author.

E-mail address: christopher.h.warner@us.army.mil (C.H. Warner).

Psychiatr Clin N Am 32 (2009) 271–281
doi:10.1016/j.psc.2009.02.006
0193-953X/09/$ – see front matter. Published by Elsevier Inc.

psych.theclinics.com

health issues.[2] This article reviews several of the common challenges that current military psychiatrists face in performing their duties with overlapping roles (as psychiatrist and military physician) and in resolving potential conflicts between these two positions. Examples of such challenges are provided for consideration as case vignettes. The key ethical considerations encountered by military psychiatrists and discussed herein include confidentiality, informed consent, dual agency, boundaries, dealing with detainees, determining fitness for deployments, treatment in combat, and separation from the military.

VIGNETTE 1: CASE OF CONFIDENTIALITY

Private First Class L is currently a patient who reports in session that she is having an extramarital affair with one of her senior supervisors in the unit during a deployment to a combat zone. She reports during the sessions that she is receiving special treatment and that on multiple occasions less qualified soldiers have been sent on dangerous missions by this supervisor in place of her. The psychiatrist, who is also in the unit, is aware that there have been recent mission failures and casualties associated with the poor performance of her section.

VIGNETTE 2: CASE OF MAINTAINING BOUNDARIES

Captain B is the psychiatrist working at a medical aid station in a small remote outpost in Iraq where he is the only mental health care provider. He has worked in the clinic for 3 months and routinely socializes with the rest of the clinic medical staff. One day while in clinic, Colonel X, who is the chief medical officer for the clinic and the psychiatrist's primary supervisor, pulls the psychiatrist aside and states that he would like to discuss his anxiety problems and is requesting a refill of his selective serotonin reuptake inhibitor and his benzodiazepine medication.

VIGNETTE 3: CASE OF DEALING WITH A SOLDIER'S DISPOSITION FROM THE MILITARY

Private First Class M is a 20- year-old woman who just returned from a successful 12-month deployment to Afghanistan, where she served as a medic working in an emergency trauma facility. She has no prior history of mental health issues. Since her return, she has been undergoing treatment for 1 to 2 months for posttraumatic stress disorder. During a visit with the psychiatrist, she expresses that she no longer desires to remain in the military and requests a chapter separation, although she has 2 years remaining on her obligation. The psychiatrist is unclear at this time as to the extent the conditions impact her fitness for continued service and her level of potential need for disability. The psychiatrist tells the soldier that he is not able to recommend a chapter at this time because he wants to ensure that she receives optimal medical care. Three days later, the soldier is admitted to the psychiatric ward with suicidal thoughts and a plan to harm herself if she is not released from the military.

VIGNETTE 4: CASE OF DETERMINING FITNESS FOR DEPLOYMENT

Sergeant S is a 27-year-old man with a history of posttraumatic stress disorder that has been well controlled through a selective serotonin reuptake inhibitor for his anxiety symptoms and the use of low-dose neuroleptic for improved sleep. He has not required any hospitalization, has no reports of substance abuse, and his job performance as mission analyst in the unit headquarters has been outstanding. The psychiatrist sees this patient at his predeployment evaluation. The soldier and his unit leader express desire to deploy, and during the interview the soldier specifically discusses plans that he and his wife have made for spending the additional money that he will make during deployment. The psychiatrist notes, however, that per the Minimum Mental Health Standards for Deployment, this soldier is unfit.

KEY TOPICS
Confidentiality

Military psychiatrists come into contact with service member-patients through two general routes. The most common route is self-referral by the service member who identifies a need for mental health care. The second route is through a process by which service members are referred for treatment by their supervisor or commanding officer (a "command referral") for evaluation. Both of the routes "in" to the military psychiatrist have ethical safeguards to protect the confidentiality of the service member-patient, but the safeguards differ in the two referral circumstances and differ from the confidentiality privilege guidelines that exist in clinical care settings outside of the military.

When service members self-refer, they generally enter treatment through a clinic setting in which they first sign privacy and disclosure statements as part of the intake process. Most clinicians also explicitly discuss the nature and the limits of confidentiality when they first meet with service member-patients. Records of clinical encounters may be stored in local paper files, but nearly all military treatment facilities currently use an electronic treatment record. The different services and facilities may have different control processes to regulate the degree to which these electronic records can be accessed by other health care providers. This said, unit commanders have no direct access to the treatment records for self-referred service member-patients.

Under conditions of self-referral, unit commanders are notified of service member mental health conditions only under rare circumstances. Most common conditions, such as moderate depression, adjustment disorders, anxiety disorders (including posttraumatic stress disorder), life circumstance problems (eg, marital discord), and work-related problems, do not significantly impair function and are not reported. Exceptions to this rule exist in some specialty communities, such as flight crews, personnel in submarine service, and personnel working with nuclear weapons. In those communities, regulations may require that the unit command be notified whenever a service member is treated with psychiatric medications. Service members are generally aware of this notification requirement and its potential impact on the employment before self-referring.

One common misconception regarding confidentiality in the care of service member-patients is that a psychiatric diagnosis of any sort results in an automatic removal of a security clearance. Psychiatrists do not disclose psychiatric treatment to commanders or security officials unless the condition is so serious as to preclude the patient's ability to safeguard national security information. Conditions that might lead to such a breach in confidentiality would include psychotic disorders and bipolar disorder if severe enough to lead to significantly impaired judgment or uncontrolled impulsivity.

Other matters that would lead to command notification in the context of a self-referred service member-patient would include ongoing suicidal ideation, homicidal ideation, severe psychiatric conditions that impair cognitive function and judgment (eg, severe major depression or bipolar disorder), psychotic disorders, and unstable conditions that may lead to periods of hospitalization. All such conditions would significantly impair work performance and potentially endanger the safety of others. A lower threshold for notification exists for service members in high-profile positions (eg, unit commanders) and personnel in a status of pending or ongoing deployment because of the access to and availability of mechanisms of lethal force.

A military psychiatrist also may come into contact with a service member-patient through a process by which service members are referred for treatment by their supervisor or commanding officer (a "command referral") for evaluation. Unlike self-referral, which is more common and has different confidentiality boundaries, with command referrals there is an expectation of some disclosure of patient information. There are statutory and regulatory provisions to rigorously protect the rights of services members in the event of command-directed psychiatric evaluations, however.[3,4] Among other protections, commanders must document the specific behaviors that have given cause for such an evaluation, the evaluation must be conducted in the least restrictive environment allowed, the service member must have access to legal counsel if desired, and if continued involuntary hospitalization is required, an independent review of necessity must be conducted every 72 hours. These safeguards assure a high level of accountability in the process of dealing with the complex issues that arise in the evaluative and treatment process. In the event of a command-directed evaluation, it is clear to all parties that a fitness-for-return-to-duty recommendation is forwarded to the command at completion of the evaluation.

Informed Consent

Psychiatric care for service member-patients adheres to the legal and ethical doctrine of informed consent, which honors an individual's ability to make a knowledgeable and free decision about his or her health and treatment. Informed consent is itself based on three elements.[5] The first element is a process of accurate and careful information-sharing in which the service member-patient is given information about his or her illness, its nature and outcome with and without recommended intervention, the risks and benefits of the care that is offered, and the alternatives to the treatment under consideration. Second, it is predicated on the sound decision-making ability of the service member-patient, that is, the ability to communicate, comprehend salient factual information relevant in the situation, reason through these facts in a logical fashion, and appreciate the meaning and implications of the decision in the context of the individual's life. Third, it depends on consent (or refusal) for treatment being authentic and voluntary, based on the genuine values and preferences of the individual and not coerced.

The third element of voluntarism has been subject to discussion and represents a potential ethical vulnerability for a service member-patient who may feel unable to seek treatment or decline recommended treatment. This perception of diminished self-determination may occur because of, for example, the legitimate and previously agreed-to constraints on freedoms in a military situation or perceived concerns that seeking care may negatively impact the service member-patient's career. Examples in which duty to military service may supersede the needs of the patient are rare but may include limitations on medication choices because of impact on service member-patient's fitness for deployment or continued service or involuntarily separating a service member-patient from the military despite his or her desire to continue service. It is imperative that the military psychiatrist address these potential limitations early in the therapeutic relationship with the service member-patient to help minimize refusal of service and optimize informed consent.

Dual Agency

Military psychiatrists play many roles related to prevention of mental health issues and crises, ongoing education of service members and colleagues, and consultation to leaders in the military related to broad and specific issues. Military psychiatrists also must balance these roles related to their overall contribution to the military along with their therapeutic interactions with patients. As physicians, they attend directly to the needs of their patients, maintain confidentiality, and protect the privacy of the information conveyed to them in clinical settings. At the same time, military psychiatrists serve the organization in ensuring that the unit is able to optimally perform its mission without undue danger to service members or others. At times these overlapping roles, each with significant responsibilities and duties, create a sense of "dual agency," which in turn can lead to real and perceived conflicts.

Although in common practice civilian psychiatrists adhere to a policy of maintaining nearly universal confidentiality, there are exceptions to that policy when the courts or legislative bodies have established criteria for a greater public good through disclosure of otherwise confidential information. Common exceptions in all fields of medicine include the reporting of suspected child abuse and—in some jurisdictions—suspected spousal or elder abuse. In mental health care there is also a "duty to protect" individuals and society at large from potential actions of persons with mental disturbances. This duty may be met through treatment, hospitalization, or notification of potential victims or law enforcement agencies, depending on the specifics of the threats.

Similarly, flight surgeons (military and civilian) also hold an obligation to report to employers and governmental agencies conditions they detect that would impair a pilot's ability to safely operate an aircraft. The military services have at their disposal weapons of extreme lethal force, and in the common performance of their daily duties, many service members have ready access to weapons ranging from small arms to large-scale weapons of destruction. Much of the equipment used by the military, such as high-performance aircraft and naval ships, also require careful routine maintenance to ensure safe operation even in a noncombat setting. Conditions that may impair cognitive abilities, judgment, and impulse control can potentially lead to devastating outcomes.

When making recommendations about treatment, duty limitations, and separation or evacuation, the mental health care provider must keep in mind the service member's ability to perform his or her assigned job in a combat environment. This assessment becomes more difficult in the case of service members who are struggling with the psychological effects of combat. The health care provider may find it difficult to determine the proper time to recommend that a unit commander remove a service member from continued combat exposure while keeping in mind the unit's mission and current needs. These situations must be examined carefully, and as with many ethical issues, there is no single right answer. Discussion with colleagues or senior mental health care providers is recommended and can be helpful in processing the issues and arriving at a course of action.

Boundaries

When providers live and work in a small community, many complex issues related to professional and personal role boundaries also arise. Military psychiatrists, more than other physicians and military physicians, need to exercise great care in establishing social relationships—not unlike mental health care providers in frontier communities.[6] Military psychiatrists are wise to maintain social relationships with fairly stable, resilient service members who are not likely to become patients in the future, something that is difficult to assure. This issue is further compounded at small, remote installations and in the deployed environment, in which no other psychiatrist may be available for referral. Perhaps the most challenging request a deployed military psychiatrist may face is when a previous nonpatient, such as a tent mate, exercise partner, or friend, needs mental health care. Changing the social relationship can be awkward and isolating for a provider and the new patient.

Senior officers and supervisors of the military psychiatrist may request treatment, and providing treatment may be not only in the senior officer's best interest but also the entire unit's. Although referral in these cases is preferable, strategies should be prepared when a lack of referral options and the potential for dual relationships is likely. Again, this circumstance resembles the concerns that arise in mental health care in small and isolated communities; it is different, however, in that the consequences of failure to attend to these issues may be more serious because of the special roles and responsibilities of military psychiatrist and service members in protecting the interests of the country.[6]

Boundaries must be discussed clearly at the outset of treatment, separating the treatment from the professional or personal relationship and establishing expectations for both parties. The military psychiatrist should, whenever possible, arrange a specific time and place for therapy sessions even if they are not in an office setting. Great care must be taken to ensure that service members recognize when they are in a therapeutic encounter. This recognition emphasizes the importance of differentiating therapeutic from social encounters. At the beginning of treatment, the psychiatrist should discuss how both parties will handle daily interactions, such as seeing each other at the dining facility, the gym, or in the general living area. Key areas to be discussed include whether and how each party would like to be recognized and greeted in a nonclinical setting and appropriate times to approach with nonemergent questions or concerns. If not discussed, these boundaries can negatively impact the therapeutic alliance between the service member and the military psychiatrist.

Ethical Considerations Related to Detainees

The Geneva Conventions of 1949 addresses principles of medical care for the sick and wounded on land, prisoners of war, and civilian populations.[7] Additional Protocol I to the Geneva Conventions provides that medical personnel "shall not be compelled to perform acts or to carry out work contrary to the rules of medical ethics."[8] Although the additional protocol has not been ratified by the United States, it may be construed as evidence of international law.

Army Regulation 190-8, Enemy Prisoners of War, Retained Personnel, Civilian Internees, and Other Detainees and the more recent Medical Program Principles and Procedures for the Protection and Treatment of Detainees in the Custody of the Armed Forces of the United States articulate the principles of humane treatment for detainees regardless of their status as lawful or unlawful combatants, noting that all detainees should be provided with humanitarian care and specifically prohibiting acts of torture, sensory deprivation, and threats or acts of violence.[9,10] Practically speaking, current regulations have been interpreted as necessitating the provision of medical care, including psychiatric assessment and treatment essentially equivalent to that provided to our own military forces. Beyond the language barrier between detainee and care provider, differences in beliefs surrounding the meaning of mental illness, the underpinnings of symptoms such as hallucinations, and cultural expectations surrounding appropriate treatment are issues to consider in treatment planning, care delivery, and resource allocation.

One immediate challenge faced by military psychiatrists treating detainees is the potential conflict between allegiance to professional ethics and the primacy of mission in military ethics. The American Medical Association and the American Psychiatric Association have articulated positions precluding physicians, including psychiatrists, from participating in coercive interrogation.[11,12] As of the writing of this issue, US military regulations preclude physicians (or any service members) from participating in torture or any cruel or inhumane acts, but US Department of Defense policy allows for psychiatric consultation to interrogation teams. The psychiatrist may not participate in cruel, inhumane, or degrading acts and has a lawful and ethical obligation to report any suspicion or observation of cruel or inhumane treatment to the appropriate authority. This may include the medical chain of command or the Inspector General. Department of Defense policy draws a distinction between physicians serving in consultative roles and those acting as care providers and dictates that these functions should be served by different persons. Many people believe that a physician's ethics may not vary as a function of the role he or she is serving, however.[13]

Detainees may participate in hunger strikes. At times this behavior may reflect an individual's decision to protest some aspect of his or her confinement; at other times refusal may be coerced by the threat of harm from others. Failure to maintain nutritional status also may result from depression or psychotic illness. US policy provides for the force feeding of detainees to preserve life. As part of the procedures for assessing detainees who refuse to eat, military psychiatrists may be asked to assess for mental illness (eg, depression or psychosis) or explore issues of mental status or environmental factors that may lead to a diminished capacity to make a voluntary decision to refuse nutrition. The Declaration of Malta and other international ethical writings have exhorted physicians to not participate in the force feeding of competent prisoners or seek to prevent this practice.[14,15] There are ethical arguments on either side of this issue. Currently, a sufficient number of US physicians agree to voluntarily participate in humane force feeding enacted with respect for detainee dignity, without threat or violence, and with minimal use of restraint that the wishes of those who decline to participate in this practice are respected.

Minimum Mental Health Standards for Deployment

Before a deployment, military units conduct medical evaluations to ensure that service member-patients are capable of performing their duties during the deployment and to make sure that continued medical care can be provided for their condition. In recent international conflicts, such as the operations in Iraq and Afghanistan, media reports began to assert that military psychiatrists and medical providers were clearing service members to deploy to a combat zone who were mentally unfit to meet the needs of the military.[16]

In 2006, the US Department of Defense developed a minimum mental health standard for deployment. This policy provides the military psychiatrist with conditions that can be managed in theater and what level of treatment can be provided during a deployment.[17] Other than psychosis and bipolar disorder, this policy does not identify specific mental health diagnoses as preventing an individual from being deployed. Instead, this decision is based on symptom severity, time under treatment, stability of the psychiatric condition, and the level of care required.

To determine if service members meet the minimum mental health standards for deployment, deploying units are incorporating mental health screening into their predeployment medical screening process. That process allows the deploying unit's medical personnel to be aware of all service members who have active neuropsychiatric diagnoses, are currently undergoing treatment, or are taking a psychotropic medication. This tracking allows the medical team to develop a continuation of treatment plan, assist in linking the service member to the necessary mental health resources during the deployment, and put in place measures to ensure that appropriate safety precautions are enacted. For example, service members who are identified as taking a benzodiazepine, a potentially sedating medication, may be deployed but restricted to duties within a headquarters facility where they can have a more consistent routine and not be expected to make rapid decisions about rules of engagement or determine whether an individual is an enemy or noncombatant.

Medical personnel also can ensure that service members have continued access to appropriate mental health care and can monitor them to ensure they remain in care. Establishing continuity of care between military mental health care providers at home and during deployment can help prevent mental health conditions from deteriorating and help ensure service member and unit safety. Failure to perform these actions can be detrimental to the service member and the unit as well as consume inordinate amounts of time for deployed military psychiatrists.

Use of Psychotropic Medications in Combat

The attitude toward using psychotropic medication in the combat theater has evolved significantly in the last 20 years. The initial Army *Field Manual on Combat Stress Control* (FM 8-51), published in 1994, focused on triage and nonpharmacologic interventions aimed at normalizing and minimizing combat stress.[18] Little guidance was provided on the role and usage of psychotropic medications, and most of these references focused only on the use of medications in emergency situations when medication might be needed to calm an agitated service member. The manual also stated that medication should be "prescribed sparingly and only when needed to temporarily support sleep or manage disruptive symptoms."[18]

A change in perspective emerged in 2006, when the US Army mental health community updated its doctrine on combat operational stress control based on lessons learned from the operations in Afghanistan and Iraq. The new guidance recommended using medications when appropriate, emphasizing the importance of considering side effects, limited availability of laboratory monitoring, and continued application of the forward psychiatry principles.[19] This policy change has led to debate about whether the use of psychotropic medications in the combat theater is ever appropriate. Persons against the policy argue that service members cannot be monitored sufficiently and are receiving amounts of medication that are in excess to that which is of standard practice within the United States.

When considering whether to prescribe a service member psychotropic medications in the combat environment, the military psychiatrist should consider several factors. Providers need to ensure that they are able to follow-up with individuals who are started on medications and that resupply is available. The method for dispensing psychotropic medications in theater is determined by several factors, including the service member's access to mental health care services, service member reliability, and the proximity of other pharmacy services. In general, service members are not to be provided more than a 1-month supply of medication to ensure adequate follow-up.

Military psychiatrists also must make decisions regarding the extent of services they can safely and effectively provide their units. Providers must recognize the limitations of their resources, capabilities, and situation and make the decision to treat in theater, return the service member to home station, or delay treatment until the service member returns home as scheduled. The decision to continue to treat in theater or to evacuate service members depends on which medications are available, how significant the symptoms are, how the service member initially responds to treatment, how significantly the symptoms may interfere with the service member's assigned duties, and what duties and responsibilities the service member is expected to perform.

Separation from the Military

At times soldiers may have mental health conditions that do not require a medical disability discharge but may make a soldier unfit for duty. These conditions are defined in Army Regulation 635-200 (Enlisted Separations).[20] Predominantly, military psychiatrists are involved with chapters 5-13 (personality disorders) and 5-17 (other mental or physical disorders).[20] Both of these chapters require that the soldier not have a condition that would require a medical discharge and disability evaluation, such as bipolar disorder, posttraumatic stress disorder, or schizophrenia. Both chapters also require that the soldier be formally counseled and afforded "ample opportunity to overcome those deficiencies."[20] They should not be used in lieu of judicial actions or other administrative separations, and military psychiatrists must be cognizant of their appropriate use and potential for misuse.

Chapter 5-13 states that a soldier can be separated for personality disorder if the condition severely impairs the soldier's ability to function in the military environment (ie, potentially jeopardizes the health and safety of others and/or key operations of the military). The policy further states that the disorder must be longstanding and deeply ingrained.[20] This is particularly important when dealing with the postdeployment soldier who may have confounding posttraumatic stress issues, mild traumatic brain injuries, or acute situational issues. It is expected that a military psychiatrist considering this separation has documented a longstanding pattern of dysfunctional behavior that clearly has impaired social and occupational relationships but is not the result of military service.

Chapter 5-17 deals with physical or mental issues not covered under other areas of the separation regulations that "potentially interfere with assignment to or performance of duty."[20] This includes conditions such as claustrophobia, disturbances of perception, emotional control or behavior, dyslexia, sleepwalking, or other disorders that may significantly impair military duties.

In recent years, the military has been accused of using these separations to withhold disability benefits from service members. Although such separations are primarily decided by commanders, an evaluation and diagnosis by an appropriately credentialed provider is required. A good working knowledge of these chapters and the separation process enables military psychiatrists to counsel commanders—some of whom may be junior in rank and experience or may be facing other pressing issues—in the appropriate and judicious use of these actions. Such knowledge and counsel help to avoid unnecessary delays, misdiagnosis, inappropriate separations, and potential procedural errors.

At times, military psychiatrists may perceive pressure to recommend use of these chapter separations as opposed to a fitness-for-duty and disability evaluation. This pressure often comes from the patient, the unit, or both who are primarily trying to expedite a rapid exit from the military for varying reasons. These "chapter separations" are often more expedient, require less paperwork and levels of review, and generally lead to a quicker separation from the military. Soldiers who are chapter separated are not afforded medical disability benefits, however, and may re-enter military service as early as 6 months after discharge. It is imperative that the military psychiatrist conduct a thorough evaluation and ensure appropriate disposition as defined by the current military regulations. It is also important for the service member to understand the meaning and consequences of the evaluation and rationale for separation. This understanding ensures the best care for the patient, the military, and the society that the soldier may be returning to upon discharge from the military.

SUMMARY

Military psychiatrists are faced with multiple, difficult questions that shape the context for ethical patient care. These questions are difficult to answer,r and future efforts, including policy and evidence-based treatment practices, should aim at reducing the ambiguity faced by military psychiatrists. New research should focus on issues as diverse as optimal approaches to informed consent, evidence-derived approaches to protecting confidentiality, outcomes of care for individuals in widely varying military roles, and medication use in the field. Training for mental health care providers who deal with military patients should be provided not only in military graduate medical education but also in job-specific courses and in ethics. This should include specific training for personnel who will be dealing with specific populations, such as the US Army's current "Dealing with Detainee course" and the Army Medical Department's "Combat Operational Stress Course" for deploying military psychiatrists and psychologists.

REFERENCES

1. Camp NM. The Vietnam war and the ethics of combat psychiatry. Am J Psychiatry 1993;150:1000–10.
2. United States Department of Defense. Department of Defense active duty military personnel by rank/grade. December 31, 2008. Available at: http://siadpp.dmdc.osd.mil/personnel/MILITARY/rg0812.pdf. Accessed February 6, 2009.
3. Department of Defense. Directive 6490.1. Mental health evaluations of members of the armed forces. Washington, DC: Department of Defense; 1997.
4. Department of Defense. Instructions 6490.4. Requirements for mental health evaluations of members of the armed forces. Washington, DC: Department of Defense; 1998.
5. Roberts LW. Informed consent and the capacity for voluntarism. Am J Psychiatry 2002;159:705–12.
6. Roberts LW, Battaglia J, Epstein RS. Frontier ethics: mental health care needs and ethical dilemmas in rural communities. Psychiatr Serv 1999;50:497–503.
7. Geneva Convention (III) relative to the treatment of the prisoners of war: article 17. August 12, 1949. Available at: http://www.icrc.org/IHL.nsf/0/6fef854a3517b75ac125641e004a9e68?OpenDocument. Accessed January 11, 2009.
8. Additional to the Geneva Conventions of 12 August 1949, and relating to the Protection of Victims of International Armed Conflicts (Protocol 1)Adopted on 8 June 1977 by the Diplomatic Conference on the Reaffirmation and Development. Available at: http://www.unhchr.ch/html/menu3/b/93.htm. Accessed January 11, 2009.
9. Army Regulation 190–8/OPNAVINST 3461.6/AFJI 31-304MCO 3461.1. Available at: http://www.apd.army.mil/pdffiles/r190_8.pdf. Accessed January 11, 2009.
10. Assistant Secretary of Defense for Health Affairs. Medical program principles and procedures for the protection and treatment of detainees in the custody of the armed forces of the United States [memorandum for the secretaries of the military departments]. Available at: http://www.cageprisoners.com/download.php?download=227. Accessed January 10, 2009.

Table 1	
Principles of medical ethics applied to addiction	
Concept	**Application**
Autonomy or self-determination	A patient in the medical ICU for her fifth admission for an upper gastrointestinal bleed in 1 year refuses admission to an inpatient addiction psychiatry unit.
Beneficence	An addiction therapist is counseling a patient from a rural area who must travel several hours to the sessions. He believes it is in the best interest of the patient to be admitted to a residential program, which is restricted to patients who have failed outpatient treatment. The therapist advocates for the patient's admission.
Nonmaleficence	A patient who has ADHD and methamphetamine dependence asks his psychiatrist to prescribe a stimulant so he won't self-medicate with illicit drugs.
Justice	A patient who has cocaine dependence who has failed outpatient treatment several times is denied admission to a long-term residential program because his insurance company states it is not clinically indicated.
Respect for people	An Iraq veteran who has PTSD and chronic pain from an intermittent explosive device requests a refill of his opioids 2 days early and is told he is a "drug addict."
Truth-telling	A nurse on a geriatric ward is abusing opioids and promises she will enter monitored treatment if her nurse manager does not report her to the nursing board.

Abbreviations: ADHD, attention deficit hyperactivity disorder; PTSD, posttraumatic stress disorder.

Part 2 of Title 42 (Public Health Code) of the Code of Federal Regulations (CFR). The second is the Health Insurance and Portability and Accountability Act of the 1996 (HIPAA), Parts 160 and 164 of Title 45 (Public Welfare) of the Code of Federal Regulations. These regulations have precedence over all other state, federal, local and institutional rulings and policies.[13–15] The rationale for these tighter safeguards is to encourage patients to discuss their substance use and its deleterious consequences fully and honestly as a means of facilitating accurate diagnosis and effective treatment. Without protection of confidentiality, disclosure of substance abuse information could lead to criminal action, loss of employment or insurance, disruption of close relationships, or family conflicts. It is incumbent upon mental health professionals working in the area of addictions to familiarize themselves with these regulations and applicable state law and to have ready access to legal advice for instances in which the regulations are unclear or contradict other legal requirements.

At first glance the rigor of these regulations may seem to impede high-quality clinical care, which requires obtaining collateral information, coordinating mental health and medical treatment, and obtaining social services for people who have addiction. Clinicians may also wonder how they are to manage competing ethical demands, such as respect for people and autonomy, nonmaleficence, truth-telling, beneficence, and justice, because these principles apply to both the patient and the public. Cognizant of these competing demands, the regulations do allow for the type of public health exceptions that mental health clinicians expect, such as reporting of the abuse of children and incompetent elders, suicidal and homicidal threats, true medical emergencies, and infectious disease reporting. The standard HIPAA provisions that apply to medical care, such as appropriately authorized research, program auditing or evaluation, disclosure to a qualified service organization assisting the program, communication among treatment staff for purposes of care, and communication with outside entities that support the program, are permitted for substance abuse information as well.[16]

Many ethical dilemmas can be avoided or at least attenuated if practitioners educate and counsel patients at the start of treatment regarding the limitations of confidentiality particularly when the legal system is involved. Such a dialog can build a spirit of trust while honoring the letter of the law. Similarly, when releasing substance abuse information, even with patient consent, awareness of the greater stigma and potential adverse impact of such releases cautions the provider to document with prudence and discretion and to report only those data necessary to achieve the purpose of the disclosure. Collaborating with patients at the initiation of treatment and on the occasion of any significant disclosure to determine the content of disclosures, alternative treatment options, and means of minimizing the harm respects patient interests even when the involvement of third parties limits privacy and autonomy. Patients who have security clearances, high-profile social or professional positions, or those who have strained family relationships may at times request that clinicians keep a "shadow chart" or "doctor the record." While empathizing with the patient's concerns, professionals should avoid such "work-arounds" because they render the professional legally vulnerable and ethically suspect. Important medical and psychiatric information that directly affects clinical care should always be documented in the medical record in a nonjudgmental and factual manner.[17]

The most ethically problematic disclosures involve exceptions specific to addictions treatment. Once a patient initiates contact with a substance use treatment facility, his identity as a person with an addictive disorder cannot be disclosed unless the circumstances meet the exceptions mentioned earlier. This restriction applies even if the patient does not appear for the initial intake or subsequently leaves the program. One of the most difficult confidentiality situations is when a client of a substance abuse program threatens a staff member or commits a crime on the premises of the facility. In such cases the identity of the patient and his status as a patient in substance abuse treatment can be reported to law enforcement. But no past criminal activity can be disclosed even if the information pertains to unsolved cases.[16] Another problematic and all too common situation occurs when patients present intoxicated to substance use programs and staff must balance privacy considerations with the need to protect the public from impaired drivers. Patients can be given the opportunity to stay at the facility until safe to drive or be provided with safe transport home. Should patients refuse all reasonable options, staff can report patients to the local motor vehicle department or notify police without revealing that the patients suffers from an addictive disorder.[18]

This legally heightened duty to respect the confidentiality of substance-abusing patients frequently comes into conflict with the equally important obligation to truth telling. Nowhere are these conflicts more challenging than in the intersection with the criminal justice system. Here the regulations provide immense help to clinicians because they protect even patients whose treatment is mandated unless a prior formal waiver of the restrictions is obtained as part of the judicial process in adjudication, probation, or parole. To safeguard the integrity of the therapeutic relationship, clinicians are well advised to limit disclosures to criminal justice entities to treatment participation reports or homicidal or suicidal threats.[13] Clinicians often experience moral distress when confronted with patients for whom failure to adhere to treatment, whether through positive toxicology screens or missed appointments, results in adverse personal, occupational, social, or legal consequences. In attempting to resolve such ethical dilemmas, it is often helpful for health professionals to remember that their primary commitment is to the good of the patient, whereas the primary obligation of police and the courts is to protect public safety and enforce the law. This recognition allows practitioners to approach lapses in treatment in a therapeutic context while not inappropriately shielding patients from the short-term ramifications of their own behavior that may in fact benefit them their recovery in the long run.[19]

INFORMED CONSENT AND DECISIONAL CAPACITY

The legal and ethical mandate to obtain informed consent from patients for all medical treatment, including psychotherapy and counseling, is grounded in the ethical principles of respect for people and autonomy. True informed consent requires the clinician provide adequate patient-centered information, including at minimum the diagnosis, proposed treatment with its attendant risks and benefits, and alternatives to the treatment, including no intervention. Informed consent also necessitates that patents have intact decision-making capacity and voluntarism to process and act on the information.[20] The traditional model of decisional capacity assesses the patient's ability to communicate a choice, to comprehend information, to reason about options, risks, and benefits, and to appreciate the effect of choices on their life course and values.[21] The patient must also possess voluntarism, the capacity to exercise self-determination without undue internal or external coercion.[22] SUDs present specific challenges for this established formulation of informed consent in the key areas of cognitive deficits related to information processing and neurobiologic and psychosocial threats to decisional capacity and voluntarism.

Research is increasingly recognizing addiction as a biobehavioral disorder that calls into question the long-held moral view of addiction as either a character flaw or a social problem, each with its own ethical valence.[23] Although this medicalizing of substance abuse does have the potential to reduce personal stigma and social shame, it also calls into question the assumptions of autonomy and personal responsibility that underlie many forms of treatment and recent drug control policy with its forensic emphasis. These advances in the biology and psychology of addiction also suggest that individuals who use substances chronically or heavily may have cognitive and volitional impairments that reduce their ability to provide informed consent or refusal for treatment and research, and may even diminish their free will to reduce or stop abusing substances despite recognition of their devastating consequences.[24-26]

In a 2007 presentation, Nora Volkow, director of the National Institute of Drug Abuse, discussed the results of a 2006 study published in the *Journal of Neuroscience*, which explored craving and conditioned responses to drugs of abuse operating on the reward pathway.[27] Eighteen subjects who had cocaine addiction were tested using PET scanning and a dopamine D2 receptor radioligand that competes with endogenous dopamine. Comparative changes in specific dopamine binding when subjects watched a video of people smoking cocaine were measured to elucidate further the mechanisms of cocaine cuing triggering dopamine release and craving. Binding of the radioligand in the dorsal, but not ventral, striatum was significantly reduced in the cocaine cue condition, indicating increased dopamine receptor binding, and the degree of reduction correlated with self-reported craving. Volkow and others have demonstrated that subjects with the highest scores on measures of withdrawal symptoms and addiction severity had the most dramatic changes in dopamine.

In commenting on these and similar findings of earlier studies Dr. Volkow stated, "We have come to see addiction as a disease that involves the destruction of multiple systems in the brain that are more or less able to compensate for one another." Volkow further commented that, "When the pathology erodes the various systems, you disrupt the ability to compensate, and the addictive disease erodes and destroys the life of the individual."[28] Chronic addiction may diminish, and even perhaps eliminate, the individual's capacity for rational and voluntary choice so critical for informed consent and the motivation and ability to change integral to addiction treatment.

Compounding these deficits in cognition are many of the behavioral manifestations of addiction that may adversely affect motivations and choices underlying patient participation in treatment and research, calling into serious question the degree to which participation is voluntary or susceptible to coercion. Craving, sensitization, withdrawal states, and habituation all can reduce subjects' ability to exercise free will.[29] Various potentially coercive forces impinge on people with addictions, including legal pressure, family and social stressors, uncontrollable craving, withdrawal symptoms, desperation, feelings of powerlessness with respect to authority figures such as care providers and researchers, social stigmatization, depression, anxiety, and poverty. At least four studies have examined participants' reasons for participation in addiction treatment, shedding some light on the question of voluntarism in consent. Wild and colleagues[30] surveyed 300 participants entering SUD treatment. Not all mandated participants experienced their participation as coercive, whereas many self-referred participants did identify coercive psychologic factors. The degree of substance dependence did not correlate with the level of coercion perceived. The authors concluded that coercion has multiple determinants, including social and psychologic variables that undermine individual autonomy. Marlowe and colleagues[31] developed a coding algorithm for reasons for addiction treatment participation. A total of 260 cocaine-dependent participants were interviewed using open-ended questions about advantages of quitting cocaine, disadvantages of continuing to use, and reasons for seeking treatment. The study found that 69% of responses represented non-coercive reasons, and that there were highly significant differences in the proportion of coercive pressures among the psychosocial domains.

Understanding how coercive factors may affect the voluntarism of patients in addiction treatment is salient for the development of assessments to detect impairments in self-determination and for the formulation of procedures to maximize patient autonomy that may contribute to the success of addiction treatment. One study in a substance abuse rehabilitation program investigated characteristics of patients who consented to randomization versus those who refused. Patients who consented had a longer history of drug abuse, less occupational stability at intake, and poorer outcomes after treatment than those who refused randomization but continued in the experimental assessment.[32] Identifying and understanding how these and other patient and clinician factors influence informed consent is the first step to designing approaches to individualize and optimize consent for addictions treatment.

The ancient philosophical controversy regarding free will and determinism[33] has been recast in neurobiologic terms as philosophers and neuroscientists debate whether and to what degree people addicted to substances of abuse are responsible for their disorders and those detrimental actions resulting from addiction. Among the most controversial implications of this paradigm shift is in the areas of court-ordered treatment of addiction and involuntary commitment for SUDs. The controversy is reflected in the wide variety of state laws regarding the matter.[34] Some jurisdictions permit the involuntary commitment of people who have drug addiction and alcohol dependence who are a danger to themselves or others under either mental health codes or separate statutes. Other states do not allow commitment for inpatient treatment of SUDs but do permit protective custody of acutely intoxicated individuals.

The inconsistency of the legal response underscores the need for clinicians to be familiar with the statutes of their local jurisdiction and to have access to legal counsel.

An allied and equally contentious ethical debate surrounds mandated treatment of SUDs often as an alternative to incarceration or as a condition of probation or parole. Even experts in the field disagree about the effectiveness of enforced treatment and whether external coercion to receive addiction treatment can and does eventually produce internal motivation to change choices and behaviors.[35,36] Under the social construction of addiction as a character flaw and even to some extent in the disease model people should be responsible for the consequences of their actions, such as losing their license for drunk driving or being fired for using drugs in the workplace, precisely because they have free will and choose to exercise poor judgment.[37,38] Under the same philosophical assumptions, however, drinking and using drugs are voluntary actions of a person who has decision-making capacity, and respect for autonomy, privacy, and individual rights means the only warrant for clinical or forensic intervention is to prevent harm to others, with the exception of explicit suicidality.[39]

The emerging neurobiologic discoveries regarding the intensity of craving and the power of compulsion in addiction suggest that analogous to other serious mental illnesses, such as schizophrenia, people who have severe addiction may have extremely diminished capacity to choose any other priorities over substances even in the face of the most deleterious medical and personal consequences, including death. The fiduciary duty of the clinician, the principle of beneficence, the doctrine of *parens patriae* would argue that mandated or even enforced treatment maybe necessary to protect the life and health of the person who has such advanced addiction. Autonomy, although operative in the early stages of the disease process, may become so damaged that the control of substances over self-determination can only be released through coerced treatment. Kaplan and others have argued that the soundest ethical warrant for enforced treatment is not a public health justification but the potential to recover self-determination. "It may be possible to justify compulsory treatment for finite periods of time that could rectify this situation and restore the capacity for autonomy."[39]

The quote from Kaplan is from an article arguing for the mandated use of the opioid antagonist naltrexone in people who have opioid and perhaps alcohol addiction, because its anti-craving properties may free patients who have addiction from coercive habits and thus free them for more autonomous and healthy choices.[39] This novel ethical issue underscores that the past decade has seen the advent of exciting and effective treatments for addictions, including new psychopharmacologic interventions. The research reviewed here highlights that many important questions remain concerning the ethical participation of patients at various stages of addiction in clinical treatment. There are almost no data that address these issues directly, however, and the few published studies related to informed consent and addiction are drawn from research rather than clinical contexts. McCrady and colleagues[40] surveyed 91 federally funded clinical investigators conducting research in addictions. Fifty-seven percent of investigators reported recruiting subjects who were susceptible to coercion. At least half of the subjects possessed vulnerabilities, and researchers reported dealing with suicidal and intoxicated subjects. Two thirds of the investigators used objective assessments of decisional capacity and comprehension of consent forms. Only half of the investigators who obtained data from collateral sources obtained informed consent from those sources. The paper recommended that informed consent guidelines for substance use research be developed.[40]

In addition, almost nothing is known about the actual informed consent processes that are used in research settings and the knowledge and attitudes of clinicians of various disciplines about informed consent in the context of addiction research. One of the few extant studies was conducted with the National Institute on Drug Abuse Clinical Trials Network. A total of 115 staff members from community-based addiction treatment programs participated in an educational session on human subject protections in addiction research, which covered informed consent among other topics. On the pretest 56% of respondents agreed or were unsure whether a patient could participate in a clinical trial without understanding what would ensue in the protocol. After a 90-minute education presentation, 24% of the participants still concurred or were uncertain that a patient could be involved in a clinical trial without understanding what would occur.[41] The study does indicate instructional interventions can be modestly beneficial once deficits are identified.

Because human subject protections are more strenuous and structured in research than clinical care, it is likely that similar or more serious knowledge and attitude deficits are present in that context. A 2005 background article on informed consent to undergo substance abuse treatment[42] documents the paucity of information on informed consent in addictions treatment and the need to develop an empiric ethics understanding of the nature and degree of informed consent issues in clinical care. Currently the professional organizations for psychologists and addiction counselors require a prescribed number of ethics hours, as do some state medical licensing boards, all testimony to broad concern about inadequate understanding and adherence to ethical practices among clinicians.

Closely related to the issue of voluntarism in informed consent are studies suggesting that interventions to enhance patient autonomy can have a positive influence on engagement in, and outcome of, treatment. A study examining the determinants of treatment climate in 89 psychiatric and substance abuse programs found that emphasis on autonomy improved the program milieu and client adjustment.[43]

To our knowledge no formal guidelines have been issued regarding appropriate informed consent for addictions treatment and there is little evidence-based guidance for practicing psychiatrists and other mental health professionals on how to identify clinically and address constructively diminished or impaired decisional capacity and voluntarism. Assessment instruments, educational approaches, and safeguarding strategies drawn from the clinical ethics and research literature provide the best practice guidance available at this juncture. These are summarized in **Box 1**.

PARITY AND SOCIAL JUSTICE

Parity may be defined as equitable treatment and access to resources according to some consistent criterion. Parity is thus primarily related to the ethical principle of fairness. In this context, the resources in question are those related to allocation of resources treatment of addictions, although it is also possible to consider parity related to allocation of prevention and research dollars.

Unfortunately there is no general agreement about what constitutes fairness in health care, because there are several approaches that different people might consider fair, for example, the utilitarian principle of maximizing benefit to individuals and to society; prioritization on the basis of need, with care going preferentially to those with more severe disorders or urgent treatment needs; or allocation determined by ability to pay (for insurance or directly for services). The current health care system in the United States includes elements of all three of these models, without a coherent organizing principle.[46]

It is difficult to justify discrimination against treatment of SUDs because they represent valid, treatable disorders that often have a genetic basis.[47] Outcomes for SUDs

---

Box 1
Best practices to enhance decisional capacity and voluntarism

Evaluate for diminished capacity to provide informed consent when impaired decisional capacity is likely.[44]

Reassess decisional capacity when clinically indicated or when patients are preparing to enter more intensive or demanding phases of treatment.

Use educational and counseling interventions to enhance ability to provide informed consent in patients who have impairments in decisional capacity.[45]

Regularly and systematically evaluate for diminished voluntarism and means of enhancing autonomy.[12]

Provide ethics training and continuing medical education for all staff in the area of addiction ethics.[15]

---

are as good if not better than many other chronic diseases.[48] Historically insurance plans have not offered coverage for mental health and SUDs equal to that provided for medical and surgical problems. In the past substance abuse treatment was often not covered, and when benefits were offered they tended to require higher out-of-pocket costs and more restrictive treatment provisions than benefits related to medical care. In recent years many states have implemented parity laws. On October 6, 2008, President Bush signed into law a mental health parity bill requiring most health plans to cover psychiatric disorders (including SUDs) at the same level as other medical disorders.[49] This law takes effect a year after it was signed and is intended to end the inequity among health insurance benefits. The act amends the Mental Parity Act of 1996 to require that a group plan of 51 or more employees that provides health benefits must ensure that the financial requirements and treatment limitations are no more restrictive for substance abuse and mental health disorders than for medical or surgical conditions.[49] Although significant gaps remain, this law goes a long way toward eliminating disparities in health insurance coverage for addictions and other psychiatric disorders.

Even with the significant move toward equity and fairness, which the Mental Health Parity Act represents, there remain many unjust areas of substance use disorder policy and care delivery in the United States that present formidable obstacles to the provision of adequate access and treatment. The first is an education deficit in health professions training regarding the diagnosis and treatment of SUDs. This lack of knowledge and associated skills in working with patients who have SUDs leads to missed opportunities to constructively intervene,[50] especially in general hospital, primary care, or emergency department settings where most addiction patients are seen.[51] Research shows that educational initiatives can improve the attitudes and behaviors of trainees, enhancing respect for people and improving quality of care.[52]

Closely related to the question of adequate training is the dissemination of evidence-based treatments for SUD. More than ever before, safe and effective pharmacotherapies, such as buprenorphine for opioid dependence and naltrexone for alcohol dependence, are available and yet still not widely accessible. A 2006 study found that use of medications for alcohol use disorders was less likely for programs lacking integrated treatment of patients who had co-occurring psychiatric disorders, criminal justice involvement, or lack of commercial insurances, all conditions with considerable relevance for social justice.[53] Illicit drug use and HIV are highly stigmatized and underserved conditions in the United States, and studies have shown that although this is a marginalized population that could greatly benefit from buprenorphine, there are substantial barriers to its use in this population.[54]

Other examples of ethical problems in the delivery of SUD care are the low rates of available treatments in the criminal justice system despite continued drug policy that considers drug use a crime rather than a disease. A 2007 study of state addiction programs for adult offenders found that less than a quarter of inmates in prisons and jails and less than 10% of those in community correctional facilities have daily access to SUD services, and most of these programs offer only drug treatment, not comprehensive clinical care.[55] Other vulnerable groups that do not receive equitable treatment of abuse of substances are patients living in rural areas,[56] certain minority groups, and women. Ethically it is to be noted that all of these cohorts have overlapping and multiple vulnerabilities that warrant more, not less, intervention. Roberts and colleagues in a study of 1558 medical and mental health providers in New Mexico and Alaska identified significant ethical challenges in the treatment—including substance abuse treatment—of rural and minority patients because of health disparities. The study found four areas of ethical relevance, all of which are highly salient for SUD: attaining treatment adherence, assuring confidentiality, establishing therapeutic alliances, and engaging in informed consent practices.[57]

There is also a concerning gender gap in the delivery of addiction services for women, with marked failure to provide child-care options and to recognize the lower socioeconomic status of women and the role of intimate partner violence and trauma in women's use of substances.[58,59] Few programs adopt feminist approaches to treatment that may prioritize relationships and values of caring over considerations of strict autonomy and a legalistic sense of accountability.[60] Women who are mothers or pregnant and abuse substances confront intense social discrimination, compounded by obstacles to obtaining both prenatal care and addiction treatment, and in some jurisdictions even legal action.[60] More than half of surveyed obstetricians, pediatricians, and family practitioners endorsed the presumption that women have a legal and moral responsibility to protect the health of newborns, and a similar number supported a statute to remove children from a women abusing drugs or alcohol even if there was no direct evidence of neglect.[61] Such attitudes may have an adverse effect on the trust between physician and patient and deter women from seeking prenatal care but they reflect doctors' legitimate concerns about how to negotiate the often conflicting obligations to mother, fetus, and society.[62]

These views reflect a deep underlying social valuation that the life and health of the unborn and of children must be protected. These salient values poignantly conflict with the equally important need to respect the self-determination, confidentiality, and human dignity of pregnant women abusing substances. Studies have shown significant discrimination in the reporting of positive toxicologies for pregnant women, with 10 times as many African American as compared with white women being reported.[63] Research indicates that the threat of criminal charges, incarceration, or transfer of children to foster care are not effective deterrents, particularly when compared with allowing women to retain custody and providing parenting assistance and treatment, which has been demonstrated to benefit mother and child.[64] Several legal rulings have overturned statutes requiring mandatory reporting of toxicology tests obtained without patient permission or criminal charges of child abuse brought against substance-abusing women. The courts have so far upheld a woman's right to privacy and confidentiality within the physician–patient relationship.[65]

The American College of Obstetrics and Gynecologists (ACOG) Committee on Ethics does not support legally mandated testing reporting or other punitive measures.

The position of the ACOG committee is that "Such measures endanger the relationship of trust between physician and patient, place the obstetrician in an adversarial relationship with the patient, and possibly conflict with the therapeutic obligation."[66] The report emphasizes primary and secondary prevention through universal screening, brief interventions, and referral for comprehensive treatment as the most ethical means of safeguarding the welfare of the unborn and children.[66]

These and many other examples indicate that passing of the Parity Act is only the first step to obtaining truly equitable, accessible, and appropriate treatment for disadvantaged populations. It behooves all those involved in health care and especially those in the addiction community to work through their professional organizations, specialty societies, and the legislative process to continue the momentum to make addiction treatment an integrated aspect of mainstream medical care.

EMERGING ETHICAL ISSUES IN ADDICTIONS

The previous discussion presents several areas, such as the need for parity in treatment and stricter confidentiality protections, in which professional and legal resolution is emerging. There are other questions, such as the moral status of addiction and to what extent the burgeoning neurobiology of choice and compulsion affect decisional capacity and personal responsibility and the associated legal and political responses, about which there is still considerable controversy. There are other ethical issues in addictions, which for lack of space cannot be covered here, for which the differing perspectives and ethical valences are only now developing (**Table 2**). These dilemmas will only reach equilibrium in the coming decades as the relevant ethical values and principles, their specification, weighting, and contextualization are clarified through empiric evidence, stakeholder dialog, and conceptual progress.

Table 2 Evolving ethical issues in addictions	
Issue	**Ethical Tensions**
Cocaine vaccine[67]	Prevention of harm to individual and society from drug use versus possible coercion, uncertain safety of vaccine, and need for informed consent
Genetic testing for addiction[68]	Ability to do good for patients at risk for developing SUDs through screening and primary prevention versus stigmatization and compromised privacy and confidentiality
Forced medication treatment with disulfiram or naltrexone[36]	Time-limited use of the medication to restore autonomy and enhance motivation versus coercion and lack of true informed consent
Harm reduction approaches, such as controlled drinking and methadone replacement[69]	Overall reduction of adverse consequences and compassion for suffering versus achieving abstinence and respect for the law
Use of opioids for chronic pain patients who have a history of or current SUDs[70]	Relief of suffering and improved function versus risk for addiction and diversion

SUMMARY

The coming decades will see exciting breakthroughs in the treatment of SUDs, such as further elucidation of the genetic mechanisms of addiction. Yet if the past is any guide to the future, each new discovery will bring with it new challenges to the core ethical obligations of honoring informed consent, protecting confidentiality, and respecting justice, while also protecting the public from harm and ensuring the good of the individual patient. For the emerging scientific shift to a biobehavioral model of addiction to transform cultural attitudes and enhance treatment and research will require the scientifically rigorous and ethically sound agency of ethicists and addiction professionals to influence public policy. The growing body of neurobiologic evidence that contests traditional assumptions about free will and responsibility will evoke more deliberate and nuanced approaches to informed consent and treatment participation and dispute the forensic orientation in drug policy. If this unprecedented paradigm change can influence health care decision making in a reasoned and balanced fashion, there is real hope that the cultural stigma, which has warranted highly stringent confidentiality protections, and the disenfranchisement underlying health disparities in addiction treatment may move in the direction of compassionate and competent care for all those who suffer from addiction.

REFERENCES

1. Substance Abuse and Mental Health Services Administration. 2006 National survey on drug use and health. Rockville (MD): Office of Applied Studies; 2007.
2. Lewin Group. The economic costs of drug abuse in the United States 1992–2002. Washington, DC: Executive Office of the President, Office of National Drug Control Policy; 2004.
3. Harwood H. Updating estimates of the economic costs of alcohol abuse in the United States: Estimates, update methods and data. Report prepared by the Lewin Group for the National Institute on Alcohol Abuse and Alcoholism, 2000. Based on estimates, analyses, and data reported in Harwood, H., Fountain, D., Livermore, G. (1998). The economic costs of alcohol and drug abuse in the United States, 1992., in, 2000.
4. McGinnis JM, Foege WH. Mortality and morbidity attributable to use of addictive substances in the United States. Proc Assoc Am Physicians 1999;111:109.
5. National Institute of Drug Abuse. Drug abuse and addiction: one of America's most challenging public health problems. Rockville (MD): National Institute of Drug Abuse; 2008.
6. National Strategy for Suicide Prevention. Mental illness and suicide facts. Rockville (MD): U.S. Department of Health and Human Services; 2001.
7. Beauchamp TL, Childress JF. Principles of biomedical ethics. 5th edition. New York: Oxford University Press; 2001.
8. Jonsen AR, Seigler M, Winslade WJ. Clinical ethics. 4th edition. New York: McGraw-Hill, Inc.; 1998.
9. White WH. Slaying the dragon: the history of addiction treatment and recovery in America. Chicago: Chesnut Health Systems; 1998.
10. Link BG, Struening EL, Rahav M, et al. On stigma and its consequences: evidence from a longitudinal study of men with dual diagnoses of mental illness and substance abuse. J Health Soc Behav 1997;38:177.
11. Crisp AH, Golder MG, Rix S, et al. Stigmatisation of people with mental illnesses. Br J Psychiatry 2000;177:4.

12. Roberts LW, Dunn LB. Ethical considerations in caring for women with substance use disorders. Obstet Gynecol Clin North Am 2003;30:559.
13. Brooks MK. Legal aspects of confidentiality and patient information. In: Lowinson JH, Ruiz P, Millman RB, et al, editors. Substance abuse: a comprehensive textbook. 4th edition. Philadelphia: Lippincott Williams & Wilkins; 2005. p. 1361.
14. Clark WH, Brooks MK. Ethical issues in addiction treatment. In: Graham AW, Schultz TK, May-SMith MF, et al, editors. Principles of addiction medicine. 3rd edition. Chevy Chase (MD): American Society of Addiction Medicine; 2003.
15. Geppert C, Roberts LR. Ethical foundations of substance abuse treatment. In: Geppert C, Roberts LR, editors. The book of ethics for addiction professionals. Center City (PA): Hazelden; 2008. p. 18.
16. U.S. Department of Health and Human Services. Treatment improvement protocol 8: intensive outpatient treatment for alcohol and other drug abuse in Treatment Improvement Protocol (TIP) series. Rockville (MD): Substance Abuse and Mental Health Services Administration; 1994. Chapter 7.
17. Dwyer J, Shih A. The ethics of tailoring the patient's chart. [see comments]. Psychiatr Serv 1998;49:1309.
18. Felthous AR. Substance abuse and the duty to protect. Bull Am Acad Psychiatry Law 1993;21:419.
19. Bogenschutz MP. Caring for persons with addictions. In: Roberts LW, Dyer AR, editors. Concise guide to ethics in mental health care. Washington, DC: American Psychiatric Publishing; 2004.
20. Roberts LW. Psychiatry: informed consent and care. In: Smelser NJ, Baltes PB, editors. International encyclopedia of the social and behavioral sciences. Amsterdam: Elsevier; 2001.
21. Appelbaum PS. Clinical practice. Assessment of patients' competence to consent to treatment. N Engl J Med 2007;357:1834.
22. Roberts LW. Informed consent and the capacity for voluntarism. Am J Psychiatry 2002;159:705.
23. Kleiman M. The "brain disease" idea, drug policy and research ethics. Addiction 2003;98:871.
24. Bates ME, Voelbel GT, Buckman JF, et al. Short-term neuropsychological recovery in clients with substance use disorders. Alcohol Clin Exp Res 2005; 29:367.
25. Koob GF. Neurobiology of addiction. Toward the development of new therapies. Ann N Y Acad Sci 2000;909:170.
26. Lundqvist T. Cognitive consequences of cannabis use: comparison with abuse of stimulants and heroin with regard to attention, memory and executive functions. Pharmacol Biochem Behav 2005;81:319.
27. Volkow ND, Wang GJ, Telang F, et al. Cocaine cues and dopamine in dorsal striatum: mechanism of craving in cocaine addiction. J Neurosci 2006;26:6583.
28. Moran M. In: Drug addiction erodes "free-will" over time, vol 42. Washington, DC: Psychiatric News; 2007.
29. Miller NS, Goldsmith RJ. Craving for alcohol and drugs in animals and humans: biology and behavior. J Addict Dis 2001;20:87.
30. Wild TC, Newton-Taylor B, Alletto R. Perceived coercion among clients entering substance abuse treatment: structural and psychological determinants. Addict Behav 1998;23:81.
31. Marlowe DB, Merikle EP, Kirby KC, et al. Multidimensional assessment of perceived treatment-entry pressures among substance abusers. Psychol Addict Behav 2001;15:97.

32. Seraganian P, Brown TG, Tremblay J. Randomization in a substance abuse treatment study: participants who consent vs those who do not. Can J Psychiatry 2003;48:388.

33. Geppert CM. In: Aristotle. Augustine and Addiction, vol. 25. Darien (CT): Psychiatric Times; 2008.

34. Layde JB. Forensic issues in the treatment of addictions. In: Geppert CM, Roberts LW, editors. The book of ethics: expert guidance for professionals who treat addiction. Center City (PA): Hazelden; 2008.

35. Klag S, O'Callaghan F, Creed P. The use of legal coercion in the treatment of substance abusers: an overview and critical analysis of thirty years of research. Subst Use Misuse 2005;40:1777.

36. Sullivan MA, Birkmayer F, Boyarsky BK, et al. Uses of coercion in addiction treatment: clinical aspects. Am J Addict 2008;17:36.

37. Cohen PJ. Addiction, molecules and morality: disease does not obviate responsibility. Am J Bioeth 2007;7:21.

38. Morse SJ. Medicine and morals, craving and compulsion. Subst Use Misuse 2004;39:437.

39. Caplan AL. Ethical issues surrounding forced, mandated, or coerced treatment. J Subst Abuse Treat 2006;31:117.

40. McCrady BS, Bux DA Jr. Ethical issues in informed consent with substance abusers. J Consult Clin Psychol 1999;67:186.

41. Forman RF, Bovasso G, Woody G, et al. Staff beliefs about drug abuse clinical trials. J Subst Abuse Treat 2002;23:55.

42. Walker R, Logan TK, Clark JJ, et al. Informed consent to undergo treatment for substance abuse: a recommended approach. J Subst Abuse Treat 2005;29:241.

43. Timko C, Moos RH. Determinants of the treatment climate in psychiatric and substance abuse programs: implications for improving patient outcomes. J Nerv Ment Dis 1998;186:96.

44. Dunn LB, Nowrangi MA, Palmer BW, et al. Assessing decisional capacity for clinical research or treatment: a review of instruments. Am J Psychiatry 2006;163:1323.

45. Moser DJ, Reese RL, Hey CT, et al. Using a brief intervention to improve decisional capacity in schizophrenia research. Schizophr Bull 2006;32:116.

46. Woolfolk RL, Doris JM. Rationing mental health care: parity, disparity, and justice. Bioethics 2002;16:469.

47. Barry CL, Sindelar JL. Equity in private insurance coverage for substance abuse: a perspective on parity. Health Aff (Millwood) 2007;26:w706.

48. McLellan AT, Lewis DC, O'Brien CP, et al. Drug dependence, a chronic medical illness: implications for treatment, insurance, and outcomes evaluation. JAMA 2000;284:1689.

49. Paul Wellstone and Pete Domenici Mental Health Parity and Addiction Equity Act of 2008, in H.R. 6983, ed 2d, 2008.

50. Kaner EF, Beyer F, Dickinson HO, et al. Effectiveness of brief alcohol interventions in primary care populations. Cochrane Database Syst Rev 2007;2:CD004148.

51. Lindberg M, Vergara C, Wild-Wesley R, et al. Physicians-in-training attitudes toward caring for and working with patients with alcohol and drug abuse diagnoses. South Med J 2006;99:28.

52. Karam-Hage M, Nerenberg L, Brower KJ. Modifying residents' professional attitudes about substance abuse treatment and training. Am J Addict 2001;10:40.

53. Ducharme LJ, Knudsen HK, Roman PM. Trends in the adoption of medications for alcohol dependence. J Clin Psychopharmacol 2006;26(Suppl 1):S13.

54. Cunningham CO, Kunins HV, Roose RJ, et al. Barriers to obtaining waivers to prescribe buprenorphine for opioid addiction treatment among HIV physicians. J Gen Intern Med 2007;22:1325.
55. Taxman FS, Perdoni ML, Harrison LD. Drug treatment services for adult offenders: the state of the state. J Subst Abuse Treat 2007;32:239.
56. McAuliffe WE, LaBrie R, Woodworth R, et al. State substance abuse treatment gaps. Am J Addict 2003;12:101.
57. Roberts LW, Johnson ME, Brems C, et al. Ethical disparities: challenges encountered by multidisciplinary providers in fulfilling ethical standards in the care of rural and minority people. J Rural Health 2007;23(Suppl):89.
58. Bhatt RV. Domestic violence and substance abuse. Int J Gynaecol Obstet 1998; 63(Suppl 1):S25.
59. Stewart D, Gossop M, Trakada K. Drug dependent parents: childcare responsibilities, involvement with treatment services, and treatment outcomes. Addict Behav 2007;32:1657.
60. Marcellus L. Feminist ethics must inform practice: interventions with perinatal substance users. Health Care Women Int 2004;25:730.
61. Abel EL, Kruger M. Physician attitudes concerning legal coercion of pregnant alcohol and drug abusers. Am J Obstet Gynecol 2002;186:768.
62. Plambeck CM. Divided loyalties. Legal and bioethical considerations of physician-pregnant patient confidentiality and prenatal drug abuse. J Leg Med 2002;23:1.
63. Chasnoff IJ, Landress HJ, Barrett ME. The prevalence of illicit-drug or alcohol use during pregnancy and discrepancies in mandatory reporting in Pinellas County, Florida. N Engl J Med 1990;322:1202.
64. Svikis DS, Reid-Quinones K. Screening and prevention of alcohol and drug use disorders in women. Obstet Gynecol Clin North Am 2003;30:447.
65. Gostin LO. The rights of pregnant women: the Supreme Court and drug testing. Hastings Cent Rep 2001;31:8.
66. ACOG Committee Opinion. Number 294, May 2004. At-risk drinking and illicit drug use: ethical issues in obstetric and gynecologic practice. Obstet Gynecol 2004;103:1021.
67. Hall W, Carter L. Ethical issues in using a cocaine vaccine to treat and prevent cocaine abuse and dependence. J Med Ethics 2004;30:337.
68. Hall W, Carter L, Morley KI. Neuroscience research on the addictions: a prospectus for future ethical and policy analysis. Addict Behav 2004;29:1481.
69. Christie T, Groarke L, Sweet W. Virtue ethics as an alternative to deontological and consequential reasoning in the harm reduction debate. Int J Drug Policy 2008;19:52.
70. Geppert CM. To help and not to harm: ethical issues in the treatment of chronic pain in patients with substance use disorders. Adv Psychosom Med 2004;25:151.

Ethics in Psychotherapy: A Focus on Professional Boundaries and Confidentiality Practices

Shaili Jain, MD[a,b,*], Laura Weiss Roberts, MD, MA[b,c]

KEYWORDS

• Ethics • Psychotherapy • Boundaries • Professionalism
• Confidentiality

Mr. B gives his cognitive-behavioral therapist, Dr. M, a nice and not inexpensive watch. Dr. M wonders whether he should accept the gift, concerned about the feelings of Mr. B, who has only recently begun to make progress in his treatment.

Ms. Y has chronic suicidal ideation and takes an overdose, resulting in her admission to a medical intensive care unit. Her therapist, Dr. T, whom she sees weekly for supportive psychotherapy, feels guilty for not taking her threats more seriously. Dr. T visits Ms. Y and sits with her at the bedside in the MICU.

Dr. C, struggling with his own feelings of depression after a divorce, begins to daydream about "a new life" with a young woman patient whom he sees four times a week for psychoanalysis.

Dr. J is a resident physician in a small community-based training program. She is learning to provide psychotherapy and notices that two of her new patients go to the same coffee shop and grocery store she frequents. She asks her psychotherapy supervisor whether this is a "boundary problem."

Dr. G, an ambitious faculty member at a prestigious medical school, plans to write up case material for an academic journal but wonders if she should obtain her patients' permission first.

These case vignettes illustrate the myriad ways in which ethics issues can present themselves in the therapist-patient dyad. Even the subtlest ethics issue may greatly

[a] Aurora Psychiatric Hospital, 1220 Dewey Avenue, Wauwatosa, WI 53213, USA
[b] Department of Psychiatry and Behavioral Medicine, Medical College of Wisconsin, Milwaukee, WI, USA
[c] Department of Population Health, Medical College of Wisconsin, Milwaukee, WI, USA
* Corresponding author.
E-mail address: shaili.jain@aurora.org (S. Jain).

Psychiatr Clin N Am 32 (2009) 299–314
doi:10.1016/j.psc.2009.03.005
0193-953X/09/$ – see front matter

influence the therapist's ability to establish a safe, effective, and beneficent framework for treatment. There is wide agreement that ethically sound conduct by the therapist is an essential precondition for clinically sound care for the patient.[1] The tight link between ethics and psychotherapy is affirmed by the American Psychiatric Association (APA), which binds its members by the ethical code of the medical profession specifically defined in *Principles of Medical Ethics of the American Medical Association* and the APA's *Principles of Medical Ethics with Annotations Especially Applicable to Psychiatry,*[2] which takes into account the special ethical problems in psychiatric treatment.

The inextricable link between good ethics and good therapeutic practice is clear; that said, *how* to provide psychotherapy ethically has been the subject of intense academic discussion spanning several decades.[3–7] The ethical issues of greatest concern in psychotherapy practice relate to what are referred to as "professional boundaries" and the confidentiality protections in the therapeutic relationship. Consider the practical matter of gifts in treatment. Is it always unethical for a psychotherapist to accept a gift from a patient? Is the "rule" more relaxed when it is an "inexpensive" gift when compared with an expensive gift? Are philanthropic gifts to an institution the same as other gifts? Is it "as unethical" when the item is a handmade gift from a seriously mentally ill client in the course of supportive therapy or from an adolescent who has reached a significant milestone in treatment? How, exactly, is a gift different from compensation?

Consider the practical matter of confidentiality in treatment. How does a therapist respond to patients who wish to supplement their face-to-face sessions with e-mail or other electronic interactions? Under what circumstances is it ethical or unethical to "use" confidential material drawn from clinical experience with a specific patient to develop scholarly pieces, which ultimately advance the therapist's academic career? What about confidentiality issues that arise in encountering patients outside of the usual setting of the psychotherapy office? How about interactions that occur in a small town, as opposed to a larger community that affords more role separation? Depending on the exact context and circumstances of care, some might argue that the ethical responses of the therapist to these professional boundary and confidentiality issues may differ across situations. If "rules" are not absolute in how they are understood and applied, how much latitude may an individual therapist exercise without sliding into patterns of actual or apparent ethical misconduct? What distinguishes an action that is ethical from one that is ambiguously or straightforwardly unethical?

This article examines two key ethics topics in psychotherapy: professional boundaries and confidentiality. These topics pertain to all therapeutic modalities, encompassing supportive and cognitive-behavioral therapy, psychoanalysis, psychodynamic and combined medication management, and related psychotherapy approaches undertaken by psychiatrists. Far from esoteric concepts, the discussion demonstrates a continued relevance to the contemporary therapist. The nature of the dilemmas may have changed (eg, how to use e-mail communication in therapy), but the need for the therapist to display ethical competence remains vital. In light of the issues of the medical profession in relation to the public trust,[8,9] the ethics of psychotherapy may be more critical than ever before.

PROFESSIONALISM AND THERAPEUTIC BOUNDARIES

Professionals have special expertise and are given privileges in our society to serve the public as a whole and to serve people as individuals through the use of this expertise. By virtue of this basic social contract, a professional must possess and

Recognizing Boundary Issues

Gutheil and Brodsky[13] stated that the therapeutic boundary creates "the physical, psychological, and/or social space occupied by the patient in the clinical relationship." How to define this space is a more complex matter and depends on the type of therapy being conducted and the requirements of the individual patient.[17] Another useful approach to understand the meaning of boundaries is to conceptualize a therapeutic frame, that is, "an envelope or membrane around the therapeutic role that defines the characteristics of the therapeutic relationship."[18,19] The therapist decides the elements of the frame, which include practical issues such as establishing the length and rhythm of regular appointments, negotiating fees for treatment, and defining the context of care, such as the office setting, the inclusion of electronic communication or not, the participation of others in treatment, and the limits regarding privacy and confidentiality. It is imperative to note that the frame is constructed by the therapist, not by the patient, whose expectations of the therapeutic relationship may be more naïve, more forgiving, or more flexible.[3]

Boundary transgressions by the therapist can be divided into two broad categories: "boundary crossings," in which there is a clear step away from usual therapeutic practice with an uncertain impact on treatment, and "boundary violations," in which the deviation from expected practice is clearly harmful to or exploitative of the patient. The tight link between ethics and therapeutic boundaries is illustrated well by Gutheil and Simon[20] in **Tables 2** and **3**; these examples show how boundary violations contradict ethical principles fundamental to the doctor-patient relationship.[3,17]

The concept of boundaries can be clearer in theory than actual practice. For example, some self-disclosure by a therapist caring for a chronically ill patient in the context of supportive therapy may be a way of fostering rapport and encouraging the therapeutic alliance, whereas this same action by a psychoanalyst would be more ethically questionable in the care of a physician-executive in his third year of treatment. In other words, partial gratification of transference wishes may ethically be associated with supportive psychotherapy, whereas it would be discouraged in psychoanalysis. Similarly, a therapist who visits a patient in the hospital to appease

Table 2	
Ethical principles and boundary violations	
Ethical Principles	**Related Boundary Violations**
Respect for the dignity of the patient	Taking advantage of the patient
Respect for the patient's authentic (healthy) goals	Aiming for one's own goals
Autonomy	Undue influence/coercion toward one's own goals and not the patient's goals
Self-determination	Fostering dependency
Fiduciary relationship	Exploitative relationship for personal gratification
Neutrality	Personal investment
Abstinence	Intrusion
Altruism	Using the patient for one's own gratification
Beneficence	Failure to act in the patient's interest
Nonmaleficence	Doing harm to the patient
Compassion	Exploiting the patient's vulnerability

From Gutheil TG, Simon RI. Non-sexual boundary crossings and boundary violations: the ethical dimension. Psychiatr Clin North Am 2002;25:585–92; with permission.

Term	Definition and Example	Characteristics
Boundary	The physical, psychological, and social space occupied by the patient in the clinical relationship	Not hard or fast, movable, context dependent
Boundary crossing	A departure from the usual norms of therapy, that is, the verbal and physical distances normally maintained in a therapeutic interaction (eg, the physical contact involved in extending a hand to help a patient who has stumbled or fallen)	Frequently occurs, benign deviation from standard practice, harmless, nonexploitative, may even support or advance therapy, may be initiated by either the patient or the therapist
Boundary violation	A boundary crossing of which the intent involves extra therapeutic gratification for the therapist; there is no benefit to the patient but significant risk of harming the patient (eg, a therapist engaging in a sexual relationship with a patient)	Takes the therapist out of the professional role, benefits the therapist more than the patient, transgresses an ethical standard, responsibility lies only with the therapist

Table 3
Boundaries, boundary crossings, and boundary violations: definitions, examples, and characteristics

Data from Gutheil TG, Brodsky A. Preventing boundary violations in clinical practice. New York: Guilford Press; 2008.

his or her guilt after the patient's suicide attempt may well be overstepping the proper bounds of the therapeutic relationship, whereas a psychiatrist who visits a terminally ill patient in the hospital and offers comfort by holding the patient's hand may well be within the bounds of acceptable behavior ethically. Adapting the technique to fit the needs and health of the patient is clinically important and acceptable.[21,22] The key is whether the patient's well-being and interests are demonstrably and unambiguously served by the behavior—that is the ethical "litmus test."[7,11]

Nonsexual and Sexual Boundary Issues

Historically, the boundaries of the therapeutic relationship and the characteristics of acceptable technique have been highly subjective and lacked standardization.[3,18] To remedy this, researchers in the area of boundaries[3,13,17] have proposed viewing the issues in categories of role, time, place and space, money, gifts, clothing, language, and physical contact.

A healthy therapeutic process has clarity and relative consistency regarding these specific domains for professional interaction. Careful attention and predictability with respect to role, time, place and space, money, gifts, clothing, language, and physical contact help establish a pattern that allows for the development of greater trust in interactions between therapist and patient. Establishing a "stable framework" for treatment with explicit approaches to conduct in each of these domains creates fewer opportunities for missteps by the therapist in serving the needs of the patient.

Nonsexual boundary violations may be difficult to discern; however, they are damaging and do not place the well-being of the patient above other interests. One example would be the psychiatrist who boasts of his celebrity patients, revealing or suggesting intimate details that can be traced back to the individuals. This is a violation of the patient's trust, regardless of whether the actual disclosure causes damage to the patient's reputation. Another example would be the psychiatrist who accepts financial favors of a patient or who routinely extends the length of sessions with a prestigious or particularly attractive patient. Although these actions do not seem nearly as egregious as sexual exploitation of a vulnerable patient, for example, these behaviors are expressions of the unchecked, unmonitored desires or hopes of the therapist and may well undermine the health of the patient. **Table 4** provides several clinical illustrations of nonsexual boundary violations.

Sexual contact between therapists and patients or former patients is always a professional boundary violation and always ethically unacceptable. Sexual contact in the therapeutic relationship is an irrefutable boundary violation because it inherently exploits the real or potential vulnerability of the patient and inherently gratifies the therapist. As stated by the APA[2]:

> *The requirement that the physician conduct himself/herself with propriety in his or her profession and in all the actions of his or her life is especially important in the case of the psychiatrist because the patient tends to model his or her behavior after that of his or her psychiatrist by identification. Further, the necessary intensity of the treatment relationship may tend to activate sexual and other needs and fantasies on the part of both patient and psychiatrist, while weakening the objectivity necessary for control. Additionally, the inherent inequality in the doctor-patient relationship may lead to exploitation of the patient. Sexual activity with a current or former patient is unethical.*

Understanding and Preventing Sexual Boundary Violations

It is widely acknowledged that the most serious ethical transgressions in psychotherapy are in the context of patient-therapist sexual contact. These transgressions cause great suffering, have become major sources of ethics complaints to professional societies, and give rise to serious malpractice litigation. National surveys have suggested that 0.9% to 12% of male therapists and 0.2% to 3% of female therapists have had sexual contact with patients.[23,24] Surveys analyzing responses of different mental health care practitioners have found no differences in incidence among psychiatrists, psychologists, and social workers.[25] Data from other specialty fields of medicine suggest higher rates of sexual contact between physicians and patients.[26,27] It is important to recognize that the severe professional and legal repercussions of such transgressions make it difficult to estimate the true prevalence of such behaviors based on self-report data (**Box 2**). These actions and the resultant intense media scrutiny have jeopardized the image of mental health care providers.[28]

Gabbard and colleagues[29–35] researched the origins of such boundary violations extensively. Sexual misconduct usually begins with relatively minor boundary violations or crossings, such as transitioning from using last names to first names, personal conversations intruding on the clinical work, and some body contact (eg, a pat on the shoulder), to meeting outside the office, sharing a meal, and finally a physically intimate relationship.[36]

Researchers have aimed to develop psychodynamic themes from cases in which boundary violations of a sexual nature have occurred. It is apparent that reductionistic attempts to oversimplify such situations seriously undermine the complex dynamics involved. A more useful approach would be acceptance of the universal vulnerability of all therapists to such misconduct.[28,30,33–35] Virtually all therapists struggle with erotic countertransference at times, which is distinct from actual boundary crossings and violations.[32]

Table 4
Nonsexual boundary issues with clinical examples and comments

Boundary Type	Clinical Example	Comments
Role	A patient becomes distressed while recalling childhood abuse and asks the therapist for a hug	The therapist must differentiate between "libidinal" demands, which cannot be gratified without entering into ethical transgressions and damaging enactments, and "growth needs," which prevent patient growth if not gratified to some extent[53]
Time	A therapist seeing a patient for weekly, highly expressive therapy routinely spends 15 minutes more than the allotted session time	Consistent departure from the therapeutic frame requires self-scrutiny on the part of the therapist
Place and space	A patient and his therapist meet for lunch at a cafe	Whether a boundary crossing or a boundary violation has occurred depends on the particular therapeutic ideology in each case[13]; for example, it would not be a boundary violation for a behaviorist to accompany a patient in a public place
Money	A therapist allows a patient's unpaid bills to mount without bringing them up in sessions	The therapist's resistance to addressing this fact requires some scrutiny
Gifts and services	A therapist accepts an expensive holiday souvenir from a grateful patient	Gifts that are regarded as "safe" include token objects such as a handmade craft[54]. "It is far easier to refuse a gift but one must know how and when to accept a gift"[55]
Clothing	To provoke a reaction, a patient starts to disrobe during a session	In such extreme circumstances, direct approaches are appropriate[56], for example, "This behavior is inappropriate, and it is not therapy; please put your clothes on"
Language	A patient routinely addresses the therapist by his or her first name	The patient may experience the use of first names as misrepresenting the professional relationship as a social friendship[38]
Self-disclosure	A therapist, worried and anxious about the breakup of a relationship with a significant other, starts to divulge details to a patient going through a similar problem	Any self-disclosure is an indication for careful self-scrutiny regarding motivation for such departure from the usual frame[13]
Physical contact (nonerotic touch)	A therapist is taking a 12-week maternity leave and her patient gives her a "good luck" hug at the last session before the leave	The therapist must consider clinical, ethical, and cultural factors, as well as patient characteristics (eg, diagnosis, developmental history, abuse history)[57]

Data from Gutheil TG, Gabbard GO. The concept of boundaries in clinical practice: theoretical and risk-management dimensions. Am J Psychiatry 1993;150:188–96.

Box 2
Consequences for therapists who transgress sexual boundaries with patients[29]

- Censure from state licensing boards
- Possible dismissal from professional organizations through the actions of ethics committees
- Malpractice litigation
- Possible criminal prosecution

Common dynamics in the development of therapist-patient sexual relations include confusion of a therapist's need to be loved with that of the patient, fantasy that love itself may be curative, susceptibility of the therapist-patient dyad to re-enact incestuous sexual involvement from the patient's past, and the tendency of some therapists to act out of latent hostility through sexual exploitation of a patient.[29,33] A relatively small percentage of such therapists can be found to have psychopathologic conditions. They often have a personal history of profound childhood abuse or neglect, and their cruel exploitation of their patients is a form of identification with the aggressor and an attempt to "turn the tables" and achieve mastery in relation to their childhood experiences.[29,32] In the case of "lovesickness," the therapist believes that he or she is in love with the patient. A typical scenario is a middle-aged male therapist in love with a much younger female patient.[29,37,38] Situational factors of an analyst or therapist who engages in sexual misconduct with only one patient include going through a life crisis such as divorce, illness, malpractice litigation, or bankruptcy.[37] Narcissistic or masochistic psychopathology has also been noted. Depression, omnipotence, and grandiosity may all play a role.[35]

It is suggested that all patients may be potentially vulnerable to manipulation, mistreatment, and sexual exploitation. In the clinical case studies encountered by Gabbard,[37] characteristics of patients who have had sexually intimate interactions with therapists may include being actively suicidal at the time, having a history of severe childhood trauma, and being more likely to have a cluster B personality disorder or a dissociative disorder.[35] It is critical to note, however, that a truly sociopathic therapist—as opposed to one who is "lovesick"—may create a situation in which it may be possible to sexually exploit a patient without prior trauma or severe psychopathology.

The therapist is culpable in situations of patient-therapist sex, not the patient. The assignment of moral blame solely on the therapist is appropriate, regardless of how "seductive" or "loving" or "in need" the patient is. Therapists, by engaging in sexual contact with patients, violate professional norms and accepted professional standards.[30] Therapists also have an ethical obligation to expose colleagues who sexually abuse their patients. This obligation may conflict with the therapist's duty to preserve confidentiality (eg, a therapist may come to know of the sexual boundary violation from a current patient, who has seen the offending therapist in the past). The systematic use of consultation may be a means to address ethical and clinical responsibilities.[39]

Preventing Boundary Problems in the Therapeutic Relationship

There are many practical strategies for preventing boundary transgressions and violations. It is important to engage in ongoing self-critique and reflection, monitor one's wishes and hopes in the care of patients to make certain that they are focused on the patient's needs and well-being, and seek supervision in complex or emotionally challenging clinical cases. Practitioners also may find certain tools, such as the

"Exploitation Index,"[38] to help support that self-evaluative process. The Exploitation Index, developed by Richard Epstein, is most suited to an urban, long-term, dynamic therapy context and is, in essence, a list of questions therapists can ask themselves about their current behavior with patients to evaluate if they are touching, crossing, transgressing, or violating expected professional boundaries in the care of their patients.

Throughout all fields of medicine, consulting a colleague or considering referring a patient elsewhere may be other safeguards that can be used to help support appropriate boundaries in the care of patients.[7,11,29] Gabbard[29] specifically warned that when the therapist begins to feel that "love" will cure a patient and, in particular, that the therapist is uniquely able to offer that love to the patient, it is imperative that patient transition occur. After the therapeutic relationship is terminated, it is not possible for the therapist and the patient to enter into an intimate personal relationship, however. It is critical to note that the vulnerability experienced by the patient, actually or potentially, endures beyond the discontinuation of the professional connection.

Beyond use of supervision for complex cases, the routine practice of supervision and peer case review is an excellent "best practice" that may help prevent boundary issues from ever becoming problems.[11] These supervisory sessions are most helpful if there is ready discussion of issues that the therapist is inclined to keep "secret."[33] Conversation in such professional settings regarding boundaries as flexible standards of good practice—rather than lists of generically forbidden behavior[17]—may be valuable, as long as clear "rules" regarding absolutely exploitative sexual or other behavior (eg, financial) are explicitly recognized.

CONFIDENTIALITY AND PRIVACY

Psychiatric records, including even the identification of a person as a patient, must be protected with extreme care. Confidentiality is essential to psychiatric treatment. This is based in part on the special nature of psychiatric therapy as well as on the traditional ethical relationship between physician and patient. Growing concern regarding the civil rights of patients and the possible adverse effects of computerization, duplication equipment, and data banks makes the dissemination of confidential information an increasing hazard. Because of the sensitive and private nature of the information with which the psychiatrist deals, he or she must be circumspect in the information that he or she chooses to disclose to others about a patient. The welfare of the patient must be a continuing consideration.[2]

Confidentiality in the therapist-patient relationship is defined as the therapist's clear commitment to nondisclosure of information revealed by the patient—or observations made by the clinician—in the context of the professional encounter without permission from the patient and in the absence of a legal requirement to reveal specific information.[7,11,40] Unlike the ideal of privacy, which is seen as more absolute, confidentiality is not recognized as an inherent right accorded to patients. Instead, in our society it is viewed as a privilege, and it may be superseded by the requirements of the law. For instance, a physician must disclose what is known to formal authorities when a patient reveals information suggesting that a child or dependent elder is being neglected, exploited, or abused.[7,11,41]

From an ethical perspective, respect for confidentiality is crucial because of the inherently personal nature of communications and observations that occur in psychotherapy.[4,11] In the United States, this ethical commitment is supported in law with the doctrine of privilege—the right accorded patients/clients by courts to safeguard their communications in therapy sessions.[5] Most recently, the Health Insurance Portability and Accountability Act (HIPAA) specified that psychotherapy notes may be kept separate from the general medical file and are not subject to third-party review based on a general consent signed in advance of the psychotherapy.[42,43]

The very act of a patient's self-disclosure in therapy makes the patient emotionally "exposed," which, in turn, emphasizes why confidentiality is so integral to the therapy's success.[5] Offsetting this principle are legal rulings that limit privilege and can present dilemmas to therapists who want to offer confidentiality to their patients, however.[5] Current factors in health care delivery involving third-party payers who may have access to information about patient encounters, diagnoses, and treatment impact the degree of confidentiality a therapist can offer.[7] Patients who use insurance to pay for their psychotherapy typically "sign away" their confidentiality safeguards, sadly opening themselves to subsequent stigma and potential discrimination. Modern therapists must meet demands for detailed recordkeeping in anticipation of the requirements and wishes of third-party payers and peer review organizations, which often means the domain for potential communication (ie, who is privy to the information) and the risk of a violation are increased.[4]

A therapist's disclosure of requested confidential information must be undertaken only after careful consideration of legal, ethical, and practical considerations (**Table 5**).[43] Of relevance to the current practice environment is the split model arrangement, in which a patient is typically seen by a therapist for psychotherapy on a frequent basis and by a physician for management of psychotropic pharmacotherapy less frequently. In this instance, it is imperative that the patient sign a formal release of information so that the therapist and psychiatrist can share communications about the progress of the patient. Such disclosures, performed regularly in a two-way manner, provide an essential cohesiveness in the delivery of care to the patient.

Special Confidentiality Issues: Electronic Records, Technology-Based Communication, and the Publication of Case Material

Psychiatric data and therapy-related information are increasingly being entered into electronic medical records. This phenomenon has caused many to worry greatly over the potential for breaches of confidentiality, and designers of electronic medical records have worked diligently to offer safeguarded products. It should be understood that personal information cannot be fully protected once it is entered into a record of this sort, and patients should be given accurate information about this "modern" problem in health care. As Mark Siegler[44] wrote more than two decades ago, when he counted the dozens of people who had access to a paper chart of a "VIP" inpatient, confidentiality is a "decrepit concept," and at the very least, patients should be made aware of the limits of confidentiality. On a more optimistic note, HIPAA permits the sequestering of psychotherapy process notes, which may offer some greater protection than the general medical record.[43]

The American Medical Association[45] has proffered the opinion that most mental health issues remain inappropriate for e-mail communications. Psychiatrists who provide care for patients across distances suggest that newer technology, including electronic media, may play a vital role in psychotherapy, ranging from video communication to e-mail correspondence.[46] For example, rural outreach programs may incorporate videophone conferencing to "shut in" or remotely located clients; innovative efforts have attempted to help support group/peer counseling efforts with severely and persistently mentally ill patients. In traditional, dynamically oriented psychotherapy, the use of e-mail and other means of electronic communication may require significant safeguards for the patient's privacy to be adequately protected. Many

Table 5
Ethical and legal implications of Jaffee v Redmond and the HIPAA medical privacy rule for psychotherapy and general psychiatry

Consent Status	Example	Legal Implications	Ethical Implications	Practical Issues
The patient consents	Consent to disclose to third-party payers, disability agencies, court proceedings	Not affected directly by privilege rules as patient consents (ie, provides a waiver); HIPPA allows patients to authorize release	Therapists have an ethical obligation to disclose only the minimum amount of information needed to satisfy the request	The waiver of privilege must *not* be coerced
The patient does not consent	Reporting communicable diseases, gunshot wounds, child abuse, or elder abuse; protecting a third party from harm, which is legally stipulated by Tarasoff: "protective privilege ends where public peril begins"	A serious matter; HIPPA protection means that subpoenas and other requests for information should not result in the disclosure of confidential information unless the patient has declined to exercise privilege	Before warning a third party, the therapist should first seek to involve the patient in the process of protecting an intended victim rather than act against the patient's wishes	If therapists are concerned about the potential for patients to harm someone, they may consider offering hospitalization as a way of simultaneously preserving confidentiality and protecting the other party

Data from Mosher PW, Swire PP. The ethical and legal implications of Jaffee v Redmond and the HIPAA medical privacy rule for psychotherapy and general psychiatry. Psychiatr Clin North Am 2002;25:575–84.

technical factors in the way e-mail accounts are set up and how messages are sent mean that such communication is not private. To use e-mail in psychotherapy, careful consideration should be given to the parameters of its use, which should be communicated to patients accordingly.[47] Patients should provide informed consent for this therapeutic modality, with proper attention to issues of risk, benefit, and alternatives.

It is difficult to wholly protect patient confidentiality in case reports in the literature, yet psychiatrists may wish to contribute to generalizable knowledge through discussions of especially complex or valuable clinical cases. The appropriate professional aim of enhancing expertise in the field must be balanced against the potential harm that may occur if a patient's identity is inadvertently revealed in a published report. Historically, this ethical dilemma has been resolved by permitting authors to mask or "disguise" clinical material to obscure the patient's identity. An emerging ethical standard in medical journals is the practice of *not* disguising clinical accounts of patients but, rather, obtaining informed consent from patients to publish such reports.

Psychoanalysts have argued that such a standard is too rigid to apply to psychoanalytic material, however. Other options that protect patients but also meet the scientific need to maintain integrity of clinical reporting have been proposed.[48,49]

If the therapist's goal is not to advance knowledge but to advance his or her career by "using" case material to "get publications," there is a conflict of interest that may distort the decisions and judgment of the therapist. This distorting pressure may interfere with appropriate efforts to maintain the duty of confidentiality to patients. This duty includes not only protecting patients' personal information but also preserving respectful appreciation of them and their trust.[50] As with many ethical dilemmas, there is no "one size fits all" solution, and each case must be reviewed carefully before a specific approach is chosen. The aims in seeking to publish case material must be honestly assessed, as should the potential risks of breached confidentiality. Ethical concerns about the protection of the patient's privacy must take precedence over the therapist's need to publish.[48–50] **Table 6** illustrates some factors that therapists should consider before publishing case material.

Table 6
Preserving confidentiality in writing case reports

Method of Preserving Confidentiality	Advantages	Disadvantages	Additional Points
Disguise superficial details of the patient's external life so that the patient is essentially unrecognizable to a reader	Preserves confidentiality	The disguise may impact the scientific integrity of material	Disguise can be minimized if the primary emphasis is on internal wishes, fantasies, and conflicts rather than the external details of the patient's life
If writing about clinical syndromes, a composite of several patients may be appropriate	Preserves confidentiality	—	—
If writing about technique or theory, the "process approach," which includes dialog but not biographical features of the patient, may be appropriate.	Preserves confidentiality	—	If consent is sought *in addition* to disguising, the impact of this request must be rigorously analyzed, discussed, and explored
Vignettes may be used rather than extended case reports	Preserves confidentiality	—	Consider getting written consent

Data from Gabbard GO, Williams P. Preserving confidentiality in the writing of case reports. Int J Psychoanal 2001;82:1067–8.

SUMMARY

The practice of psychotherapy gives rise to many ethical dilemmas. In this article we offered a "primer" on the most commonly cited ethical concerns in psychotherapy related to professionalism and therapeutic boundaries and confidentiality. There is no single answer to the varied and complex ethical issues that therapists may encounter in their treatment of patients. Such dilemmas are dynamic, nuanced, complex, and highly context dependent. Although professional codes offer guidance on optimal standards of conduct, they do not always offer clear answers; hence, therapists need to be able to critically evaluate and interpret such codes in relation to their daily practice.

The contemporary therapist continues to face new dilemmas in an ever-evolving and dynamic twenty-first-century practice environment. Ethical therapists serve the well-being of their patients above all other interests or commitments. Therapists who are attentive to the professional obligations they possess can adopt several strategies to increase their ethical competence, including constantly evaluating their own attitudes and behaviors in addition to those of their patients, engaging in dialog and developing expertise in relation to ethics issues, having a solid grasp of relevant professional codes of conduct, and demonstrating an openness to consultation with peers and exposure of their work to peer review.

ACKNOWLEDGMENTS

The authors wish to thank Laura Grabowski and Ann Tennier for their help in the preparation of this article.

REFERENCES

1. Roberts LW, Hoop JG, Dunn LB. Ethical aspects of psychiatry. In: Hales RE, Yudofsky SC, Gabbard GO, editors. The American psychiatric publishing textbook of psychiatry. 5th edition. Washington, DC: American Psychiatric Publishing; 2008. p. 1601–36.
2. American Psychiatric Association. The principles of medical ethics with annotations especially applicable to psychiatry. Arlington (VA): American Psychiatric Association; 2008.
3. Gutheil TG, Gabbard GO. The concept of boundaries in clinical practice: theoretical and risk-management dimensions. Am J Psychiatry 1993;150:188–96.
4. Karasu TB. The ethics of psychotherapy. Am J Psychiatry 1980;137:1502–12.
5. Lakin M. Coping with ethical dilemmas in psychotherapy. New York: Pergamon Press; 1991.
6. Redlich F, Mollica RF. Overview: ethical issues in contemporary psychiatry. Am J Psychiatry 1976;133:125–36.
7. Roberts LW, Dyer AR. Concise guide to ethics in mental health care. Washington, DC: American Psychiatric Publishing, Inc.; 2004.
8. Cohen JJ. Professionalism in medical education, an American perspective: from evidence to accountability. Med Educ 2006;40:607–17.
9. Kohn LT, Corrigan J, Donaldson MS. To err is human: building a safer health system. Washington, DC: National Academy Press; 2000.
10. Green SA, Bloch S. Working in a flawed mental health care system: an ethical challenge. Am J Psychiatry 2001;158:1378–83.
11. Roberts LW, Hoop JG. Professionalism and ethics: Q & A self-study guide for mental health professionals. Washington, DC: American Psychiatric Pub; 2008.

12. Malmquist CP, Notman MT. Psychiatrist-patient boundary issues following treatment termination. Am J Psychiatry 2001;158:1010–8.
13. Gutheil TG, Brodsky A. Preventing boundary violations in clinical practice. New York: Guilford Press; 2008.
14. Appelbaum PS. Informed consent to psychotherapy: recent developments. Psychiatr Serv 1997;48:445–6.
15. Beahrs JO, Gutheil TG. Informed consent in psychotherapy. Am J Psychiatry 2001;158:4–10.
16. Croarkin P, Berg J, Spira J. Informed consent for psychotherapy: a look at therapists' understanding, opinions, and practices. Am J Psychother 2003;57:384–400.
17. Gutheil TG, Gabbard GO. Misuses and misunderstandings of boundary theory in clinical and regulatory settings. Am J Psychiatry 1998;155:409–14.
18. Langs R. The bipersonal field. New York: J. Aronson; 1976.
19. Spruiell V. The rules and frames of the psychoanalytic situation. Psychoanal Q 1983;52:1–33.
20. Gutheil TG, Simon RI. Non-sexual boundary crossings and boundary violations: the ethical dimension. Psychiatr Clin North Am 2002;25:585–92.
21. Eissler KR. The effect of the structure of the ego on psychoanalytic technique. J Am Psychoanal Assoc 1953;1:104–43.
22. Gabbard GO. Psychodynamic psychiatry in clinical practice. Washington, DC: American Psychiatric Press; 1990.
23. Holroyd JC, Brodsky AM. Psychologists' attitudes and practices regarding erotic and nonerotic physical contact with patients. Am Psychol 1977;32:843–9.
24. Pope KS, Levenson H, Schover LR. Sexual intimacy in psychology training: results and implications of a national survey. Am Psychol 1979;34:682–9.
25. Borys DS, Pope KS. Dual relationships between therapist and client: a national study of psychologists, psychiatrists, and social workers. Prof Psychol Res Pr 1989;20:283–93. Available at: http://dx.doi.org/10.1037/0735-7028.20.5.283. Accessed March 17, 2009.
26. Coverdale J, Bayer T, Chiang E, et al. National survey on physicians' attitudes toward social and sexual contact with patients. South Med J 1994;87:1067–71.
27. Bayer T, Coverdale J, Chiang E. A national survey of physicians' behaviors regarding sexual contact with patients. South Med J 1996;89:977–82.
28. Gabbard GO, Menninger WW. An overview of sexual boundary violations in psychiatry. Psychiatr Ann 1991;21:649–50.
29. Gabbard GO. Psychodynamics of sexual boundary violations. Psychiatr Ann 1991;21:651–5.
30. Gutheil TG, Gabbard GO. Obstacles to the dynamic understanding of therapist-patient sexual relations. Am J Psychother 1992;46:515–25.
31. Gabbard GO. Reconsidering the American Psychological Association's policy on sex with former patients: is it justifiable? Prof Psychol Res Pr 1994;25:329–35.
32. Gabbard GO. Transference and countertransference in the psychotherapy of therapists charged with sexual misconduct. Psychiatr Ann 1995;25:100–5.
33. Gabbard GO. Lessons to be learned from the study of sexual boundary violations. Am J Psychother 1996;50:311–22.
34. Gabbard GO. Post-termination sexual boundary violations. Psychiatr Clin North Am 2002;25:593–603.
35. Celenza A, Gabbard GO. Analysts who commit sexual boundary violations: a lost cause? J Am Psychoanal Assoc 2003;51:617–36.

36. Simon RI. Sexual exploitation of patients: how it begins before it happens. Psychiatr Ann 1989;19:104–12.
37. Gabbard GO, Lester EP. Boundaries and boundary violations in psychoanalysis. New York: Basic Books; 1995.
38. Epstein RS, Simon RI. The exploitation index: an early warning indicator of boundary violations in psychotherapy. Bull Menninger Clin 1990;54:450–65.
39. Stone AA. Sexual misconduct by psychiatrists: the ethical and clinical dilemma of confidentiality. Am J Psychiatry 1983;140:195–7.
40. Fennig S, Secker A, Levkovitz Y, et al. Are psychotherapists consistent in their ethical attitude to patient confidentiality? Isr J Psychiatry Relat Sci 2004;41:82–9.
41. Simon RI. Clinical psychiatry and the law. Washington, DC: American Psychiatric Press; 1992.
42. Phillips J. Philosophical and ethical issues in psychotherapy. Curr Opin Psychiatry 2003;16:685–9. Available at: http://dx.doi.org/10.1097/00001504-200311000-00014. Accessed March 17, 2009.
43. Mosher PW, Swire PP. The ethical and legal implications of Jaffee v Redmond and the HIPAA medical privacy rule for psychotherapy and general psychiatry. Psychiatr Clin North Am 2002;25:575–84, vi–vii.
44. Siegler M. Sounding boards: confidentiality in medicine. A decrepit concept. N Engl J Med 1982;307:1518–21.
45. Lewers DT. Guidelines of patient-physician electronic mail: report to the board of trustees, American Medical Association. Available at: http://www.ama-assn.org/ama/pub/category/2386.html. Accessed March 17, 2009.
46. Hilty DM, Yellowlees PM, Cobb HC, et al. Use of secure e-mail and telephone: psychiatric consultations to accelerate rural health service delivery. Telemed J E Health 2006;12:490–5.
47. Kassaw K, Gabbard GO. The ethics of e-mail communication in psychiatry. Psychiatr Clin North Am 2002;25:665–74.
48. Gabbard GO. Disguise or consent: problems and recommendations concerning the publication and presentation of clinical material. Int J Psychoanal 2000;81: 1071–86. Available at: http://dx.doi.org/10.1516/0020757001600426. Accessed March 17, 2009.
49. Gabbard GO, Williams P. Preserving confidentiality in the writing of case reports. Int J Psychoanal 2001;82:1067–8.
50. Kantrowitz JL. Writing about patients: responsibilities, risks, and ramifications. New York: Other Press; 2006.
51. Nishizono M. Ethical issues in psychotherapy. Jpn J Psychiatry Neurol 1994; 48(Suppl):33–8.
52. Gutheil TG. Radical victimology and the retreat from patients. Newsl Am Acad Psychiatry Law 1994;19:10–1.
53. Casement PJ. The meeting of needs in psychoanalysis. Psychoanal Inq 1990;10: 325–46.
54. Knox S, Hess SA, Williams EN, et al. "Here's a little something for you": how therapists respond to client gifts. J Couns Psychol 2003;50:199–210.
55. Stein H. The gift in therapy. Am J Psychother 1965;19:480–8.
56. Berne E. What do you say after you say hello? The psychology of human destiny. New York: Grove Press; 1972.
57. Bonitz V. Use of physical touch in the "talking cure": a journey to the outskirts of psychotherapy. Psychother Theor Res Pract Train 2008;45:391–404. Available at: http://dx.doi.org/10.1037/a0013311. Accessed March 17, 2009.

A Basic Decision-Making Approach to Common Ethical Issues in Consultation-Liaison Psychiatry

Mark T. Wright, MD[a,b],*, Laura Weiss Roberts, MD, MA[a,c]

KEYWORDS

- Ethics • Consultation-liaison psychiatry
- Psychosomatic medicine • Four topics method
- Psychiatry training • Clinical cases

Psychosomatic medicine is the subspecialty of psychiatry that deals with biologic, social, and psychologic issues arising in clinical medicine. Psychosomatic medicine resides at the interface of physical and mental illness. The clinical practice of psychosomatic medicine, or, as it is more commonly called, consultation-liaison (C-L) psychiatry, in general medical settings has long entailed dealing with ethical issues.[1] Indeed, C-L psychiatrists are called on to provide expertise and skill in highly clinically and ethically complex situations, assisting colleagues, patients, and families in life-threatening, life-ending, and life-restoring situations.[1,2] Given psychiatry's devotion to the humanistic side of medicine, moreover, physicians and other health care providers frequently expect C-L psychiatrists to be able to resolve ethical dilemmas, even in institutions in which ethics committees and clinical ethics consult services exist.[3,4]

Unfortunately, psychiatrists often receive no more substantive training in clinical ethics than their nonpsychiatric colleagues. The entities that oversee psychiatric training have yet to prescribe specific training, either in content or in methods, in clinical ethics areas important to psychiatry. The Accreditation Council for Graduate Medical Education (ACGME),[5] for instance, currently requires only that psychiatry

[a] Department of Psychiatry and Behavioral Medicine, Medical College of Wisconsin, 8701 Watertown Plank Road, Milwaukee, WI 53226, USA
[b] Department of Neurology, Medical College of Wisconsin, 8701 Watertown Plank Road, Milwaukee, WI 53226, USA
[c] Department of Population Health, Medical College of Wisconsin, 8701 Watertown Plank Road, Milwaukee, WI 53226, USA
* Corresponding author. Department of Psychiatry and Behavioral Medicine, Medical College of Wisconsin, 8701 Watertown Plank Road, Milwaukee, WI 53226, USA.
E-mail address: mwright@mcw.edu (M.T. Wright).

Psychiatr Clin N Am 32 (2009) 315–328
doi:10.1016/j.psc.2009.03.001
0193-953X/09/$ – see front matter © 2009 Elsevier Inc. All rights reserved.

residents demonstrate professionalism, mentioning aspects of professionalism such as respecting patient privacy and autonomy, maintaining appropriate professional boundaries, and cultural sensitivity. The ACGME guidelines[5] refer to the Principles of Medical Ethics with Annotations Especially Applicable to Psychiatry,[6] now many years old, as "an integral part of the educational process" but suggest simply distributing these guidelines to residents and operating in accordance with them. The core competencies for psychiatrists delineated by the American Board of Psychiatry and Neurology[7] speak only of a need for general psychiatrists to exhibit ethical behavior and give attention to issues of confidentiality, informed consent, and conflict of interest. A need for knowledge of standards and procedures related to involuntary psychiatric treatment is also mentioned. Likewise, the ACGME guidelines[5] state only that psychiatrists in psychosomatic medicine fellowship training should show professionalism and "adherence to ethical principles"; the only specific ethics topic mentioned is capacity to give informed consent.

Recent subspecialty guidelines in psychosomatic medicine defined by the American Board of Psychiatry and Neurology (ABPN)[8] and authors in the C-L psychiatry literature[4,9–13] suggest more rigorous expectations.

The ABPN[8] guidelines for specialists in psychosomatic medicine exceed the guidelines discussed earlier and state that practitioners should be familiar with concepts related to decision-making capacity, advance directives, right to refuse treatment, informed consent, living wills, duty to warn, withholding medical treatment, patient autonomy, and confidentiality. It is apparent that opinion leaders in psychosomatic medicine identify a chasm between the ethics training of psychiatrists and the demands of C-L practice.

Several writers[9–11,13] have brought attention to the fact that psychiatric training does not make one a clinical ethicist; these authors have contrasted the training and work of C-L psychiatrists and clinical ethicists. To help meet these educational and training goals, advocates of ethics training for C-L psychiatrists have put forth a bibliography[12] and specific recommendations for training programs.[4] Unfortunately, the demands of typically busy, hectic psychiatric consultation services will not wait until educators and practitioners design and implement curricula in ethics. Until C-L psychiatrists become more proficient in clinical ethics, consultation requests involving ethical dilemmas will continue to provoke concern, and perhaps anxiety, in consultants, and consulting caregivers will continue to be dissatisfied and frustrated when psychiatrists are unable to provide clear answers to their questions. Many C-L psychiatry services would benefit from rapid implementation of a simple ethical decision-making process.

ETHICAL DECISION-MAKING APPROACHES

Several clinical ethical decision-making models exist. They all have strengths and may be readily incorporated into clinical thinking and decision making in real time. We briefly sketch five relevant approaches that have received attention in the literature for their value in clinical settings, including one that is specifically of importance to C-L psychiatry because of its usefulness in examining dilemmas surrounding issues of informed consent and informed refusal for care. We then describe in detail a highly recognized decision-making model, the Four Topics Method, and provide illustrations of its use in cases drawn from the everyday work of psychosomatic medicine practice.

An early ethical analysis method advanced by Beauchamp and Childress,[14] in their widely-cited work on bioethics first published in 1979, defines four cardinal ethical principles in clinical care: nonmaleficence (an obligation to avoid doing harm), beneficence (an obligation to benefit patients whenever possible and to seek their good), respect for autonomy (the ability to make deliberated or reasoned decisions for oneself and to act on the basis of such decisions), and justice (fairness).[15,16] In this approach, the clinician is careful to explicitly identify the role of these principles in the clinical care needs of the patient and to identify and resolve ethical tensions that arise when these principles conflict.

Two other thinkers have proposed sequential evaluation of ethically important considerations arising in individual patient cases. Lederberg[4] has written on a "situational diagnosis" methodology. This process includes a systematic examination of patient and family issues (including any mental illness present in the patient or key significant others), staff issues, "joint" issues (eg, family–staff relationships), legal/institutional issues, and ethical issues. A thorough examination of all issues precedes ethical analysis, and this analysis can suggest educational, psychologic/psychiatric, and ethical interventions that can be implemented in a hierarchical fashion. Similarly, Hundert[17] has proposed a model for examining and acting on ethical concerns arising in specific patient care situations. This approach involves first methodically identifying each of the basic values (eg, welfare, justice, liberty) that have collided to produce an ethical dilemma. By weighing, or "computing," the relative importance of each value, as each individual does in forming his or her own moral principles, a moral action is suggested.

Each of these models may have a place in the general work of a clinician and may be helpful in the work of a C-L practitioner. Perhaps the most common ethical issues in C-L psychiatry pertain to the evaluation of decisional capacity and the provision by patients of informed consent or informed refusal for treatment. Approaches to informed consent and decisional capacity are well described in the literature[18–23] and are highlighted in other selections in this issue of *Psychiatric Clinics of North America*.[24–28] In brief, informed consent depends on three components: information-sharing processes, decision-making ability, and voluntarism capacity.[16,21] With respect to information-sharing processes, informed consent or refusal entails careful communication of information regarding the nature of an illness process, with and without recommended intervention, and information regarding anticipated risks, benefits, and alternatives relevant to the recommended treatment. Rare but severe potential complications need to be shared in this process of communication between clinician and patient. Further, the communication process ideally occurs in a manner that addresses patient concerns, enhances the patient's ability to understand and absorb what is being said, is not rushed, and permits some dialog and clarification.[19] Decisional capacity is built on four capacities that may be more or less fully intact. The first is the ability to communicate, by any means (eg, verbally or with gestures). The second is the ability to understand—literally, the ability to comprehend the factual information that is being conveyed in the consent process or "encounter." The third is the ability to reason, that is, to work rationally and flexibly with the information, and to evaluate or, in a sense, calculate the risks and benefits faced in the decision. The final element of decisional capacity is the ability to appreciate the meaning of the decision in the context of one's life history and values; this capacity is deeply shaped by an individual's life story and the neurocognitive capacity for insight. Voluntarism capacity is the ability to possess and express a free, uncoerced, authentic preference and is influenced by developmental issues, symptom-related considerations, psychologic features, and contextual factors.[21] Threats to this capacity are extraordinarily diverse and may range from manifestations of disease (eg, alexithymia in psychosis or negative cognitive distortions in depression) to setting of care (eg, treatment in a military hospital or treatment on a locked unit in a county jail).

In evaluating capacity for consent or refusal for care, a C-L psychiatrist must first clarify what the exact decision is that must be made and evaluate the patient's abilities in relation to the nature and risk of the decision. Consent for a routine procedure, such as a flu shot or a cholesterol check, is benchmarked against a different standard than consent for another routine procedure, such as a mammogram or a colonoscopy, or a more substantive and risky intervention, such as chemotherapy or a surgical procedure. Criticisms of informed consent and refusal processes are commonly focused on how a consult to evaluate capacity occurs only if a patient objects to a recommended procedure, introducing bias for compliance in patients. In an original and invaluably formative paper by Drane,[29] this criticism is dismantled because capacity is benchmarked not by compliance but by capacity to assume appropriate risks; the key consideration is whether a patient is capable of giving informed refusal for recommended care.[30] Drane's model for addressing the issue of competency to consent to, or refuse, medical care is predicated on the principle of nonmaleficence first and foremost. He has suggested that using a single, monolithic standard of competency may be inappropriate and has proposed a "sliding scale" standard of competency. In this model, decisions regarding low-risk/high-benefit care require a patient only to be aware of the general situation and to assent to the care. As the risk-to-benefit ratio of medical care increases, competency entails a more sophisticated understanding of the possible outcomes of different care options, and a greater ability to articulate preferences. In other words, if a decision is riskier, then there is a more rigorous standard in place; this is more typical of informed refusal decisions.

THE FOUR TOPICS METHOD

By far the most widely recognized clinical ethics decision-making strategy is the work of Siegler and colleagues,[31,32] who have described a Four Topics Method of systematically analyzing and resolving clinical ethical conflicts. It has been suggested that the Four Topics Method of ethical decision making could be easily taught and used in the practice of C-L psychiatry.[3] In this article, the Four Topics Method is described and used to analyze some clinical cases illustrative of ethical dilemmas commonly encountered in C-L psychiatry.

The Four Topics model is based on the idea that decisions regarding ethical dilemmas should result from a process that considers operant factors and possible outcomes in a systematic way. Jonsen and colleagues[32] have suggested that the particulars of any clinical case can be linked with moral principles through an analysis of (in their usual order of importance) medical indications, patient preferences, quality of life issues, and contextual features. This approach is based on casuistry, a pragmatic and concrete approach in moral philosophy that is most elegantly described by Stephen Toulmin.[33] Traditional ethical rules, or moral principles, such as beneficence, nonmaleficence, autonomy, loyalty, and fairness, are applied to issues as they arise in the analysis. This approach examines the situation in an organized, global fashion and allows those involved to weigh and prioritize considerations in the four areas. Just the process of separating the issues in this manner can quickly result in a reasonable and practical solution.

The Four Topics Method begins with an analysis of medical indications, which entails looking at a patient's diagnosis, treatment options, and prognosis in the usual ways of clinical medicine. An examination of treatment options includes a discussion of goals, potential risks and benefits, and probable outcomes for each. The principles of beneficence and nonmaleficence are often the most important moral principles considered at this stage of analysis. In C-L psychiatry in particular, the basic issues related to the primary physical illness are critical to evaluate for their potential impact on the psychologic presentation or the cognitive functioning of the patient. The presence or absence of psychiatric disease processes must also be assessed carefully as one element of the medical indications component of the patient's case.

Understanding patient preferences comes next in the Four Topics approach. Patients' preferences regarding medical care are determined by their own values and their assessments of the risks and benefits of care. Before these preferences can be fully understood, a consultant must know what clinical information the patient has been given by his or her caregivers, and this is the reason this step follows an analysis of medical indications. Incapacitation (eg, because of cognitive dysfunction) makes appreciating and respecting patient preferences difficult, or impossible, and necessitates the involvement of surrogates (such as advance directives and significant others) in the analysis. At this stage, autonomy is often the most important ethical principle to consider. Complex issues can arise, particularly in the context of mental illness, when the expressed preferences of an individual are obscured, distorted, or produced by symptoms of disease, such as impulsivity in a poststroke or delirious patient, the expansiveness and recklessness of a person experiencing manic symptoms, or ominous feelings, hopelessness, mental anguish, or sense of foreboding due to trauma-related or affective processes.

Illness, injury, and medical treatments can affect a patient's quality of life. Ethical analysis of quality-of-life issues needs to examine the possible residual physical and mental deficits a patient may have with, or without, treatment of the illness. Discussion of quality-of-life issues mainly focuses on the patient's opinions but also includes the thoughts of the patient's caregivers and significant others. Quality-of-life considerations are usually most important in situations in which a patient's prognosis is poor and his or her preferences are unclear. Decisions regarding forgoing treatment and beginning palliative care are considered at this stage. Ethical analysis of quality-of-life issues again entails consideration of the principles of beneficence, nonmaleficence, and autonomy.

Numerous contextual (situational) factors influence illness and its diagnosis and treatment, and conversely, a patient's illness can have wide-ranging environmental effects. A thorough analysis of an ethical dilemma must include examination of caregiver, family, financial, religious, cultural, legal, and other factors surrounding the clinical situation. Possible benefits and burdens to caregivers and significant others should be examined. The moral principles of loyalty and fairness are often considered at this stage of analysis.

FOUR ILLUSTRATIVE CASES

Although a C-L psychiatrist's typical cases can vary infinitely in details, a few specific ethical themes and issues are encountered repeatedly, as in other areas of medicine. This limited scope of ethical concerns seems to have been codified in the 2008 ABPN[8] guidelines for specialists in psychosomatic medicine and can serve to limit and simplify ethics education somewhat. Although a competent C-L psychiatrist needs the ability to address other ethical dilemmas, such as questions of duty to warn and involuntary psychiatric hospitalization, an initial step toward proficiency in clinical ethics might entail developing the ability to address the dilemmas regarding patients' decision making that commonly arise in C-L work.

The following clinical scenarios are based on actual cases from several institutions known to the authors and serve as examples of ethical dilemmas commonly encountered by the busy C-L psychiatrist. Concerns regarding patient decision making are highlighted, but other ethical issues are included. Following each case is an analysis and discussion using the Four Topics Method.

Case 1: A "Legitimate" Desire to Die?

A 70-year-old woman was admitted to the surgical intensive care unit with a self-inflicted gunshot wound. The patient used a gun belonging to her husband to shoot herself in her cardiac pacemaker. The patient developed third-degree heart block and sustained a small right lung laceration and pneumohemothorax as a result of her gunshot wound. Despite heart rates in the 30s to 50s, the patient remained asymptomatic. Her thoracic injuries necessitated placement of a chest tube for a short time, and the patient passively cooperated with this. Early in the hospitalization, when the patient said intractable pain from metastatic cancer had made her suicidal, some staff members believed that care should be withheld and the patient should be allowed to die because she was in severe pain and dying was "what she really wanted."

When the patient was later evaluated by the C-L psychiatry service, she said she had been planning to kill herself for several weeks. She said she shot herself in her pacemaker because it was her understanding that she would die immediately if the pacemaker ever malfunctioned. The patient said she wanted to die because cancer had spread throughout her body and she could no longer stand the pain. When pressed, the patient could not provide details regarding her cancer. The psychiatry consultants diagnosed depression and wondered if the patient's claim of having metastatic cancer was, in fact, a mood-congruent delusion. The psychiatrists cautioned that psychotic depression was likely governing the patient's choices regarding her overall health care. When the patient continued to express a desire to die and refused implantation of a new pacemaker, the psychiatry service was asked to comment specifically on her capacity to make medical decisions.

Discussion

Medical indications The patient has a chronic cardiac arrhythmia. The patient's cardiologists believe that she does not need emergency, immediate implantation of a new pacer but say that one should be placed in the next 48 hours. They say the patient will need to be monitored in the ICU until the pacer is replaced. The cardiology team tells the patient and her family that cardiac pacemaker implantation is a low-risk procedure and that her prognosis after replacement of the pacer will be good. Failure to replace the pacemaker is associated with significant risks, however, including sudden death. Further medical evaluation fails to reveal any evidence of cancer. More extensive psychiatric evaluation does reveal that the patient has major depression with psychotic features, however. The medical team, advised by the psychiatric consultants, implements strict suicide precautions. Psychiatric hospitalization after the acute medical issues have resolved is found to be indicated and treatment with medications (antidepressants, antipsychotics) is recommended.

Patient preferences The patient expresses her wishes to die and to decline necessary medical treatment. The psychiatrists note that the patient's capacity to make medical decisions is significantly impaired by a severe and clearly life-threatening neuropsychiatric disease, major depression. The decision regarding life-saving and quality-of-life–preserving intervention, in particular, is distorted by delusional beliefs. Her appreciation of the risks of the procedure, and of declining this intervention, is compromised; her active suicidality colors her medical decision making. For these reasons, the need for a surrogate decision maker during this acute period is emphasized by the psychiatric consultants. When her mental illness has improved or entered remission, her capacity for informed consent or informed refusal may be restored, and her enduring preferences may be more clearly discerned.

Quality of life The cardiology team tells the patient's family that she could die without a pacer, but they say she should lead a normal life if the pacer is replaced. The psychiatry team tells the family the patient will remain at high risk for suicide unless her psychotic depression is treated.

Contextual features The patient's elderly husband is overwhelmed by her situation and can offer little in the way of past history or treatment suggestions. The patient's two adult children, who live in another city, do not know the details of her history, but they are in favor of treating the patient against her will, if necessary. Despite clarification of the patient's initial statements and situation, the ICU nurses caring for the patient continue to insist that the patient wants to die and wonder if she should be allowed to do so. In discussing the patient's case, some of the care team members express the notion that depression is a "natural" part of aging. With discussion, they acknowledge that caring for a patient who is refusing care is unusual for them, and difficult. At a conference involving the patient's children, ICU nurses and physician, cardiologist, and psychiatrist, it is decided that her children will obtain temporary guardianship and her pacer will be replaced.

This patient's age and dramatic initial statements and presentation led some of her caregivers to rush to the conclusion that her suicidality was somehow appropriate. Diagnosis of the patient's severe mental illness did not fully dissuade some of the caregivers from their view that the patient's desire to die was rational. This circumstance represents an important opportunity to talk with colleagues about the existence and seriousness of mental illness and the imperatives to treat neuropsychiatric disease just as one would treat cardiovascular, gastrointestinal, genitourinary, or musculoskeletal conditions. Failure to do so may be based on prejudicial attitudes or lack of medical/psychiatric sophistication, giving rise to disparities in medical care provided for people who have neuropsychiatric diseases. A thorough exploration of quality of life and contextual issues in this case revealed transferential issues and misconceptions about aging in some staff members that could have resulted in suboptimal care being given to the patient. This case provided an excellent opportunity for the psychiatrist to work with complex and challenging issues with the staff on the case and to talk through the complexities that arise in medical decision making when a patient has severe mental illness.

Case 2: A Patient Refusing Evaluation and Treatment

A 72-year-old man was admitted to the hospital from the emergency department with a 3-month history of severe anorexia, weight loss, and epigastric pain. Physical examination revealed a cachectic, jaundiced, elderly man with a stage II pressure ulcer over his sacral area. Laboratory studies showed markedly elevated bilirubin and alkaline phosphatase levels and a prealbumin level of less than 5 mg/dL, indicating significant malnutrition. An abdominal CT scan revealed a possible mass in the head of the pancreas. Suspecting pancreatic cancer, the patient's physicians discussed the diagnosis with him. When told he may have cancer, the patient flatly insisted he did not, without any apparent consideration of the information provided by his doctors. He seemed suspicious of his doctors' motives. Later, when his physicians again tried to discuss cancer and get his consent for an endoscopic retrograde cholangiopancreatogram, the patient vaguely acknowledged possibly having cancer but said he needed no further evaluation or treatment because God had always healed him.

The patient stated his wish to leave the hospital, but did not try to leave his room or even his bed, saying he was "tired" and would "go later."

Family members, who acknowledged that they had been "estranged and distant" for many years, reported the patient had always been "odd," "paranoid," and "a loner" and had never been able to hold jobs for long. The patient had never been married and had no children. Family members said he recently had been "speaking more and more" about God but said he never attended any church. They said he had never seen a mental health professional. The patient reportedly sought basic medical care from a trusted internist in the remote past, but after this physician's retirement, the patient received little or no health care. The patient had no history of impulsive or erratic behavior and had never been violent toward others.

The patient's relatives believed that the physicians should respect the patient's wishes to leave the hospital. The psychiatric consultant was asked by the primary physician to assess the patient's competence. When the psychiatrist asked the patient why he had been hospitalized, he said "they say I have cancer" and refused further questioning.

Discussion

Medical indications The physicians strongly suspect the patient has pancreatic cancer but would like to do further studies before commenting definitively on diagnosis, treatment options, and prognosis. If the patient has pancreatic cancer, the goals of treatment would be cure versus palliation, depending on the type and extent of the cancer. The sense of the medical team was that the patient had advanced disease with a poor prognosis. The C-L psychiatrist develops the working hypothesis that the patient may suffer from a chronic psychotic illness such as schizophrenia or a Cluster A personality disorder,[34] although he points out that pancreatic cancer can present with diverse neuropsychiatric phenomena. Irrespective of the proximal or distant cause, the patient's mental status is found to be compromised with evidence of significant cognitive deficits, impairment of insight, overvalued ideas and paranoid beliefs, and denial, which may have been part of a chronic mental illness or more immediate psychologic issues associated with a new and devastating medical illness.

Patient preferences The psychiatrist is satisfied that the patient has received adequate information regarding the medical diagnosis and needed tests, and the psychiatrist carefully approaches the issue of an existing condition affecting his thinking at this time. After speaking with the patient, the psychiatrist determines that he lacks the capacity to make his medical decisions based on neurocognitive deficits and other illness-related factors. The psychiatrist indicates that, although the patient may have some basic understanding of the facts of his case, he does not demonstrate an appreciation of the personal implications of these facts.[35] The psychiatrist wonders whether it is possible that nonpathologic religious beliefs—a true sense of faith and optimism associated with a positive and enduring religious life experience—could be the cause of this failure to acknowledge the severity of his situation, rather than psychosis. There is evidence from the patient's past history, however, that his religious beliefs were not part of a larger personal, family, or cultural life context. The psychiatrist suggests that some restoration of the patient's decisional capacity could occur with treatment with an antipsychotic medication. When he realizes the patient will not accept medication and that a court would not likely order medication treatment in the absence of a clear diagnosis and imminent dangerousness, the psychiatrist initiates a discussion regarding surrogate decision makers. The patient has no advance directives.

Quality of life The patient's oncologists say there is a high probability he has pancreatic cancer and that his prognosis for long-term survival is poor, with or without treatment. They say the patient's quality of life will be extremely poor because of anorexia, weakness, and pain.

Contextual features As the doctors thoroughly discuss the patient's situation with his estranged brother and sister, the siblings say he has "never liked doctors" and believe it is unlikely he will voluntarily cooperate with care. When asked about the patient's religious comments, the siblings reiterate that the patient has no history of clear spiritual or religious interest, and they believe his comments about being healed by God were simply an excuse to leave the hospital. The siblings continue to believe that the patient's wishes to leave the hospital without treatment should be respected. They refuse to be involved in treating the patient against his will, and in discussing this they admit that they fear the patient might become angry and aggressive with them. With further open discussion, the oncologists admit they do not relish the idea of aggressively treating such a "low-functioning" and uncooperative patient, especially one with such a poor prognosis. When the psychiatrist raises the danger of giving suboptimal care to the patient because he is mentally ill, the oncologists and other members of the treatment team agree that they will treat the patient in accordance with their standard treatment protocols if appropriate consents are obtained.

Given the patient's poor medical prognosis and severely compromised quality of life, with or without further evaluation and treatment, coupled with his refusal of care and his family's support of his position, the treatment team and the patient's siblings decide he will be discharged from the hospital to the care of his sister. He is to be given symptomatic and palliative treatments as he will accept them. A treatment guardian is arranged for the supportive care process.

This case is difficult, and the ultimate decision of the clinical care team is governed by the medical indications, which are that this patient has advanced disease for which there is no cure and an inevitable terminal outcome. The patient's preferences, although influenced by psychiatric disease, were honored with sufficient ethical safeguards put in place (eg, family involvement, follow-up care, treatment guardian for supportive care processes). If the C-L psychiatrist had responded to this request for a competency evaluation in a focused way, the result might have been a simple finding of incapacity and likely forced intervention and treatment, with still a poor outcome. The C-L psychiatrist's first duty is to evaluate the role and contribution of psychiatric disease to the patient's clinical presentation. In addition, broader analysis using the Four Topics Method moved understanding of the case beyond the basic medical facts and patient preferences. In keeping with Drane's[29] model, because the decision to intervene or not was not going to dramatically affect prognosis and quality of life, a less rigorous standard of competency was seen as acceptable; still, a treatment guardian was secured to help ensure appropriate supportive and, ultimately, palliative care and to give sufficient safeguards in the situation.

Case 3: A Question Regarding Capacity to Live Independently

A 26-year-old man who had a history of alcoholism dating back to his teens sustained a traumatic brain injury in a motor vehicle crash at age 25. A brain MRI scan done a few days after the crash revealed hemorrhagic contusions in the orbitofrontal and anterior temporal lobes. The patient required hospitalization for 3 weeks, and after hospital discharge the patient spent a month in a traumatic brain injury rehabilitation program. Despite excellent rehabilitation care, the patient was left with significant personality changes (disinhibition and occasional agitation) and cognitive deficits (slowed processing, recent memory impairment, and executive dysfunction). The rehabilitation specialists determined that the patient would not be able to return to his previous job in construction. The patient was discharged to a supported living apartment where his parents and professional caregivers would help with meal preparation, home cleaning, and managing finances. After rehabilitation discharge, the patient began to drink alcohol supplied by a sibling and developed severe problems with impulse control. Two months after discharge, the patient began to refuse help from his caregivers. When the patient's parents did not hear from him for 3 weeks, they called police, who found the patient thin and living in an unkempt home with no food. He was brought to the hospital by police and was admitted for "failure to thrive."

Discussion

Medical indications The patient's consultant psychiatrist and other physicians give him diagnoses of alcohol dependence and dementia due to traumatic brain injury. The physicians tell the patient's parents his prognosis is guarded: they say his relatively young age and the relatively short period of time since the crash bode well for him, but his alcoholism and the extent of his brain injury are poor prognostic factors. They suggest the patient might show cognitive and behavioral improvement with abstinence from alcohol and with treatment with medications (eg, a cholinesterase inhibitor, and divalproex sodium for impulse control problems) but say that, even with appropriate treatment, the patient will not be capable of independent living in the near future.

Patient preferences The patient believes he has no mental problems or functional impairment and refuses to cooperate with his care. The patient's physicians believe his cognitive impairment is incompatible with independent living at this time, and his parents are advised to seek guardianship.

Quality of life The patient's parents ask if his drinking and disinhibited behaviors are due to "immaturity" and wonder if "he just needs to grow up." They express concern that a guardianship will "rob him of his independence." Some members of the care-giving team share this view and believe it is a "really tough ethical problem" to take away a "young man's rights." The physicians explain that the patient's drinking and other behaviors are not "normal, expected behaviors" of a young man but are being driven and reinforced by his disinhibition and poor impulse control and will lead to more serious health issues in the future. They tell the parents that, even with medication treatment and cessation of drinking, the patient's prognosis for a return to independent living is guarded. The dangerousness of the patient's inability to care for himself is emphasized.

Contextual features With further discussion, the parents say they both grew up in "strict" families in rural communities and had "little freedom" until they were married and on their own. They say their upbringing led them to discipline the patient very little when he was growing up, and they admit they would be uncomfortable now in the role of guardian. The parents and treatment team decide to pursue guardianship but to ask for a court-appointed, professional guardian.

This case is another in which a minimalistic psychiatric consult focused on the patient's decisional capacity might have led to an unsatisfactory outcome. If the psychiatric consultant had simply recommended that the patient's parents become legal guardians for their son, they probably would have been granted this by the courts but would have been uncomfortable, and probably ineffective, in this role. A broader survey of the case that included the developmental histories of the parents and the patient revealed important potential problems that could be addressed more constructively through the approach recommended by the psychiatrist.

Case 4: Unclear Motivation

A 44-year-old woman who had no history of mental illness wished to anonymously donate a kidney for transplantation (ie, to be an "altruistic donor"). When she was hospitalized for presurgical testing, mild hypertension was diagnosed. When told by the transplant team that hypertension was a risk factor for future renal disease, the patient persisted with her wish to donate a kidney. While the patient was hospitalized, the C-L psychiatry service was consulted for an organ donor evaluation. The patient said she had worked as a librarian for 20 years. She said she was happily married and had no children. When asked about having no children, the patient said she and her husband, an airline pilot, decided not to have children because of his frequent work-related absences from the home. When asked about her history of altruistic behavior, the patient reported only making some financial donations to charities. When asked why she wanted to donate a kidney now, the patient spoke of wanting to "give something back to humanity." She also said she was intrigued by the idea of part of her "living on" in someone else. She said she would prefer that a woman receive her kidney but said she wanted to donate "with no strings attached." The patient expressed special interest in a case of transvaginal kidney donation reported in the news recently.[36] When interviewed by phone, the patient's husband expressed concern about her donating a kidney because he believed the surgical risks were significant, but he said he would allow her to make her own decision. The transplant nephrologist praised the patient for her "selfless" act. On outpatient follow up, the patient reported some symptoms of depression to the psychiatrist and attributed this to arguments she had with her husband over many years, primarily related to her desire to have children and to his lack of supportiveness. He recently has threatened to have a vasectomy to "settle the issue." The issue of kidney donation has now become a "bone of contention" between them, she acknowledges. Further questioning led to the patient disclosing a sense of emptiness, and she was somewhat receptive when the psychiatrist suggested that she was trying to correct this by donating a kidney. She continued to insist, though, that she wanted to donate.

Discussion

Medical indications The patient is found to be a medically suitable donor. In an extensive evaluation, the C-L psychiatrist diagnoses mild depression. No prior psychiatric disease is identified in the history.

Patient preferences After being advised of the risks associated with kidney donation, including future hypertensive nephropathy, the patient demonstrates good understanding and reiterates her desire to donate her kidney.

Quality of life The transplant psychiatrist identifies depression in the patient and key psychologic issues that may affect the outcome of the case and the patient's suitability as a donor. It seems that the patient is distressed about the issue of whether or not to have children, and whether to remain in her marriage. The psychiatrist believes the patient may be sublimating her desire for children into a desire to donate a kidney and has an unstable psychosocial context. The psychiatrist fears that, left unaddressed, these issues could lead to posttransplant disappointment, worsened depression, and more severe marital problems.

Contextual features When interviewed a second time by the transplant psychiatrist, the patient's husband expresses concern that he will not be home to help the patient if she has postoperative complications. He goes on to express resentment and says he believes the patient is trying to make him "feel guilty for not wanting a family." When the transplant psychiatrist expresses concern regarding dynamic issues to the nephrologist, the nephrologist insists the patient is "fine" and says she already has a "great" recipient for the kidney. A conference involving the patient, her husband, the nephrologist, and the transplant psychiatrist brings to light the patient's regrets and the marital conflicts. After this, all of the concerned parties agree that kidney donation should be deferred until the patient and her husband have a chance to further explore things in psychotherapy.

This situation, like many others encountered in C-L psychiatry practice, is one in which the psychiatrist is a "double agent"; the psychiatrist is asked to serve competing interests.[1] A well-meaning nephrologist with a very ill patient who has end-stage renal disease could, explicitly or implicitly, pressure a psychiatrist to quickly approve what seems to be an ideal donor. Such an evaluation, though, would not be in the best interest of the donor. Using the Four Topics Method in this case prompted a thorough evaluation of the patient's thoughts and those of her husband, and this revealed problems that could have led to a negative outcome had the patient been allowed to donate.

SUMMARY

Ethical dilemmas are found throughout the daily work of C-L psychiatrists. Unfortunately, most psychiatrists have no more training in ethics than their nonpsychiatric colleagues. Psychiatric consults spurred by ethical dilemmas can provoke anxiety in psychiatrists and leave anxious colleagues without the clear recommendations they seek. C-L psychiatrists, and probably all psychiatrists, need more training in clinical ethics. C-L psychiatrists do not need to become clinical ethicists, but competence in handling the ethical issues most commonly seen in C-L work is needed. The 2008 ABPN[8] guidelines for specialists in psychosomatic medicine mention specific ethics topics important in C-L work, and ways of attaining competence in these areas have been discussed in the C-L literature.

The four cases discussed here illustrate the high level of complexity often seen in situations in which ethical dilemmas arise in C-L psychiatry. Given the sometimes furious pace of hospital work, it can be easy for C-L psychiatrists to be seduced by the idea of the quick, focused consult that simply responds to a simple question with a simple answer. Because cases involving ethical dilemmas often involve multiple stakeholders, each with his or her own set of concerns, a brief consult focused only on the patient often leads to errors of omission. A wider approach, such as that suggested by the Four Topics Method, is needed to successfully negotiate ethical dilemmas. Busy C-L psychiatry services may struggle at first to find the time to do the type of global evaluations discussed here, but increasing familiarity with approaches such as the Four Topics Method should lead to quicker ways of gathering and processing the needed information.

REFERENCES

1. Murray GB. Ethical problems in liaison psychiatry. Psychiatr Ann 1979;9:75–9.
2. Roberts LW, Geppert CM, Warner TD, et al. Bioethics principles, informed consent, and ethical care for special populations: curricular needs expressed by men and women physicians-in-training. Psychosomatics 2005;46:440–50.

3. Hayes JR. Consultation-liaison psychiatry and clinical ethics: a model for consultation and teaching. Gen Hosp Psychiatry 1986;8:415–8.
4. Lederberg MS. Making a situational diagnosis. psychiatrists at the interface of psychiatry and ethics in the consultation-liaison setting. Psychosomatics 1997; 38:327–38.
5. Accreditation Council for Graduate Medical Education. Psychiatry program requirements. Available at: http://www.acgme.org/acWebsite/RRC_400/400_prIndex. asp. Accessed February 26, 2009.
6. American Psychiatric Association. The principles of medical ethics with annotations especially applicable to psychiatry. Arlington (VA): American Psychiatric Association; 2008.
7. American Board of Psychiatry and Neurology. Publications - core competencies outlines: core competencies outline for psychiatry and neurology. Available at: http://www.abpn.com/competencies.htm. Accessed February 26, 2009.
8. American Board of Psychiatry and Neurology. Publications - core competencies outlines: core competencies outline for psychosomatic medicine. Available at: http://www.abpn.com/competencies.htm. Accessed February 26, 2009.
9. Powell T. Consultation-liaison psychiatry and clinical ethics. representative cases. Psychosomatics 1997;38:321–6.
10. Steinberg MD. Psychiatry and bioethics. An exploration of the relationship. Psychosomatics 1997;38:313–20.
11. Youngner SJ. Consultation-liaison psychiatry and clinical ethics. historical parallels and diversions. Psychosomatics 1997;38:309–12.
12. Preisman RC, Steinberg MD, Rummans TA, et al. An annotated bibliography for ethics training in consultation-liaison psychiatry. Psychosomatics 1999;40: 369–79.
13. Leeman CP. Psychiatric consultations and ethics consultations. Similarities and differences. Gen Hosp Psychiatry 2000;22:270–5.
14. Beauchamp TL, Childress JF. Principles of biomedical ethics. New York: Oxford University Press; 1979.
15. Beauchamp TL, Childress JF. Principles of biomedical ethics. 6th edition. New York: Oxford University Press; 2009.
16. Roberts LW, Hoop JG, Dunn LB. Ethical aspects of psychiatry. In: Hales RE, Yudofsky SC, Gabbard GO, editors. The American Psychiatric Publishing textbook of psychiatry. 5th edition. Washington, DC: American Psychiatric Pub; 2008. p. 1601–36.
17. Hundert EM. A model for ethical problem solving in medicine, with practical applications. Am J Psychiatry 1987;144:839–46.
18. Grisso T, Appelbaum P. Assessing competence to consent to treatment: a guide for physicians and other health professionals. London: Oxford University Press; 1998.
19. Sugarman J, McCrory DC, Powell D, et al. Empirical research on informed consent. An annotated bibliography. Hastings Cent Rep 1999;29:S1–42.
20. U.S. Advisory Committee on Human Radiation Experiments. The human radiation experiments: final report of the president's advisory committee. New York: Oxford University Press; 1996.
21. Roberts LW. Informed consent and the capacity for voluntarism. Am J Psychiatry 2002;159:705–12.
22. Roberts LW, Geppert CM, Bailey R. Ethics in psychiatric practice: essential ethics skills, informed consent, the therapeutic relationship, and confidentiality. J Psychiatr Pract 2002;8:290–305.

23. Roberts LW. Mental illness and informed consent: seeking an empirically derived understanding of voluntarism. Curr Opin Psychiatry 2003;16:543–5.
24. Belitz J, Bailey RA. Clinical ethics for the treatment of children and adolescents: a guide for general psychiatrists. Psychiatr Clin North Am 2009;32:243–57.
25. Dunn LB, Misra S. Research ethics issues in geriatric psychiatry. Psychiatr Clin North Am 2009;32:395–411.
26. Barry LK. Ethical issues in psychiatric research. Psychiatr Clin North Am 2009;32: 381–94.
27. Walaszek A. Clinical ethics issues in geriatric psychiatry. Psychiatr Clin North Am 2009;32:343–59.
28. Warner CH, Appenzeller GN, Grieger T, et al. Ethical considerations in military psychiatry. Psychiatr Clin North Am 2009;32:271–81.
29. Drane JF. Competency to give an informed consent. A model for making clinical assessments. JAMA 1984;252:925–7.
30. Roberts LW, Dyer AR. Concise guide to ethics in mental health care. Washington, DC: American Psychiatric Publishing, Inc.; 2004.
31. Siegler M. Decision-making strategy for clinical-ethical problems in medicine. Arch Intern Med 1982;142:2178–9.
32. Jonsen AR, Siegler M, Winslade WJ. Clinical ethics: a practical approach to ethical decisions in clinical medicine. 6th edition. New York: McGraw Hill, Medical Pub. Division; 2006.
33. Jonsen AR, Toulmin SE. The abuse of casuistry a history of moral reasoning. Berkeley (CA): University of California Press; 1988.
34. American Psychiatric Association. Diagnostic and statistical manual of mental disorders: DSM-IV-TR. Text Revision. 4th edition. Washington, DC: American Psychiatric Association; 2000.
35. Appelbaum PS, Grisso T. Assessing patients' capacities to consent to treatment. N Engl J Med 1989;319:1635–8.
36. Johns Hopkins Medicine. Hopkins transplant surgeons remove healthy kidney through donor's vagina. Available at: http://www.hopkinsmedicine.org/Press_releases/2009/02_02_09.html. Accessed February 26, 2009.

Ethics in Contemporary Community Psychiatry

Anita Everett, MD, DFAPA[a],*, Charles Huffine, MD[b]

KEYWORDS

- Ethics • Community psychiatry • Beneficence
- Nonmaleficence • Autonomy • Boundaries
- Dual agency • Universal application

The practice of community psychiatry has evolved tremendously over the last four decades since the era of the Community Mental Health Services Act in 1963. A hallmark of contemporary clinical community psychiatry is work with patients and consumers in traditional and nontraditional settings and in multidisciplinary team settings. Community psychiatry often involves working within publicly funded, organized systems of care. Community psychiatrists often play a role in advocacy for increased access to effective services.

Medical ethics guidelines for psychiatry historically have been written to address clinical practice—mostly the types of dyadic patient/physician relationships with a psychodynamic emphasis practiced in private practice settings. One of the commonest ethical problem areas for practicing psychiatrists and in fact all physicians is that of maintenance of professional boundaries in practice settings. Much of the psychiatric guidance on ethics includes highly developed attention to boundary crossings and violations in traditional therapeutic dyadic relationships.[1] This article builds on the existing values and ethical foundations of medical ethics and develops them such that they are applicable to community psychiatry. We address ethical foundations that apply to clinical settings and administrative and advocacy roles. This article has two central goals: (1) to provide community psychiatrists a framework in which to approach a novel ethical situation and (2) to provide general psychiatrists with a broadened understanding of applied ethics in the many novel situations encountered in contemporary community psychiatry practice.

WHAT IS COMMUNITY PSYCHIATRY?

Contemporary community psychiatry can be characterized as including expertise with three practice elements that are consistent with the original scope of service as defined

[a] Community and General Psychiatry, Johns Hopkins School of Medicine, Bayview Campus, Baltimore, MD, USA
[b] Child and Adolescent Programs, King County Mental Health, Chemical Abuse and Dependency Service, Seattle, WA, USA
* Corresponding author.
E-mail address: aeveret4@jhmi.edu (A. Everett).

Psychiatr Clin N Am 32 (2009) 329–341
doi:10.1016/j.psc.2009.03.006
0193-953X/09/$ – see front matter © 2009 Elsevier Inc. All rights reserved.

in the Community Mental Health Services Act of 1963.[2] These elements include: (1) expertise in the treatment of persons with serious and persistent mental illnesses, (2) expertise in the psychiatric treatment of individuals who are socioeconomically disadvantaged, and (3) expertise in working with and developing programs for the general community, especially populations at risk. Common to each of these areas is the necessity to understand the complex relationship between individual vulnerabilities and an individual's social context.

In its beginnings, community psychiatry distinguished itself from private psychiatry in terms of place of work. Public and community psychiatrists worked at state or local government operated clinics that were funded primarily through public funds or grants administered by local and state governments. This was in contrast to private psychiatry that was usually practiced in inpatient settings and private offices. Individuals who had private insurance were seen in these settings on a fee-for-service basis and typically received individual psychotherapy with medications as indicated. Over the last 20 years, Medicaid programs have funded an increasing percentage of mental health services provided to the US population.[3] This has blurred the distinction between public and private clinics and clinicians because Medicaid can be accepted by providers from private and public providers. While some Medicaid mental health services are managed directly by state offices, many Medicaid programs are managed by private managed care companies which further blur the distinction between public and private settings. A fundamental component of Medicaid is patient choice to receive medical services from the physician and system of one's choice. For public mental health systems, this often resulted in a breakup of traditional catchment area boundaries and increased privatization of services. This has further blurred the distinction between public and private practice settings. Community psychiatry practice cannot now be strictly defined in terms of funding sources or work site settings. A preferred, more progressive definition of community psychiatry is a psychiatrist who has expertise in the following primary areas.

Treatment of Enduring Mental Illnesses

A contemporary definition of community psychiatry includes expertise in the range of clinical, rehabilitative, and pharmacologic treatments that facilitate recovery and resilience in individuals with enduring mental illnesses. It includes expertise in assessment and diagnosis of major, disabling mental illnesses and technical knowledge of the relative risks and benefits of pharmacologic interventions. Often community psychiatrists are the physicians most committed to the treatment of these individuals, and a good working knowledge of the diagnosis and treatment approaches for common medical conditions is useful.

It is usual for the doctor-patient relationships in contemporary community psychiatry to be multi-dyadic. A simple doctor-patient dyad is not common. Physicians, professionals, and paraprofessionals may be organized into well-defined teams, such as with the assertive community treatment (ACT) model, or a more loosely associated grouping of professionals, such as a patient with schizophrenia who has a psychiatrist, therapist, job coach, and peer support specialist involved in his or her recovery and treatment. These professionals may work within the same organization or may be employed by entirely distinct agencies. Persons with serious mental illness commonly experience one or multiple comorbid medical and psychiatric illnesses that complicate diagnosis and treatment. They often require coordination with a range of non–mental health care professionals.

Treatment of Mental Health Conditions in Persons with Socioeconomic Disadvantage

Persons with enduring mental illnesses often are disabled such that sustaining full-time employment with private health insurance benefits is difficult. Medicaid is an insurance mechanism that is available for US citizens who live below the federal poverty level. Another group of patients live in poverty but have incomes that are just above state Medicaid eligibility limits. States have different mechanisms for providing care to uninsured citizens, and community mental health care centers are often part of the public safety net that serves uninsured and underinsured individuals. Another group of individuals that may seek services in community mental health care settings because of socioeconomic disadvantage are new immigrants in the United States, with or without documentation. Other special populations of disadvantaged individuals that may be served by community mental health care centers include mentally ill offenders who are in jails or prisons, individuals with mental retardation or severe learning disabilities, and transitional age youth and young adults with residual problems from a troubled childhood.

Persons who live at or near poverty bring challenges to treatment. The protective factors experienced in more economically stable families are often absent in families of unstable means. They typically have lower health and mental health literacy, pay, less attention to preventive care, and rely more on emergency care for medical and psychiatric conditions. Health issues often have progressed from early and more readily treatable conditions to late-stage conditions and less treatment-responsive states. Community mental health centers often consider program development or advocate for programs that include prevention, early intervention, and health and mental health literacy. In recent years, many prominent community mental health centers have become actively engaged in encouraging the development of "social capital" through community outreach and invitations to persons with social disadvantages to participate in their communities so that effective natural supports can be developed for individuals with socioeconomic deprivation and mental illness.

Program Development for Populations at Risk

The history of community mental health includes a strong relationship with public health care. Many early community mental health centers were created in county public health departments. Community mental health centers may include universal preventive services in their range of services. Such progressive programs provide early intervention as well as treatment of established and persistent mental illnesses. Community mental health care centers may serve older adults who require coordination with medical and social services for health and mental health conditions. Transitional age youth with limited family and community resources who are vulnerable to homelessness and substance abuse problems are best served by preventive and early intervention services familiar with specific methods and resources to help them address their interface with adverse social and community conditions. Whether the range of services offered by a community behavioral health organization includes prevention or is limited to treatment of established illnesses; services must be planned and managed for the community as a whole. The needs of the community must be taken into account when financial resources are limited and resource distribution questions arise.

TRADITIONAL MEDICAL ETHICS PRINCIPLES AND COMMUNITY PSYCHIATRY

Western medical ethics are centered on four general principles: beneficence, nonmaleficence, autonomy, and justice. These principles are embedded in the American

Medical Association's code of medical ethics[4] and have been the basis of medical ethics guidelines since those articulated by Hippocrates in approximately 450 BC.[5] These principles inform the duties and role expectations of contemporary physicians. In this section we briefly define and discuss the general principles within these categories and how these principles apply to the contemporary practice of community psychiatry. Examples from community settings are provided.

Beneficence

Beneficence is the act of doing good. In the *Principles of Biomedical Ethics*,[6] Beauchamp and Childress discussed two aspects of beneficence. The first of these is positive beneficence; the second is utility. Positive beneficence refers to an obligation to provide benefit, and utility refers to the weighing of risks and benefits of a particular intervention and recommending the most beneficial or useful choice.

Positive beneficence is a particular challenge for community psychiatrists. Would this create an ethical obligation for psychiatrists to provide and advocate for services that promote recovery to the fullest extent possible? Throughout the 1980s, the clubhouse model was a much-heralded form of psychosocial rehabilitation. Critics of the clubhouse model suggest that it provides a holding place but does not promote recovery and positive change. In many systems this model has been replaced by the more active supported employment model, which much more aggressively promotes the self-agency of mental health consumers through the attainment of supported employment. Positive beneficence might be interpreted as an obligation for psychiatrists to provide and advocate for services that promote recovery to the fullest extent possible for each consumer (ie, that simply providing a custodial or holding environment is not ethical).

Utility refers to the weighing of risks and benefits of a particular intervention and recommending the most useful or beneficial choice. A ready example of the utility principle in contemporary community psychiatry is the process of choosing antipsychotic medications. These medications have clear benefits and present serious and clear risks or side effects. In this situation, the utility principle would obligate the psychiatrist to understand the relative risks and benefits of medication choices and make the best recommendation to the patient.

Beneficence is a central principle that arises in consideration of ethical violations related to inappropriate prescribing. The utility aspect of beneficence is operant in considering the risks of addiction versus the benefit of anxiety relief with benzodiazepines or alleviation of physical pain with narcotics.

The traditional ethical culture of US physicians includes strong emphasis on providing benefit to the autonomous patient at hand. Recent developments in medical ethics have noted the dilemmas in considering the principle of beneficence in a resource-poor environment and how to distribute (or ration) the resources. The American Medical Association ethical guidelines recently included consideration of resources; however, the priority on the individual patient remains clear. Recommending what is good for the individual patient is a familiar stance for US physicians. Consideration of what might be beneficial for a population or a given community is an unfamiliar concept and can be disconcerting to physicians, but it is an obligation for community psychiatrists. A state Medicaid policy that restricts or rations access to expensive antipsychotic medication could be in conflict with the principles of positive beneficence and utility when considering the needs of an individual, but the policy may enable all individuals in need of medications to have access to "some" medication benefit. Public payer policy may restrict access to a "most" useful treatment interfering with the physician's ethical obligation to weigh the risks and benefits of a particular treatment recommendation and recommend the best choice. Community psychiatrists are often involved in or have opportunities to influence public policy. A sound understanding of the competing interests of beneficence for the individual versus beneficence for a population is critical for physicians in leadership roles in public psychiatry.

Nonmaleficence

Nonmaleficence is the principle often encapsulated by the phrase "first do no harm." This principle is embedded in treatment culture and, on the surface, seems straightforward. For psychiatry, however, there are several examples of treatments and interventions that can cause harm and, at least retrospectively, confer no clear benefit. Several notorious treatments were used, mostly in asylums, in which the risk of harm clearly outweighed any purported benefit (eg, lobotomies, cold wraps, and insulin shock treatment). Two contemporary examples from community psychiatry in which this principle might provide guidance are the use of seclusion and restraint and the use of antipsychotic medications. Over the last several years, there has been a clear focus on reducing the use of seclusion and restraint. Part of the argument that supports this is that the use of seclusion and particularly restraint may have long-term traumatizing effects with greater negative impact on an individual than the safety benefit for a psychiatric hospital. Persons at particular risk for retraumatization by restraints include female patients who have been victims of violence and sexual assault. Although practice in community settings is not often associated with emergency restraint use, a person traumatized by this intervention may seek treatment in community settings.

One of the most common causes for claims of professional misconduct in psychiatry and all of medicine is that of professional boundary violations. Nonmaleficence is often the central principle on which allegations of boundary violations are made. The question might be: Did this relationship that the physician had a duty to manage result in harm to the patient? In considering the ethics of the situation of rigid adherence to office-based practice versus increasing flexibility to meet with patients in alternative, natural settings, the principle of positive beneficence competes with nonmaleficence.

The issue of nonmaleficence is particularly germane when considering outright exploitation of a patient (eg, taking sexual advantage of a patient or using the relationship to exploit a patient financially). It has been argued that the road to exploitation (disregard for nonmaleficence) begins with deviation in practice that leads to exploitation. Gabbard[1] called this the slippery slope. Although it may be the case that founded exploitations virtually always start with a pattern of deviation from treatment as usual, not all deviations from treatment as usual result in eventual exploitation or nonmaleficence. A consideration of the entire context and opportunities for positive beneficence of a situation balanced against a consideration of nonmaleficence in novel clinical situations is required. A hallmark of contemporary community psychiatry is working in a wide variety of nontraditional settings so that the context of boundaries is not traditional office based and dyadic psychiatric practice. Martinez classified boundary crossings from type 1 (exploitive boundary violations) to type IV, which he described as innovative and well-thought-out extensions of the treatment relationship into the treatment plan. He offered a system of graded risks emphasizing the psychiatrist's duty to constantly evaluate beneficence versus nonmaleficence.[7]

Autonomy

Autonomy is an essential ethical concept for community psychiatrists. It refers to the patient's human right to be an active participant in his or her own treatment. In most medical contexts, it is generally presumed that the individual has the mental capacity to make rational decisions regarding health care. In psychiatric contexts, most individuals also have the capacity to make rational health care decisions, but this is not always the case. Informed consent for medical procedures and certain types of treatments (long-term use of antipsychotic medications) is a formal process recognizing a patient's right to be involved in high-risk treatment decisions. Written recognition of patient autonomy in psychiatry is manifested by the requirement that individuals sign their treatment plans. Ideally, that indicates agreement to a course of treatment.

Respect for an individual's autonomy is a prominent concept in community psychiatry on many levels. In inpatient settings, patients have much less autonomy than in outpatient settings. Doors are locked, and medication is "ordered" and administered to a patient. This situation is necessary because of the nature of psychiatric illness, which may cause periods of diminished capacity to participate in rationale treatment decisions.

In comparison, outpatient services have few effective controls on a patient's behavior even if the patient is subject to an "outpatient commitment." Community psychiatric practice involves respect for the autonomy of an individual even in extreme situations, such as delusional psychosis. In the case of compromised capacity caused by a state of mental illness, it has been argued that professional paternalism is justifiable so long as its goal is the restoration of a person to a state in which he or she can again function autonomously.[8]

Two terms, "recovery" and "consumer," have become central in community psychiatry and are rooted in consideration of a patient's autonomy. The term "consumer" is used to describe persons who use mental health services. Physicians often prefer the term "patient," which connotes a special relationship and responsibility between a physician and the patient.[9] Although it has been demonstrated that most individuals are not offended by the terms patient, consumer, client, or service recipient,[10] many advocates prefer the term *consumer*. This term does include two elements that are associated with an assertion of greater autonomy for individuals. "Consumer" connotes a less dependent role than "patient." Comparing the historic stereotypical and disempowered asylum patient in an overcrowded, understaffed institution managed by authorities, a consumer of today has a much greater expectation for self-agency. A consumer in our US market-based culture is an empowered person who has purchasing power to choose between products and shopping venues. Similarly, one aspect of the term "consumer" in community psychiatry includes the idea that mental health care consumers are sufficiently autonomous that they can choose the services and providers (including psychiatrists) that are most likely to facilitate their recovery.

The word "recovery" is used to describe the course of patient-determined rehabilitation from disability caused by a mental illness. This term, often used to describe a path of successful, sober, and clean life after a period of substance addiction, has been revised for individuals with mental illness. Recovery-based treatment emphasizes a psychiatrist partnering with patients in pursuit of the patients' goals to work toward self-agency and autonomy such that they are in a position to direct own lives on a life trajectory that is meaningful to each individual. Professional staff support the individuals in this pursuit by providing accurate diagnosis and effective treatments that better equip them to pursue their recovery goals.

In considering autonomy and self-agency in community psychiatry, a common ethical dilemma is that of "allowing" consumers to fail at life activities. In preparation for discharge from traditional inpatient settings, the asylum psychiatrist often was responsible for prescribing the level of community housing that an individual would best thrive in. For instance, if the individual wanted to live with his brother and it had repeatedly resulted in decompensation in the past, the psychiatrist could override patient preference and direct that the patient either stay in the hospital or be discharged to a more structured level of care, such as a group home. The ethical principle with primacy in this scenario would be that of positive beneficence or the obligation to "do good" or offer a professional opinion regarding what would be best for the patient. Autonomy of the individual would be of relatively lesser weight in this era.

This scenario is contrasted with the not uncommon situation of a contemporary ACT team working with a consumer who insists on living with a brother, as in the previous example, despite recurrent destabilization of his illness. The reasons for instability in any housing situation are multiple and individually specific. In this example, the brother has a substance abuse problem and has repeatedly exploited the consumer for his SSI money. He also believes that psychiatric medication and attending the supported employment program recommended by the ACT are useless.

In recovery-based community psychiatry services, the autonomy of the individual has much more weight in the treatment-rehabilitation process. Rather than overriding the consumer's desire to live with his brother, a contemporary ACT team might work to assure that the consumer is fully aware of healthier housing arrangements. At the same time they would do what they could to facilitate success in his living with his brother, which would involve intensive outreach into the home, attempts to educate the brother, developing medication regimens that would be harder for the brother to undermine, and encouraging an external payee. In this situation, the community psychiatrist as leader of the team balances respect for the patient's autonomy with the beneficence principle. To support the autonomy of the patient, the team needs to have a deeper understanding of the reasons why the patient repeatedly moves back to the brother's home. Greater clinical sophistication and situation-specific problem solving is needed in contemporary mental health care to balance beneficence, nonmaleficence, and autonomy.

A criticism of recovery is that "patients can do whatever they want." It has been argued that psychiatrists working within a recovery paradigm abandon their ethical obligation to provide benefit and avoid harm; that is, they abandon the ethical primacy of beneficence and nonmaleficence in respect of the patient's autonomy. This is a spurious concern because patients in the community have rights, as do all persons, and are free to make bad decisions. The contemporary stance of community psychiatry is to balance respect for the patient's autonomy with sound professional recommendations that are based on beneficence and nonmaleficence. In practice, the community psychiatrist has a responsibility to accurately diagnose illnesses and recommend effective treatment. Respect for autonomy does not require that the psychiatrist agree with all decisions a consumer makes; neither does it create an obligation to prescribe medication or treatment that in his or her opinion will not provide benefit to the patient. The autonomy of a patient may be overridden in extreme circumstances in which the individual, because of illness, is at risk for seriously harming self or others. The authority to involuntarily commit individuals by state commitment codes (ie, to override autonomy) is based on nonmaleficence and the social justice principle that involves the state's authority to protect the incapacitated patient from harming self or others in society.

Emanuel and Emanuel[11] reviewed models for addressing the balance among beneficence, nonmaleficence, and autonomy. They made a case that using all possible skills for convincing a reluctant patient to accept a helpful treatment was ethically preferable to either invoking medical authority or passively accepting a patient's bad decision. Respect for the autonomy of individuals in need of psychiatric services is an important element in community psychiatric practice and is an ethical principle that has assumed more weight in recent years. This is manifested through the use of terms such as consumer and the adoption of the recovery paradigm as a treatment approach in community services.

Justice

The fourth of the ethical principles as conceptualized by Beauchamps and Childress is that of justice. In its simplest form, justice refers to the provision of fairness. Generally, and as it applies to health care, justice has a social comparative dimension. Two examples of a large-scale health policy question might be: Do all individuals have equal access to health care services? Should all groups have equal access or should some have more access? Physicians in the United States health care system are much more oriented toward beneficence of the individual patient and generally are not as experienced with the ethics involved with resource distribution to a population or group of individuals.

For community psychiatry, the ethical principle of justice can be a consideration at a clinical level in direct care and on a larger systems level. A classic example of a direct care justice decision would be the use of staff time for patients who do not show for appointments. How much time and effort should be allocated with outreach and encouragement for patients who consistently are not able to keep appointments and may be the most ill and most in need? Might the use of valuable clinician's time be best spent for patients who consistently do show and are making clinical gains and are possibly most likely to use the health benefit to become independent?

A justice-based, decision-making example on a systems level would be that of access to expensive antipsychotic medications. From an individual psychiatrist perspective, unfettered access to all medications regardless of cost would be ideal. This would be a perspective that would prioritize the beneficence principle over a social justice principle. A psychiatrist working in a public setting, such as a state or community mental health clinic that provides medications within a budget, might determine that some fair rationing of access to the most expensive medications would be a reasonable policy. This psychiatrist, informed by research that does not demonstrate clear increased beneficence or decreased nonmaleficence for newer and more expensive medications, might contribute to policy that creates tiers of access to medications with cost as a factor. In this situation the psychiatrist would be considering "distributive justice"—the fair distribution of resources to a group of people as a primary priority—which would be balanced against beneficence for the individual.

In some situations, psychiatrists might see a lack of resources for the mental health care needs of a population as an injustice. Strong advocacy for improved resources that preserve principles of beneficence and justice is an ethical stance. It is in this advocacy that psychiatrists often join with patients, family members, and other advocates in common cause and in new forms of relationships.

American physicians tend to be more familiar with and versed in the application of ethical principles in individual doctor-patient settings. Physicians in countries with national health care schemes work more often with the ethical issues associated with distributive justice. In order for community psychiatrists to be able to effectively assume leadership roles in the public health and mental health arena, familiarity with resource distribution principles is important. The American Medical Association emphasized a positive responsibility of physicians to participate in public health or population-based health care to some degree with the 2001 revision of American Medical Association ethical principles. Principle VII was revised to include an ethical responsibility to participate in activities that "improve the health of communities and the betterment of public health." A new principle, number IX, was added. The principle states: "A physician shall support access to medical care for all people,[12]" thus embracing a profession-wide ethical stance for improved medical resources of all types for the entire population.

SPECIAL ETHICAL TOPICS IN COMMUNITY PSYCHIATRY

In the first section of this article a definition and context for community psychiatry were provided. In the second section, four principles of medical ethics were presented and applications in contemporary community psychiatry and mental health services were discussed. In this final section, specific topics that are particularly significant to practice as a community psychiatrist are discussed. These topics were emphasized in recommendations made by the American Association of Community Psychiatry Board of Directors to the American Psychiatric Association in response to revision of the Principles of Medical Ethics with Annotations Especially Applicable to Psychiatry (2001 Edition).[13] The special topics that are covered include boundaries, dual agency, and the universality of ethics.

Boundaries

Positive professional relationships between physicians and patients are an important component of effective treatment. This is true for general medical practice, psychiatry, and all mental health care providers. "Boundary" is one of the terms used in medicine and psychiatry to characterize rules for this relationship. Mishandling professional boundaries may result in diminished benefit of treatment and possible harm to the patient through neglect or exploitation.

In the situation of an analytic psychiatric practice in which a central technical aspect of successful treatment is the promotion of intense transference, all aspects of the professional relationship are highly controlled. Maintenance of consistent boundaries is essential. Community psychiatrists see this emphasis in the analytic situation not as a matter of ethics but as adherence to a specific technique. In fact, in many situations a lack of interaction and a sense of deprivation may harm the patient.

Community psychiatrists may see patients in office settings and various community settings, such as the patient's home, school, shelter, or other community settings, such as on the street or in other public places. Engagement is a critical component in working with treatment-resistant individuals such as youth who are reluctant to enter treatment.

In many situations that arise daily on the front lines of community psychiatric practice, core ethical principles must be considered. Consider this example. An ACT team psychiatrist, at the request of a case manager, stops by a shelter at the end of the work day to visit a patient who has not been doing well. The patient knows it is after normal work hours and has heard the doctor is going through a contentious divorce. Is this a boundary crossing (ie, unwise)? If the nightshift case manager meets the physician at the shelter, does this change the potential ethics of the situation? In this situation, on a practical level, the psychiatrist may find it useful to consider the ethical principles. (1) Beneficence: Which is best for this patient, to make him wait until tomorrow or take a small amount of time to meet with someone who is not stable and is likely to benefit from a discussion about his situation with a trusted physician? (2) Nonmaleficence: Will this visit be likely to harm him or the psychiatrist's long-term therapeutic alliance with him? If the psychiatrist sees this individual, is he altering his schedule to accommodate his patient's needs or is he indulging his wish to be needed by the patient or by his team? What is driving the decision to see this individual?

(3) Autonomy: Is an after-work visit consistent with the recovery goals that the patient created when in a more stable condition? (4) Justice: Is going to the shelter after normal working hours going to set a new precedent for all other patients seen by the team? In community practice it is imperative that psychiatrists consider each of these domains of ethical practice.

In community psychiatry, the capacity to adapt to a situation at hand for the good of the patient while maintaining a professional relationship is an essential skill. It is also important to distinguish what are technical issues that may be poorly thought through and what are ethical lapses. A boundary violation is clearly an ethical issue. The term "boundary crossing" is so nebulous and laden with implications of perceived dangers that many feel the term should be dropped altogether. Strict adherence to boundary guidelines designed for inpatient or office-based outpatient settings is often not possible and may at times impede treatment or cause harm to patients.

Dual Agency

Often in community psychiatric settings, psychiatrists, patients, and staff may interact in multiple roles. For example, peer-to-peer counselors may be patients and employees of an organization; or psychiatrists may advocate in local or state government with patients or parents of patients; or psychiatrists may be involved in a community service project with consumers. The practice of contemporary community psychiatry includes the active management of dual relationships so that the patient benefits and is not exploited. Each of the four ethical principles is involved with these types of relationships.

To illustrate how each of the principles would be considered, the following scenario is presented. Dr. George is a psychiatrist in a city in the Midwest. The state psychiatric society is involved with several other advocacy groups in advocating for increased access to psychiatric services. There are long waits in the local emergency departments because of lack of services. The waiting list for an outpatient appointment in this community is 3 months. Several inpatient beds have been closed by local hospital administrators who determined that they could no longer afford to operate these beds because of the low reimbursement rates provided by the state's Medicaid program and local private carriers. Recently, the son of city council member was in the emergency department and was nearly assaulted by a manic patient waiting for a psychiatric admission. This powerful city council member called for a blue ribbon commission to study the problem and provide recommendations that the city government could enact to alleviate this situation.

Because Dr. George is a community psychiatrist and is active in his state psychiatric organization, he has been invited to participate. The CEO of his agency has agreed to let him participate in this activity and expects that he will represent the interests of the center. As the commission was being organized, it occurred to a member that having a consumer on the commission would be a good idea. Dr. George happens to have a patient, Fabio, who has bipolar disorder. He is articulate and recently had a long emergency department wait for admission during a manic episode in the context of a contentious divorce. The central conflict in the divorce is his wife's intent to sever his relationship with their children. Fabio has been a loyal patient for years at the community center. Dr George works with him on their ACT team. He is considering recommending him as a consumer representative for the commission.

Each of the four ethical principles comes into consideration in this scenario. (1) Nonmaleficence. What is the potential harm to this patient as a result of participation on this commission? Would his participation risk destabilization of his illness and perhaps inadvertently cause public exposure of sensitive family issues? Would Dr. George's nomination of Fabio represent exploitation because he is likely to speak favorably in a public forum about his treatment and Dr. George's service as his psychiatrist? Would the consumer be adversely financially impacted if the only way to attend meetings was an expensive cab ride? Would the perception of pleasing his doctor by agreeing to participate adversely impact his treatment relationship with him? (2) Beneficence. Would participation in this commission be of benefit to Fabio? This is an opportunity to engage in a valuable community effort that has the potential to positively impact services in the entire community and could be an opportunity for him to connect with many prominent community members in a good cause. (3) Justice. Would the impact of the identification of one consumer from the many others who participate in the ACT team cause resentment and be seen as unfair? Is it appropriate for the psychiatrist to identify one consumer who is likely to represent the situation well, or should there be a fair lottery or a vote by all ACT consumers on the team to choose who gets the opportunity to participate? If the community clinic wants to pay for the cab expense to get to the meeting, is this a just distribution of clinic funds? (4) Autonomy. This last consideration is perhaps the most critical issue in this situation. In considering nonmaleficence issues it was assumed that the psychiatrist had the authority to decide whether the patient should be recommended for the commission. When presenting this as a possible opportunity to the consumer, respect for the individual's autonomy would be demonstrated by engaging the consumer and discussing the pros and cons, the benefits and potential harm. It is essential that Dr. George present the opportunity to Fabio in a way that he feels no pressure and is free to make the decision to participate or not. The degree to which the psychiatrist attempts to influence his patient or in any way encroach on his autonomy must be constantly on Dr. George's mind and be carefully monitored.

Opportunities for such dual relationships are common in community practice. Avoidance of the complexities of dual relationship may limit the opportunity for beneficence and the support of an individual's recovery in his or her community. The preferred stance for contemporary community practice is to maintain awareness of all aspects of dual relationships and actively manage them. A consideration of each of the four ethical principles presented in this article may be a useful framework in working through the potential benefits versus harm in a dual relationship.

Universal Application

The term "universal application" is used to describe the application of ethical principles to other professionals or providers. For the community psychiatrist, this is an issue at two levels. At one level is the issue of medical ethics and the question of application to psychiatrists versus other physicians. A second level is that of psychiatrists versus other behavioral health care providers.

From an ethical perspective, the practice of contemporary community psychiatry may have more in common with practice in a general medical setting in a small town (where dual roles are common) than a private psychiatric practice setting in which individual psychotherapy is the modal treatment. Relationships are a vital component of treatment in all three of these settings. The style and intensity of the relationship, including attending to boundaries, is different in an intensive psychodynamic therapeutic stance than it is in a community psychiatric practice or general outpatient medical practice. Formal adherence to strict boundaries in community practice settings may be counter therapeutic.

The second level on which universal application can occur is considering the applicability of a psychiatrist's ethical principles to other providers in community mental health care settings. Community psychiatrists work with teams and groups of providers. More often than not, the professional relationship for the patient is not a simple doctor-patient dyad. Often a community psychiatrist is in either a formal or informal position of leadership on a team with nonmedical professionals in which he or she can influence the ethical practice of others. Other professionals, such as social workers and nurses, generally have a set of articulated ethical guidelines that they are taught as a part of graduate coursework and internship supervision. Similar to medical practices, these professionals are held to standards by their professional organizations and state licensing boards or authorities. Also similar to medical practice, these professional guidelines may not be particularly relevant to situations encountered by contemporary community mental health care professionals.

Other critical community service providers—paraprofessionals such as case managers, rehabilitation technicians, service coordinators, and peer support specialists—may not have had any formal training in professional ethics. Community psychiatrists often have the ability to influence and support a clinical and treatment culture that is grounded in sound ethical principles. When community psychiatrists are constrained based on a misunderstanding of boundary rules as ethical dictums versus primarily technical practice issues, they may lose their ability to lead a team that has a tradition of more flexible concepts of boundaries and dual relationships.

SUMMARY

Community psychiatry is a wonderful and rewarding career path that increasing numbers of psychiatrists are choosing to practice.[14] This article was created to provide an orientation to the characteristics of contemporary community psychiatric practice that render it distinct in terms of ethical considerations. We defined and described community practice. We provided a framework based on classical medical ethics that can be used to consider challenges in particular community practice situations. We also offered special considerations of key areas in which community practice demands novel treatment methods coupled with special clinical expertise in assessing risks and benefits. We hope to have provided a discussion that supports a broadening of existing psychiatric ethical guidelines so that they are inclusive of the kinds of situations routinely encountered by community psychiatrists and other community mental health care professionals and paraprofessionals. It is our hope that ideas presented in this article will help to equip psychiatrists and their community teams to facilitate the successful rehabilitation and recovery of the individuals they serve.

REFERENCES

1. Gabbard GO, Nadelson C. Professional boundaries in the physician patient relationship. JAMA 1995;273:1445–9.
2. Sharfstein S. What ever happened to community mental health? Psychiatr Serv 2000;51:616–20.
3. Mark TL, Coffey RM, McKusick DR, et al. National estimates of expenditures for mental health services and substance abuse treatment. 1991–2001 SAMHSA Publication No. SMA 05-3999. Rockville (MD): Substance Abuse and Mental Health Services Administration; 2005.
4. American Medical Association. Code of medical ethics. Available at: http://www. ama-assn.org/ama/pub/category/2512.html.
5. National Library of Medicine. History of medicine: Greek medicine. Available at: http://www.nlm.nih.gov/hmd/greek/greek_oath.html.

6. Beauchamps TL, Childress JF. Principles of biomedical ethics. 5th edition. Oxford: Oxford University Press; 2001.
7. Martinez R. Ethical human sciences and services. New York: Springer Publishing Co.; 2000.
8. Komrad MS. A defence of medical paternalism: maximizing patients' autonomy. J Med Ethics 1983;9:38–44.
9. Bosley W. Consumer vs patient. letter to the editor. Psychiatr Serv 1995;46(7):732.
10. Verinder S, Whitney D, Kazarian SS, et al. Preferred terms for users of mental health services among service providers and recipients. Psychiatr Serv 2000; 51:203–9.
11. Emanuel EJ, Emanuel LL. Four models of the physician-patient relationship. JAMA 1992;267:2221–6.
12. American Medical Association. Revised principles of medical ethics. Available at: http://www.ama-assn.org/ama/upload/mm/369/principlestracked.pdf. Accessed June 17, 2001.
13. Opinions of the ethics committee on the principles of medical ethics with annotations especially applicable to psychiatry. Washington, DC: American Psychiatric Association; 2001.
14. Ranz J, Vergare M, Wilk J, et al. The tipping point from private practice to publicly funded settings for early and mid-career psychiatrists. Psychiatr Serv 2006; 57(11):1640–3.

Clinical Ethics Issues in Geriatric Psychiatry

Art Walaszek, MD

KEYWORDS

• Geriatric psychiatry • Medical ethics • Informed consent
• Mental competency • Personal autonomy • Social justice

BACKGROUND AND GENERAL PRINCIPLES

The *Charter on Medical Professionalism* identifies three fundamental ethical principles embedded within medical care—patient autonomy, patient welfare, and social justice,[1] all of which are relevant to the care of older adults. Older adults face myriad medical and psychosocial issues that may impair their quality of life and their activities of daily living. Although most older adults function independently, many lose autonomy because of conditions such as dementia, depression, anxiety, visual impairment, arthritis, and chronic pain. Psychiatrists are called upon to assess the capacity of older adults to make medical decisions, to live independently, and to manage their affairs. This article focuses on the principles and evidence base involved in informed consent, capacity assessment, and surrogate decision-making, all of which relate to the ethical principle of autonomy.

The principle of patient welfare dictates that physicians must provide treatments that serve the best interest of their patients. In dementia care, a number of challenges arise in this context, including (1) genetic testing of patients and family members for irreversible, neurodegenerative conditions; (2) informing patients of the diagnosis of dementia; (3) the use of cognitive enhancing medications, which yield modest benefits at high costs; (4) the use of antipsychotic medications to address problematic behaviors, which has a controversial risk–benefit ratio; and (5) the appropriateness of artificial hydration and nutrition in advanced dementia. Older adults also are uniquely vulnerable to exploitation, a situation that has led to legislation and regulations regarding physicians' roles in identifying and reporting elder abuse. Care of patients at the end of their lives entails determining an appropriate balance of intervention and palliation.

Finally, the aging of the United States population, the ever-escalating costs of health care, and an economy that is likely to remain distressed for years converge to test the principle of social justice. Health care resources are limited and therefore should be

Dr. Walaszek has served as a consultant to Terra Nova Learning Systems, LLC.
Department of Psychiatry, University of Wisconsin School of Medicine & Public Health, 6001 Research Park Boulevard, Madison, WI 53719, USA
E-mail address: awalaszek@wisc.edu

Psychiatr Clin N Am 32 (2009) 343–359
doi:10.1016/j.psc.2009.02.004

psych.theclinics.com

allocated fairly and justly with a view not merely to extending the quantity of life but to enhancing the quality of life. Although this allocation is largely a matter of public policy, psychiatrists and their older patients and families make clinical decisions that, in the aggregate, can have a substantial impact on the distribution of resources.

AUTONOMY AND INFORMED CONSENT

Autonomy—the belief that individuals should be allowed to make choices and act independently without coercion—is a bedrock principle of medical ethics.[1,2] Physicians respect patients' autonomy by engaging them in making medical decisions through the process of informed consent. The ability to provide informed consent rests on the relevant information being available (information), the capacity to make a decision (decisional capacity), and the ability to make a free choice (voluntarism).[3] Decisional capacity, in turn, requires the following decisional abilities:

1. The ability to express a preference
2. The ability to understand relevant information about a clinical situation and about the choice to be made
3. The ability to reason about the situation by manipulating the relevant information
4. The ability to appreciate the situation, that is, to understand how the situation is personally relevant

Older adults are prone to a number of medical conditions that may affect their ability to provide informed consent. The most obvious of these conditions are dementia and delirium, which by definition impair cognition. Numerous studies have demonstrated the impact of cognitive impairment on decisional capacity in patients who have Alzheimer's disease (AD). In a prospective study comparing subjects who had mild AD and healthy older adult controls, the former showed impairments in the domains of understanding, reasoning, and appreciation at baseline. At 2-year follow-up, subjects who had AD showed further declines in these domains, and the overall proportion of subjects who had AD deemed to not have the capacity to make medical decisions increased substantially.[4] The same research group demonstrated less severe, but progressive, impairments in capacity in subjects who had amnestic mild cognitive impairment (MCI), which may be a precursor to AD.[5] Short-term verbal memory impairment, executive dysfunction, and slowed processing speed were found to be neuropsychological correlates of incapacity.[6] Another study of 48 subjects who had mild or moderate AD confirmed significant impairments in understanding, reasoning, and appreciation in this population and found that only 40% demonstrated capacity to consent to treatment with cognitive-enhancing medications; insight (awareness of symptoms, diagnosis, and/or prognosis) and higher cognitive function were correlated with maintaining capacity.[7] Cognitive performance was found to account for 78% of the variance in understanding scores, 39% of the variance in reasoning scores, and 25% of the variance in appreciation scores in a study comparing 44 patients who had mild to moderate dementia and 44 controls.[8] Parkinson's disease, with or without associated dementia, also leads to impairments in decision-making capacity.[9,10] Although there are no studies investigating decision-making capacity in the other most common causes of dementia, vascular dementia and frontotemporal dementia, it stands to reason that clinicians should be attuned to disturbances in capacity in these populations as well.

Concerns about informed consent also extend to patients who have mood disorders. Older psychiatric inpatients suffering from severe depression, including hopelessness, have been found to underestimate the benefits and overestimate the risks of life-sustaining treatment; treating depression did not affect patients' desire for such treatment.[11] This finding has been extended to depressed medical inpatients, who were more likely than nondepressed patients to refuse life-sustaining treatment and to accept hypothetical scenarios of physician-assisted suicide or euthanasia than nondepressed patients.[12]

Electroconvulsive therapy (ECT) can be a highly effective treatment for older adults suffering from severe major depression, albeit one with the potential for significant cognitive and cardiopulmonary side effects. A meta-analysis of 13 studies involving consent for ECT showed that approximately half of patients (of all ages) who had received ECT did not think that they had been given an adequate explanation regarding the treatment.[13] Thus, clinicians must assess and document carefully their patients' capacity to provide informed consent before starting treatment and then regularly during maintenance ECT.[14] In a prospective trial of an educational intervention to improve capacity, depressed older adults demonstrated lower scores than younger adults in the domains of understanding, reasoning, and expressing a choice, although all had adequate capacity to consent to ECT.[15] The literature on involuntary treatment of patients lacking capacity to accept or refuse ECT is very limited; legal requirements vary widely across different jurisdictions, and clinicians must be aware of local laws and standards of care.

The impact of schizophrenia on capacity also has been evaluated in older adults. Palmer and colleagues[16] compared the capacity to consent to antipsychotic treatment of 59 outpatients who had schizophrenia and schizoaffective disorder (mean age, 50.2 years) and normal controls. Patients fared worse than controls in the domain of understanding but not in reasoning or expressing a choice. Age and severity of psychopathology were not correlated with capacity, whereas overall cognitive function and specific cognitive domains were. The authors noted that there was substantial variability in capacity among the patients and that cognition accounted for only 25% of variance. These results are consistent with studies of younger patients who have schizophrenia that indicate that negative symptoms and cognitive dysfunction are more strongly associated with incapacity than positive symptoms (eg, see Ref.[17]).

Age and gender have not been associated with decision-making capacity, but the roles of ethnicity, cultural background, and spirituality in the assessment of the capacity of older adults have not yet been well studied.[18] Multiple studies have demonstrated that older adults who have been hospitalized and who reside in long-term care have high rates of incapacity.[18] The frequency of cognitive impairment found in patients in hospice suggests that this population may be at risk for incapacity as well.[19]

Although this article focuses on decisional capacity, cognitive impairment also may affect voluntarism, that is, the ability of an older adult to make choices freely and without coercion or manipulation.[3] Roberts argues that four "domains of influence" may affect voluntarism: developmental factors, illness-related considerations, psychological issues and cultural and religious values, and external features and pressures.[3] Patients who have cognitive impairment, specifically executive dysfunction (an illness-related factor), may have diminished impulse control and therefore may respond involuntarily to environmental stimuli.[20] Apathy (impaired initiation and execution of actions), found in both dementia and depression, can lead to the ethically troubling situation of a patient seeming to consent to an intervention without actually having the capacity to do so.[21] These neuropsychological changes, in addition to the progressive memory deficits of AD and the personality changes found in various types of dementia, lead to an erosion of the self that fundamentally affects voluntarism.[3] Older adults may face external features in the form of pressure or coercion on the part of caregivers and other family members; abuse and exploitation are discussed in greater detail later in this article. Finally, a substantial proportion of older adults live or will live in long-term care where, even in the best of circumstances, limitations on making personal choices are the norm.[22]

ASSESSING CAPACITY TO MAKE MEDICAL DECISIONS

Psychiatrists often are called upon to assess the capacity of an older adult patient to consent to or to refuse a specific medical intervention. Physicians also may participate in the evaluation of a patient's overall capacity to make medical decisions; a judgment of incapacity can result in the activation of a health care power of attorney. Readers should be aware of local laws and regulations governing the process of assess capacity and addressing incapacity; the following is a general discussion of this process.

Clinicians should maintain a high index of suspicion for incapacity in older patients who have dementia, delirium, depression, and neurological disorders that may affect cognition, although the presence of a particular diagnosis does not necessarily make a patient incapable of making medical decisions.[23] Clinicians also should be mindful of the possibility of incapacity in patients in certain settings, namely long-term care facilities, medical-surgical inpatient units, and hospice. The evaluation of a capacity is distinct from the evaluation of the overall competence to manage one's affairs, in that the latter involves a formal judicial process, including the selection of a guardian.[24] Evaluation of other capacities, such as living independently, testamentary capacity, and driving, is discussed later.

The assessment of capacity is fundamentally a clinical process: the clinician interviews the patient and then uses all available data to make a clinical judgment.[25] Unfortunately, substantial variability exists in clinical practice, with multiple studies demonstrating low levels of agreement among assessors of capacity. For example, five physicians at one medical center were asked to judge the capacity of 29 patients who had mild AD and 16 older adult controls; although agreement among physicians was high regarding capacity in the controls, agreement for the patient group was quite low ($\kappa = 0.14$).[26] The same group, however, found that agreement improved when physicians were asked to assess capacity using five specific legal standards (evidencing a treatment choice, making a reasonable treatment choice, appreciating the consequences of a treatment choice, providing rational reasons for a treatment choice, and understanding treatment situation/choices), with κ as high as 0.57.[27]

As noted earlier, neuropsychological correlates of incapacity have been investigated. Studies on the utility of bedside cognitive assessment instruments such as the Mini-Mental Status Examination (MMSE)[28] have yielded mixed results. In their review, Kim and colleagues[29] argue that the use of a single cutoff score (ie, scores above the cutoff indicate capacity and scores below the cutoff indicate incapacity) is not warranted. Scores at or below 16 or 17, however, are very specific for incapacity (low risk of false negatives), and scores at or above 24 to 27 are unlikely to be associated with incapacity; intermediate scores may indicate that further assessment of capacity is required. A subsequent study of 37 patients who had mild to moderate AD verified this approach, with specificity of 93% at an MMSE cutoff of 19 and sensitivity of 91% at a cutoff of 26.[30]

Multiple instruments have been developed to standardize the assessment of capacity, including the MacArthur Competence Assessment Tool for Treatment (MacCAT-T),[31] the Hopemont Capacity Assessment Interview (HCAI),[32] and the Competency to Consent to Treatment Interview (CCTI)[33] (**Table 1**). The MacCAT-T

Table 1		
Instruments for assessing decision-making capacity in older adults		
Instrument	**Advantages**	**Disadvantages**
MacCAT-T	Based on MacArthur model that now is the reference standard; most extensive psychometric data available; interview focuses on specific clinical situation	Training required to ensure inter-rater reliability
CCTI	Extensive database in cognitively impaired populations; specifically designed for use in Alzheimer's disease	Use of hypothetical vignette limits applicability to current clinical situation; uses a fifth legal standard (ie, "capacity to make a reasonable choice") of unclear merit
HCAI	Standardized procedure and scoring	Very little psychometric data available; use of hypothetical vignette limits applicability to current clinical situation
HCAT	Specifically designed to evaluate capacity to execute an advance directive	

Abbreviations: CCTI, Competency to Consent to Treatment Instrument;[33] HCAI, Hopemont Capacity Assessment Interview;[32] HCAT, Hopkins Competency Assessment Test;[58] MacCAT-T, MacArthur Competence Assessment Tool for Treatment.[31]

Data from Dunn LB, Nowrangi MA, Palmer BW, et al. Assessing decisional capacity for clinical research or treatment: a review of instruments. Am J Psychiatry 2006;163:1323–34; and Grisso T, Evaluating competencies: forensic assessment and instruments. New York: Kluwer Academic/Plenum Publishers, 2002.

interview process begins with discussing the patient's actual clinical situation (her or his disorder and the recommended treatment, including risks, benefits, and alternatives) and concludes with the patient's choice and her/his reasoning; the interviewer asks multiple questions to assess the patient's understanding, reasoning, and appreciation. The HCAI and CCTI use hypothetical vignettes, followed by questions probing decisional abilities. Two studies from the same group have compared these instruments directly in geriatric settings.[23,34] There was fair agreement among the instruments with regard to understanding but poor agreement for appreciation and reasoning, suggesting the instruments are not interchangeable. Dunn and colleagues,[35] having reviewed 15 capacity assessment instruments (including these three) in detail, suggested that the MacCAT-T is the best studied and has the broadest application across various clinical scenarios. Nevertheless, given the limitations of these instruments, they are best used as adjuncts to the clinical assessment rather than as replacements for the interview.

Karlawish[25] has proposed a process of evaluating capacity in older adults in which the clinician asks the patient a series of questions to assess the abilities of understanding, appreciation, choice, and reasoning, rating each answer for adequacy (**Table 2**). Based on the assessment of each decisional ability, and perhaps supplemented by a capacity assessment instrument and cognitive testing, the clinician then determines whether the patient has the capacity to consent to or refuse a specific medical intervention. A "sliding scale" approach is widely accepted: the higher the risk of an intervention (or, the higher the risk of refusing the intervention), the higher is the standard required for consent (or refusal).[36] Clinicians should familiarize themselves

Table 2	
Clinical assessment of medical decision-making capacity in older adults	
Decisional Ability	**How to Assess**
Understanding	After disclosing clinical information (eg, risks and benefits of a specific treatment), clinician asks patient to repeat, in her/his own words, the information.
Appreciation	Clinician ascertains how well the patient accepts that the facts presented actually apply to the patient by probing the patient's beliefs about her or his diagnosis and about the possible benefits from treatment.
Reasoning	Clinician assesses patient's ability to compare options, patient's ability to infer how a particular choice will affect the patient, and the logical consistency of these answers.
Expressing a choice	Clinician determines if patient can communicate a consistent decision about treatment.

Data from Moye J, Karel MJ, Azar AR, et al. Capacity to consent to treatment: empirical comparison of three instruments in older adults with and without dementia. Gerontologist 2004;44(2):166–75; and Karlawish J, Measuring decision-making capacity in cognitively impaired individuals. Neurosignals 2008;16:91–8.

with local regulations and standards of care pertaining to the practice of capacity assessment.

Although more explicitly regulated, the initiation of involuntary psychiatric treatment also involves a psychiatrist's assessment of a patient's capacity to refuse psychiatric interventions. In a geriatric setting, the scenarios include suicidality, poor self-care resulting from depression or dementia, and threat of self-harm or harm to others resulting from behavioral disturbance in dementia. Regulations vary by jurisdiction with regard to whether a surrogate decision-maker (eg, a person who has health care power of attorney) can admit patients involuntary or if a legal involuntary commitment process is required.[37]

A capacity assessment yields a dichotomous outcome: the patient is deemed able or not able to make a medical decision. In reality, however, older adult patients often collaborate with family members and other caregivers in decision-making, suggesting a third outcome: capacity to make a decision with assistance or when decision-making responsibility is shared.[38] Unfortunately, legal procedures generally are unavailable to facilitate shared medical decision-making, and patients, families, and physicians must rely on informal mechanisms.[38]

ASSESSING OTHER CAPACITIES

Dementia, delirium, and depression may affect both older adults' capacity to make medical decisions and their capacity to make other decisions necessary to function independently. To live independently, older adults must be able to make decisions about and carry out basic activities of daily living such as bathing, dressing, toileting, ambulation, and feeding themselves, and instrumental activities of daily living (IADLs) such as managing finances, driving, housekeeping, and meal preparation.[39] Accurate identification of problems with functional capacity is critical to balance the ethical imperatives of patient autonomy and welfare (**Table 3**). Clinicians should maintain a high index of suspicion for impairments in IADLs and associated decision-making capacity in older adults who have dementia, delirium, depression, and chronic medical illnesses. Psychiatrists may become involved in determining the appropriate level of

Table 3	
Assessment of other capacities in older adults	
Capacity	**How to Assess**
Everyday decision-making and ability to live independently	Structured assessments of functional abilities (eg, Kohlman Evaluation of Living Skills[44]) and executive function (eg, Executive Interview[45]) may help detect elders needing higher levels of care. The Assessment of Capacity for Everyday Decision Making assesses specific capacities.[43] Screen for self-neglect.
Finances	Both self- and informant reports of financial abilities may be inaccurate.[49] The Financial Capacity Instrument allows structured assessment of financial knowledge, skills, and judgment.[46]
Driving	Patients who have mild cognitive impairment and early dementia should be monitored carefully, and formal driving skills evaluation should be considered. Patients who have moderate or more severe dementia should not drive.[50]
Sexual relations	Evaluate the patient's awareness of the relationship, capacity to avoid exploitation, and awareness of potential risks.[53]
Voting	Patients who have severe dementia are unlikely to have capacity. The Competence Assessment Tool for Voting can be used to assess capacity in mild-to-moderate stages.[55] Ensure that older adults who have capacity actually can cast a ballot.[56]
Testamentary capacity	The Hopkins Competency Assessment is designed specifically to evaluate capacity to execute an advance directive.[58]

care of a community-dwelling elder who has declined functionally and in assessing the ability of an older adult patient to return home following a hospitalization.

Increasing age, worsening health status, and cognitive impairment all correlate with lower capacity to make everyday decisions,[40] and patients who have AD in particular have been found to perform poorly on standardized measures of everyday problem-solving.[41] Lai and colleagues[42] developed the Assessment of Capacity for Everyday Decision-Making, a semi-structured interview that, like the MacCAT-T, assesses the domains of understanding, appreciation, and reasoning. Preliminary evidence suggests that this instrument may be a valuable adjunct in the clinical evaluation of everyday decision-making capacity.[43] The Kohlman Evaluation of Living Skills may be useful in identifying patients who have impairments in the capacity to live independently severe enough to result in self-neglect.[44] In a cross-sectional study of 193 residents of a continuing care retirement community, executive dysfunction (as measured by the Executive Interview and the Executive Clock-Drawing Task) was associated with the need for higher levels of care.[45]

Moye and Marson[18] have reviewed the literature exploring older adults' capacity to manage their finances. Financial abilities vary greatly among individuals and depend on socioeconomic status, occupational attainment, and financial experience.[18] Both patients who have both MCI and those who have AD demonstrate difficulties with financial management.[46–48] The Financial Capacity Instrument (FCI) assesses a patient's financial factual knowledge, procedural knowledge, and judgment; patients who had even mild AD had high proportions of impaired capacity, and those who had moderate AD were almost uniformly incapable.[46] More recently, these investigators have found that, in MCI, both patients and caregivers misestimate patients' financial abilities, raising doubts about the validity of both self-reports and informant reports and highlighting the need for more structured evaluation tools such as the FCI.[49]

Older adults are prone to a number of conditions that may affect their driving ability, including AD, Lewy body dementia, Parkinson's disease, and cerebrovascular disease. Clinicians must balance a respect for patients' autonomy (and ability to transport themselves) with concerns about safety. An American Academy of Neurology Practice Parameter recommends that patients who have AD of moderate or greater severity (clinical dementia rating $\geq$ 1) not drive; those who have mild AD or MCI (clinical dementia rating = 0.5) should be considered for a formal evaluation of driving skills, which is more reliable than self-assessment, informant assessment, or a clinician's assessment.[50] Laws vary by jurisdiction regarding physicians' obligation to report potentially dangerous driving.[51]

Although sexual activity declines with age, a substantial proportion of older adults, including those who have cognitive impairment and those living in long-term care facilities, remain sexually active.[52] The potential for abuse or exploitation exists, but the capacity of the older adult to consent to a sexual act has been poorly studied. The most commonly cited model of capacity assessment involves evaluating the patient's (1) awareness of the relationship, (2) capacity to avoid exploitation, and (3) awareness of potential risks. Deficits in any of these areas indicate that the patient does not have capacity to consent to a sexual relationship.[53]

Laws regarding the ability to vote vary widely, with only eight states in the United States (Connecticut, Florida, Iowa, Massachusetts, New Mexico, Ohio, Oregon, and Wisconsin) explicitly referencing a capacity to vote.[54] A standard for assessing the capacity of older adults who have dementia to vote has been developed only recently.[54] Appelbaum and colleagues[55] operationalized the "Doe voting capacity standard" in the Competence Assessment Tool for Voting, which assesses whether a patient (1) understands the nature and effect of voting, (2) has the capacity to make an electoral choice, (3) can reason about that choice, and (4) appreciates the significance of voting. The authors found that, of 33 patients who had AD, those who had mild or very mild disease performed well, but those who had severe disease did not have capacity to vote.[55] Older adults in long-term care facilities face an additional barrier: many who wish to vote and are capable of doing so may not be able to because of procedural problems at facilities, suggesting that steps need to be taken to ensure that older adults are not disenfranchised.[56] Surrogate decision-makers are not allowed to cast votes for incapacitated elders.[54]

Finally, testamentary capacity, that is, the ability to execute a will (and to enact an advance directive), depends on intact cognitive functioning. For example, Gregory and colleagues[57] found that an MMSE cutoff score of 18 had a sensitivity of 87% and specificity of 82% in identifying capacity as determined by an interview assessing understanding, reasoning, appreciation, and choice. The HCAI, which also has been used to evaluate capacity to give informed consent, was designed to evaluate a patient's capacity to write an advance directive.[58] Part of the rationale for early identification of dementia is to allow patients to execute an advance directive and will when they still have the capacity to do so. Unfortunately, the execution of a will also may expose a cognitively impaired elder to financial exploitation.[59,60] Readers are referred to the review by Spar and Garb[61] for a detailed approach to assessing testamentary capacity.

ADDRESSING DIMINISHED CAPACITY

A clinician's judgment of incapacity should lead to a search for the cause of incapacity (if not known) and an attempt to improve capacity. Potentially treatable causes of incapacity include delirium, dementia, depression, and polypharmacy. Although delirium is, by definition, a transient condition, older adult inpatients who have delirium (especially those who also have dementia) have worse functional and cognitive outcomes up to 1 year after hospitalization than those without delirium.[62] This finding suggests that treating delirium may not be enough to restore capacity, especially in patients who have underlying dementia. In the case of AD, cholinesterase inhibitors and the N-methyl-D -aspartic acid antagonist memantine have been found to be modestly more effective than placebo on cognitive and functional measures;[63] it is plausible that these agents also could improve decisional capacity, but this hypothesis has not been tested. As noted earlier, treatment of late-life depression did not seem to alter older adults' desire to select life-sustaining therapies except in those suffering from severe depression.[11] Thus, the evidence that treating underlying conditions may affect decisional capacity is mixed.

An alternate approach to improving capacity is to employ cognitive and educational strategies. Sugarman and colleagues[64] surveyed the literature on methods of improving informed consent in older adults. Techniques that may be useful to improve patients' ability to comprehend and recall treatment information include simplifying information, providing it in the form of a story book or video, and disclosing information in parts.[64] Jeste and colleagues[65] found that videotapes, computer-aided instruction, touch-screen devices, and informational booklets were helpful in middle-aged and older adults in a number of medical scenarios (eg, learning about cardiopulmonary resuscitation and advance directives) but not in psychiatric settings. The studies reviewed in these reports did not necessarily include incapacitated patients and therefore may not be applicable to this population.[64,65] With regard to consenting to participate in research, Dunn and colleagues[66] found that a computerized slideshow of relevant information led to improved comprehension in middle-aged and elderly outpatients who had schizophrenia and other psychotic disorders; this work recently was extended to patients who had mild AD and MCI.[67] Roberts and Dyer[24] propose a stepwise approach to obtaining consent in patients who have capacity deficits, namely, first seeking consent for beginning treatment and then, as the patient's symptoms, functioning, and capacity improve, moving on to larger decisions.

When capacity cannot be restored or a medical decision must be made when the patient is incapable of doing so, the clinician must turn to a surrogate decision-maker. Patients who have executed advance directives (specifically, a health care power of attorney) have selected a surrogate decision-maker beforehand. Unfortunately, the proportion of older adults who have advance directives is low. For example, a study of 175 veterans age 85 years and older found that only 34% had documented care preferences, and 46% had selected surrogates.[68] Patients diagnosed as having dementia, in particular, may have a narrow window within which to execute an advance directive, given the progressive impairment in capacity caused by dementia.[57] Instruments such as the Health Care Values Survey may assist patients who have dementia in determining their end-of-life care preferences.[69] Most states have surrogate consent laws that determine a sequence of family members (eg, spouse, adult children, and so on) who can become surrogate decision-makers in the event a person becomes incapacitated and does not have an advance directive. Historically, clinicians took on this responsibility in the absence of family members, particularly in long-term care settings.[70]

Two standards govern the behavior of surrogate decision-makers: best interest and substituted judgment.[70] In the former, the surrogate makes a decision based on what the surrogate perceives is in the best interest of the patient. In the latter, the surrogate makes a decision based on the choice the patient would have made, if the patient had been able to do so. Gutheil and Appelbaum[70] describe an approach that combines both standards: "When it is clear that an incompetent would have selected a particular course of action, most courts require that the decision maker follow that choice. In the absence of such evidence, ... the decision maker is free to act in the person's best interests." A study of family members of patients who had advanced dementia confirmed that a combined approach is commonly used.[71] Surrogates face a number of additional challenges. For example, a study of 81 surrogate decision-makers found that only 73% had correctly identified their family members' resuscitation orders, and only 47% demonstrated good understanding of the clinical situation.[72] Shalowitz and colleagues[73] reviewed the literature on the accuracy of surrogate decision-makers and found that surrogates predicted patients' preferences incorrectly 32% of the time. Family members of patients who had advanced dementia identified the following barriers to surrogate decision-making: unrealistic expectations of patients, not having had discussions with patients about preferences (or waiting too long to do so), and patients' denial of dementia.[71]

When a patient's incapacity extends beyond medical decision-making to the ability to manage her or his affairs and live independently, family members (or health care providers) need to turn to the legal system for possible guardianship. Guardianship is necessary to admit to a nursing home a patient who no longer has the capacity to make this decision.[22] Disadvantages of guardianship include the patient's loss of autonomy and privacy, the high cost and time involved with formal legal proceedings, and the possibility that a guardian unfamiliar with the patient may make decisions not consistent with the patient's values and preferences.[70] Readers are referred to Moye and colleagues[74] for a detailed review of the process of evaluating a patient for guardianship and should be aware of local laws governing guardianship proceedings.

ETHICAL ISSUES SPECIFIC TO THE CARE OF PATIENTS WHO HAVE DEMENTIA

Although the capacity to make decisions is a central ethical issue in dementia care, clinicians face other ethical concerns in screening, diagnosis, management of cognitive decline, management of behavioral disturbance, and end-of-life care.[75]

The identification in the 1990s of several genetic markers associated with AD (apolipoprotein E, PS1, PS2, APP) raised concerns about the consequences of positive test results in asymptomatic people and their family members, including genetic discrimination, stigma, and effects on employability. An influential position statement argued that apolipoprotein E testing should have a limited role in diagnosis and no place in screening asymptomatic people; PS1/PS2/APP testing is useful in evaluating patients who have early-onset dementia.[76] A more recent study of the effect of genetic disclosure on adult children of patients who had autopsy-confirmed AD revealed that the persons randomly assigned to learn their apolipoprotein E status did not become more depressed or anxious (even those who had the ε4 allele, which confers higher risk of AD) and did become more engaged in activities that might reduce the chance of developing AD (eg, exercise). Subjects who had the ε4 allele also were more likely to change their long-term care insurance.[77] All subjects had extensive genetic counseling, suggesting that genetic testing in asymptomatic relatives of patients who have AD may be ethical if proper supports are in place. Anonymous genetic testing, whereby results are not placed in an individual's medical records, also may help reduce the possibility of discrimination.[78] This issue will need to be revisited regularly as other biomarkers (eg, functional neuroimaging with positron emission tomograph) become available.

Early concerns about utility of diagnosing an irreversible, terminal condition such as AD have waned as effective treatments have emerged. In fact, the ethical principle of truth-telling dictates that physicians must inform patients of the diagnosis. Post,[79] in reviewing this issue, pointedly wrote that "diagnostic truth-telling is the necessary beginning point for an AD ethics of autonomy." Early diagnosis allows advanced planning, including planning for "optimal life experiences in remaining years of intact capacities," preparing advance directives and power of attorney, considering participation in research, participating in support groups, and deciding whether to take cognitive enhancers.[79] The diagnosis of MCI is more nuanced, because no effective therapies are available as yet, and, although MCI is a risk factor for the development of AD, its prognosis is not clear.

Although cognitive enhancers (donepezil, galantamine, rivastigmine, memantine) have been found to be modestly effective in delaying cognitive and functional decline[63] and are deemed acceptable by caregivers,[80] the cost effectiveness of the medications is uncertain. In fact, the cost of donepezil may be over $120,000 per quality-adjusted year of life, and the savings resulting from delayed institutionalization may not offset the cost of medication.[81] It is not clear at what point in the course of AD cognitive-enhancing therapies should be stopped, raising concerns about both risk–benefit assessment and cost effectiveness. The rapidly increasing population of older adults in general and patients who have AD in particular also raises questions in the ethical domain of social justice: namely, concerns about the just allocation of scarce medical resources may result in policies limiting the use of these agents, as has occurred in the United Kingdom.[82]

Most patients who have dementia experience behavioral and/or psychological symptoms, including depression, anxiety, psychosis, wandering, and agitation, leading to poor patient quality of life, caregiver burden, concerns about patient safety, and institutionalization. Antipsychotics, the pharmacological agents most likely to be effective in reducing these symptoms, are associated with significant morbidity and mortality.[83] Although treatment guidelines have been updated to relegate antipsychotics to second-line treatment (after behavioral interventions), and although the use of antipsychotics in long-term care facilities is highly regulated, antipsychotics probably will remain a mainstay of managing severe behavioral disturbance. Clinicians thus face the ethical dilemma of recommending a treatment that simultaneously may reduce uncomfortable symptoms and hasten death; a further complication is that the patients themselves rarely have capacity to make this decision. This area clearly requires further empirical investigation.

Patients who have dementia are particularly vulnerable to abuse, include physical abuse, financial exploitation, neglect, and self-neglect. Forty-six states have mandatory reporting requirements when health care professionals suspect elder abuse; the remaining four states (Colorado, New York, North Dakota, and South Dakota) have voluntary reporting laws.[60] Clinicians should familiarize themselves with local laws governing the reporting of abuse. Rates of elder abuse range from 4.5 to 14.6 per 1000 elders, with an estimated 550,000 cases nationwide.[84] Self-neglect, the most common form of elder abuse, can be difficult to detect because such patients may not be able to provide accurate self-reports and often have no caregivers to report the neglect. Psychiatrists working with patients who have dementia should maintain a high index of suspicion for self-neglect. A clinician concerned about self-neglect should formally assess the patient's capacity to live independently and should contact the relevant local authority tasked with addressing elder abuse.

The terminal stage of dementia is marked by severe cognitive impairment and inanition. It is appropriate and desirable to employ a palliative care approach for patients who have severe dementia, including a focus on promoting patient comfort, avoiding hospitalization and surgery, and employing do-not-resuscitate orders.[75] Among the most challenging steps is the withholding of artificial hydration and nutrition. Feeding tubes probably do not reduce a patient's suffering and may, in fact, cause suffering; decreased oral intake is expected in terminal dementia.[85] The Alzheimer's Association Position on the Treatment of Patients with Advanced Dementia states, "if such a patient rejects and food and water by mouth, it is ethically permissible to choose to withhold nutrition and hydration artificially administered by vein or gastric tube."[86] Post[79] reframes end-of-life care in dementia as an issue of social justice; that is, the cost to society of interventions to extend the life of patients who have advanced dementia may not be just or justifiable.

ETHICAL ISSUES AT THE END OF LIFE

For end-of-life issues outside the setting of dementia, readers are referred to the thorough and detailed review by Lyness.[87] Of particular interest to psychiatrists is the intersection of depression, hopelessness, and a wish to die in end-of-life situations. Depressed and hopeless elders are more likely than controls to refuse life-sustaining treatments.[11,12,88] This refusal probably results from cognitive distortions associated with depression; successfully treating depression should restore the will to live. Sullivan,[89] however, has noted that there are circumstances in which it is reasonable to accept the decision of a patient, even one who has depression, to refuse life-sustaining treatments. He eloquently argued:

> Psychiatrists treating patients at the end of life need to look beyond competence evaluations and depression treatment to help patients expand the repertoire of hope available to them. We know a few things that we can do to help diversify hope for dying patients: palliative care that reduces symptoms, to allow for lucidity and relationship; bringing family and friends into intensive care and nursing home settings; patient life-review by writing biographies and dictating stories; and fostering reconciliation with friends, family, and community.[90]

He thus recasts patient welfare at the end of life in terms of comfort, compassion, and interpersonal connectedness.

SUMMARY

Psychiatrists face a number of ethical challenges when caring for older adults and their families. Of paramount importance is ensuring that older adults have the capacity to make decisions about their medical care and their overall welfare. Psychiatrists must remain alert for the possibility of incapacity, which, if suspected, should prompt a thorough evaluation of decisional capacities. There is a robust literature guiding clinicians conducting such evaluations. Geriatric care focuses on maintaining or improving quality of life, which is especially relevant in end-of-life situations. With the aging of the United States population, discussion must take place at a societal level regarding a fair and just distribution of medical resources. Psychiatrists must be vigilant that the mental health needs of older adults, including access to effective therapies, are addressed adequately in such discussions.

REFERENCES

1. ABIM Foundation. Medical professionalism in the new millennium: a physician charter. Ann Intern Med 2002;136(3):243–6.

2. Appelbaum PS, Grisso T. The MacArthur treatment competence study. I: mental illness and competence to consent to treatment. Law Hum Behav 1995;19(2): 105–26.
3. Roberts LW. Informed consent and the capacity for voluntarism. Am J Psychiatry 2002;159(5):705–12.
4. Huthwaite JS, Martin RC, Griffith HR, et al. Declining decision-making capacity in mild AD: a two-year longitudinal study. Behav Sci Law 2006;24:453–63.
5. Okonkwo OC, Griffith HR, Copeland JN, et al. Medical decision-making capacity in mild cognitive impairment: a 3-year longitudinal study. Neurology 2008;71(19): 1474–80.
6. Okonkwo OC, Griffith HR, Belue K, et al. Cognitive models of medical decision-making capacity in patients with mild cognitive impairment. J Int Neuropsychol Soc 2008;14(2):297–308.
7. Karlawish JHT, Casarett DJ, James BD, et al. The ability of persons with Alzheimer disease (AD) to make a decision about taking an AD treatment. Neurology 2006; 64:1514–9.
8. Gurrera RJ, Moye J, Karel MJ, et al. Cognitive performance predicts treatment decisional abilities in mild to moderate dementia. Neurology 2006;66(9):1367–72.
9. Dymek MP, Atchison P, Harrell L, et al. Competency to consent to medical treatment in cognitively impaired patients with Parkinson's disease. Neurology 2001; 56(1):17–24.
10. Martin RC, Okonkwo OC, Hill J, et al. Medical decision-making capacity in cognitively impaired Parkinson's disease patients without dementia. Mov Disord 2008; 23(13):1867–74.
11. Ganzini L, Lee MA, Heintz RT, et al. The effect of depression treatment on elderly patients' preferences for life-sustaining medical therapy. Am J Psychiatry 1994; 151(11):1631–6.
12. Blank K, Robison J, Doherty E, et al. Life-sustaining treatment and assisted death choices in depressed older patients. J Am Geriatr Soc 2001;49(2):153–61.
13. Rose DS, Wykes TH, Bindman JP, et al. Information, consent and perceived coercion: patients' perspectives on electroconvulsive therapy. Br J Psychiatry 2005; 186:54–9.
14. Greenberg RM, Kellner CH. Electroconvulsive therapy: a selective review. Am J Geriatr Psychiatry 2005;13:268–81.
15. Lapid MI, Rummans TA, Pankratz VS, et al. Decisional capacity of depressed elderly to consent to electroconvulsive therapy. J Geriatr Psychiatry Neurol 2004;17(1):42–6.
16. Palmer BW, Dunn LB, Appelbaum PS, et al. Correlates of treatment-related decision-making capacity among middle-aged and older patients with schizophrenia. Arch Gen Psychiatry 2004;61(3):230–6.
17. Stroup S, Appelbaum P, Swartz M, et al. Decision-making capacity for research participation among individuals in the CATIE schizophrenia trial. Schizophr Res 2005;80(1):1–8.
18. Moye J, Marson DC. Assessment of decision-making capacity in older adults: an emerging area of practice and research. J Gerontol B Psychol Sci Soc Sci 2007; 628(1):3–11.
19. Irwin SA, Zurhellen CH, Diamond LC, et al. Unrecognised cognitive impairment in hospice patients: a pilot study. Palliat Med 2008;22(7):842–7.
20. Workman RH Jr, McCullough LB, Molinari V, et al. Clinical and ethical implications of impaired executive control functions for patient autonomy. Psychiatr Serv 2000; 51(3):359–63.

21. Grimes AL, McCullough LB, Kunik ME, et al. Informed consent and neuroanatomic correlates of intentionality and voluntariness among psychiatric patients. Psychiatr Serv 2000;51(12):1561–7.

22. Kapp MB. 'A place like that': advance directives and nursing home admissions. Psychol Public Policy Law 1998;4(3):805–28.

23. Moye J, Karel MJ, Azar AR, et al. Capacity to consent to treatment: empirical comparison of three instruments in older adults with and without dementia. Gerontologist 2004;44(2):166–75.

24. Roberts LW, Dyer AR. Concise guide to ethics in mental health care. Washington, DC: American Psychiatric Publishing, Inc.; 2004.

25. Karlawish J. Measuring decision-making capacity in cognitively impaired individuals. Neurosignals 2008;16:91–8.

26. Marson DC, McInturff B, Hawkins L, et al. Consistency of physician judgments of capacity to consent in mild Alzheimer's disease. J Am Geriatr Soc 1997;45(4):453–7.

27. Marson DC, Earnst KS, Jamil F, et al. Consistency of physicians' legal standard and personal judgments of competency in patients with Alzheimer's disease. J Am Geriatr Soc 2000;48(8):1014–6.

28. Folstein MF, Folstein SE, McHugh PR. 'Mini-mental state': a practical method for grading the cognitive state of patients for the clinician. J Psychiatr Res 1975;12: 189–98.

29. Kim SYH, Karlawish JHT, Caine ED. Current state of research on decision-making competence of cognitively impaired elderly persons. Am J Geriatr Psychiatry 2002;10:151–65.

30. Kim SYH, Caine ED. Utility and limits of the MMSE in evaluating consent capacity in Alzheimer's disease. Psychiatr Serv 2002;53(1):1322–4.

31. Grisso T, Appelbaum PS, Hill-Fotouhi C. The MacCAT-T: a clinical tool to assess patients' capacities to make treatment decisions. Psychiatr Serv 1997;48(11): 1415–9.

32. Edelstein R. Hopemont Capacity Assessment Interview manual and scoring guide. Morgantown (WY): West Virginia University; 1999.

33. Marson DC, Ingram KK, Cody HA, et al. Assessing the competency of patients with Alzheimer's disease under different legal standards. Arch Neurol 1995;52: 949–54.

34. Gurrerra RJ, Karel MJ, Azar AR, et al. Agreement between instruments for rating treatment decisional capacity. Am J Geriatr Psychiatry 2007;15:168–73.

35. Dunn LB, Nowrangi MA, Palmer BW, et al. Assessing decisional capacity for clinical research or treatment: a review of instruments. Am J Psychiatry 2006;163: 1323–34.

36. Drane JF. Competency to give an informed consent: a model for making clinical assessments. JAMA 1984;252(7):925–7.

37. Rissmiller DJ, Musser E, Rhoades W, et al. A survey of use of a durable power of attorney to admit geropsychiatric patients. Psychiatr Serv 2001;52(1):98–100.

38. Kapp MB. Decisional capacity in theory and practice: legal process versus 'bumbling through.' Aging Ment Health 2002;6(4):413–7.

39. Lawton MP, Brody EM. Assessment of older people: self-maintaining and instrumental activities of daily living. Gerontologist 1969;9:179–86.

40. Thornton WL, Deria S, Gelb S, et al. Neuropsychological mediators of the links among age, chronic illness, and everyday problem solving. Psychol Aging 2007;22(3):470–81.

41. Willis SL, Allen-Burge R, Dolan MM, et al. Everyday problem solving among individuals with Alzheimer's disease. Gerontologist 1998;38(5):569–77.

42. Lai JM, Karlawish J. Assessing the capacity to make everyday decisions: a guide for clinicians and an agenda for future research. Am J Geriatr Psychiatry 2007; 15(2):101–11.

43. Lai JM, Gill TM, Cooney LM, et al. Everyday decision-making ability in older persons with cognitive impairment. Am J Geriatr Psychiatry 2008;16(8):693–6.

44. Pickens S, Naik AD, Burnett J, et al. The utility of the Kohlman Evaluation of Living Skills test is associated with substantiated cases of elder self-neglect. J Am Acad Nurse Pract 2007;19(3):137–42.

45. Royall DR, Chiodo LK, Polk MJ. An empiric approach to level of care determinations: the importance of executive measures. J Gerontol A Biol Sci Med Sci 2000; 60(8):1059–64.

46. Marson DC, Sawrie SM, Snyder S, et al. Assessing financial capacity in patients with Alzheimer disease: a conceptual model and prototype instrument. Arch Neurol 2000;57(6):877–84.

47. Tuokko H, Morris C, Ebert P. Mild cognitive impairment and everyday functioning in older adults. Neurocase 2005;11(1):40–7.

48. Griffith HR, Belue K, Sicola A, et al. Impaired financial abilities in mild cognitive impairment: a direct assessment approach. Neurology 2003;60(3):449–57.

49. Okonkwo OC, Wadley VG, Griffith HR, et al. Awareness of deficits in financial abilities in patients with mild cognitive impairment: going beyond self-informant discrepancy. Am J Geriatr Psychiatry 2008;16(8):650–9.

50. Dubinsky RM, Stein AC, Lyons K. Practice parameter: risk of driving and Alzheimer's disease. Neurology 2000;54:2205–11.

51. American Psychiatric Association. Practice guideline for the treatment of patients with Alzheimer's disease and related dementias. 2nd edition. Washington, DC: American Psychiatric Press, Inc.; 2007.

52. Davies HD, Zeiss AM, Shea EA, et al. Sexuality and intimacy in Alzheimer's patients and their partners. Sex Disabil 1998;16(3):193–203.

53. Lichtenberg P, Strzepek D. Assessments of institutionalized dementia patients' competencies to participate in intimate relationships. Gerontologist 1990;30: 117–20.

54. Karlawish JH, Bonnie RJ, Appelbaum PS, et al. Addressing the ethical, legal, and social issues raised by voting by persons with dementia. JAMA 2004;292(11): 1345–50.

55. Appelbaum PS, Bonnie RJ, Karlawish JH. The capacity to vote of persons with Alzheimer's disease. Am J Psychiatry 2005;162:2094–100.

56. Karlawish JH, Bonnie RJ, Appelbaum PS, et al. Identifying the barriers and challenges to voting by residents in nursing homes and assisted living settings. J Aging Soc Policy 2008;20(1):65–79.

57. Gregory R, Roked F, Jones L, et al. Is the degree of cognitive impairment in patients with Alzheimer's disease related to their capacity to appoint an enduring power of attorney? Age and Ageing 2007;36:527–31.

58. Janofsky JS, McCarthy RJ, Folstein MF. The Hopkins Competency Assessment Test: a brief method for evaluating patients' capacity to give informed consent. Hosp Community Psychiatry 1992;43:132–6.

59. Peisah C, Finkel S, Shulman K, et al. The wills of older people: risk factors for undue influence. Int Psychogeriatr 2009;21(1):7–15.

60. Tueth MJ. Exposing financial exploitation of impaired elderly persons. Am J Geriatr Psychiatry 2000;8:104–11.

61. Spar JE, Garb AS. Assessing competency to make a will. Am J Psychiatry 1992; 149(2):169–74.

62. McCusker J, Cole M, Dendukuri N, et al. Delirium in older medical inpatients and subsequent cognitive and functional status: a prospective study. CMAJ 2001; 165(5):575–83.
63. Cummings JL. Drug therapy: Alzheimer's disease. N Engl J Med 2004;351:56–67.
64. Sugarman J, McCrory DC, Hubal RC. Getting meaningful informed consent from older adults: a structured literature review of empirical research. J Am Geriatr Soc 1998;46(4):517–24.
65. Jeste DV, Dunn LB, Folson DP, et al. Multimedia educational aids for improving consumer knowledge about illness management and treatment decisions: a review of randomized controlled trials. J Psychiatr Res 2008;42:1–21.
66. Dunn LB, Lindamer LA, Palmer BW, et al. Improving understanding of research consent in middle-aged and elderly patients with psychotic disorders. Am J Geriatr Psychiatry 2002;10(2):142–50.
67. Mittal D, Palmer BW, Dunn LB, et al. Comparison of two enhanced consent procedures for patients with mild Alzheimer disease or mild cognitive impairment. Am J Geriatr Psychiatry 2007;15(2):163–7.
68. Wu P, Lorenz KA, Chodosh J. Advance care planning among the oldest old. J Palliat Med 2008;11(2):152–7.
69. Karel MJ, Moye J, Bank A, et al. Three methods of assessing values for advance care planning: comparing persons with and without dementia. J Aging Health 2007;19:123–51.
70. Gutheil TG, Appelbaum PS. Clinical handbook of psychiatry and the law. 3rd edition. Philadelphia: Lippincott Williams & Wilkins; 2000.
71. Hirschman KB, Kapo JM, Karlawish JH. Why doesn't a family member of a person with advanced dementia use a substituted judgment when making a decision for that person? Am J Geriatr Psychiatry 2006;14(8):659–67.
72. Rodriguez RM, Navarrete E, Schwaber J, et al. A prospective study of primary surrogate decision makers' knowledge of intensive care. Crit Care Med 2008; 36(5):1633–6.
73. Shalowitz DI, Garrett-Mayer E, Wendler D. The accuracy of surrogate decision makers: a systematic review. Arch Intern Med 2006;166(5):493–7.
74. Moye J, Butz BW, Marson DC, et al. A conceptual model and assessment template for capacity evaluation in adult guardianship. Gerontologist 2007; 47(5):591–603.
75. American Academy of Neurology Ethics and Humanities Subcommittee. Ethical issues in the management of the demented patient. Neurology 1996;46:1180–3.
76. Post SG, Whitehouse PJ, Binstock RH, et al. The clinical introduction of genetic testing for Alzheimer disease: an ethical perspective. JAMA 1997;277(10):832–6.
77. Roberts JS, Cupples LA, Relkin NR, et al. Genetic risk assessment for adult children of people with Alzheimer's disease: the Risk Evaluation and Education for Alzheimer's Disease (REVEAL) study. J Geriatr Psychiatry Neurol 2005;18(4):250–5.
78. Alzheimer's Association position on genetic testing. April 2008. Available at: http://www.alz.org/national/documents/statements_genetictesting.pdf. Accessed January 4, 2009.
79. Post SG. Key issues in the ethics of dementia care. Neurol Clin 2000;18(4): 1011–22.
80. Karlawish JH, Casarett DJ, James BD, et al. Why would caregivers not want to treat their relative's Alzheimer's disease? J Am Geriatr Soc 2000;51(10):1391–7.
81. Loveman E, Green C, Kirby J, et al. The clinical and cost-effectiveness of donepezil, rivastigmine, galantamine and memantine for Alzheimer's disease. Health Technol Assess 2006;10(1):iii–iv, ix–xi, 1–160.

82. National Institute for Health and Clinical Excellence. Donepezil, galantamine, riva-stigmine (review) and memantine for the treatment of Alzheimer's disease (amended). London: NICE; 2007.

83. Schneider LS, Dagerman K, Insel PS. Efficacy and adverse effects of atypical antipsychotics for dementia: meta-analysis of randomized, placebo-controlled trials. Am J Geriatr Psychiatry 2006;14:191–210.

84. Jogerst GJ, Daly JM, Brinig MF, et al. Domestic elder abuse and the law. Am J Public Health 2003;93(12):2131–6.

85. Gillick MR. Rethinking the role of tube feeding in patients with advanced dementia. N Engl J Med 2000;342(3):206–10.

86. Alzheimer's Association position on treatment of patients with advanced dementia. May 1988. Available at: http://www.alz.org/national/documents/statements_advancedementia.pdf. Accessed January 5, 2009.

87. Lyness JM. End-of-life care: issues relevant to the geriatric psychiatrist. Am J Geriatr Psychiatry 2004;12(5):457–72.

88. Menon AS, Campbell D, Ruskin P, et al. Depression, hopelessness, and the desire for life-saving treatments among elderly medically ill veterans. Am J Geriatr Psychiatry 2000;8(4):333–42.

89. Sullivan MD, Youngner SJ. Depression, competence, and the right to refuse lifesaving medical treatment. Am J Psychiatry 1994;151:971–8.

90. Sullivan MD. Hope and hopelessness at the end of life. Am J Geriatr Psychiatry 2003;11(4):393–405.

When, Why, and How to Conduct Research in Child and Adolescent Psychiatry: Practical and Ethical Considerations

Donna T. Chen, MD, MPH[a,b,c,*], Lois L. Shepherd, JD[a,b,d]

KEYWORDS

- Research ethics • Children and adolescents • Mental health
- Practice-based research • Practical clinical trials

Consider the following: A psychiatrist is asked to join a research network and wonders if she should. Another psychiatrist tries to untangle research rules about parental permission, consent, and assent for an adolescent patient who is receiving psychotherapy without her parents' knowledge. How should these psychiatrists approach the ethical challenges of the rapidly changing world of research in child and adolescent psychiatry?

Psychiatrists have, as a profession, endorsed evidence-based medicine,[1,2] and much needed research can only be done with the participation of psychiatrists practicing in real-world settings.[3] Indeed, the Child and Adolescent Psychiatry Trials Network (CAPTN) was set up primarily to facilitate large trials in real-world settings.[4] Accordingly, psychiatrists and other clinicians who treat mental health problems of children and adolescents will increasingly encounter opportunities to conduct research in their clinical practices.[5] Even if they are not directly involved in research, treating psychiatrists will be asked for advice by parents considering whether to enroll their children in a study they

[a] Center for Biomedical Ethics and Humanities, University of Virginia School of Medicine, Box 800758, Hospital Drive, Barringer 5th Floor, Charlottesville, VA 22908, USA
[b] Department of Public Health Sciences, University of Virginia School of Medicine, Charlottesville, VA, USA
[c] Department of Psychiatry and Neurobehavioral Sciences, University of Virginia School of Medicine, Charlottesville, VA, USA
[d] School of Law, University of Virginia, Charlottesville, VA, USA
* Corresponding author. Center for Biomedical Ethics and Humanities, University of Virginia School of Medicine, Box 800758, Hospital Drive, Barringer 5th Floor, Charlottesville, VA 22908.
E-mail address: dtc6k@virginia.edu (D.T. Chen).

Psychiatr Clin N Am 32 (2009) 361–380
doi:10.1016/j.psc.2009.03.003
0193-953X/09/$ – see front matter
psych.theclinics.com

have found or have been asked to participate in.[6] Finally, in determining how much confidence to give published research results, psychiatrists need to understand how research studies are conducted. For all of these reasons, it is becoming essential that all practicing psychiatrists understand the basics of research ethics.

Several excellent overviews of the ethical issues that arise in child and adolescent psychiatric research have been published in recent years and serve to focus attention on the many ethical and practical challenges inherent in this work.[7,8] This article extends these discussions by focusing on some important decision points through case discussions. Because much future research will occur in the offices of private–practice psychiatrists,[1,3,9] the following cases emphasize some of the unique ethical concerns that arise in this setting. Most of the concerns discussed, however, are also present in research conducted in other settings.

Practice-based research networks (PBRNs) create a research infrastructure across multiple real-world practice settings and exist in multiple specialties.[10–12] The CAPTN is an important example of a PBRN in psychiatry.[4] These networks generally allow physicians to participate in the creation, design, and conduct of large practical clinical trials aimed at answering questions relevant to practicing physicians and their patients. Often, these large trials compare the effectiveness of two or more common interventions or test for a response from adjunctive treatments. Generally, they are not early phase studies of safety; many do not involve a placebo control group; and frequently, they allow for open assignment of patients to treatment arms, rather than randomization or double-masking.

Other studies conducted in private practices are sponsored by pharmaceutical and device companies and performed with the help of for-profit companies called clinical research organizations (CROs) and site management organizations (SMOs), which organize and manage clinical trials involving hundreds of community-based practices.[13–16] Rather than aiming to improve clinical decision-making, industry-sponsored studies are generally designed to gain regulatory approvals from the Food and Drug Administration (FDA), which are related to marketing their products. There are a number of excellent overviews of the ethical, legal, and regulatory aspects of research conducted in practice-based research networks[17–21] or for CROs.[22–24]

The first two cases that follow (A and B) present some of the general ethical concerns (and their practical consequences) involved in decisions about whether to participate in research and if so, in what kind of research. The remaining cases provide a brief analysis of particular examples of some ethical concerns in psychiatric research with child or adolescent participants. The particular issues highlighted in each case are listed in **Box 1**.

Box 1
Issues highlighted in cases

Case A: Deciding Whether to Conduct Research
Differences between research and medical care
Conflicts of interest
Relationship of trust with patients and community
Financial incentives (including finder's fees)
Conflicts of commitment
Risk-benefit assessments
Considerations involving staff
Operational challenges of research
Separation of medical and research records

Case B: Deciding Which Studies To Conduct and Communicating with Patients About Them
Scientific, social or clinical value of research study
Scientific validity of research study

Requirement of independent review
Individual responsibility for ensuring ethical conduct
Risk–benefit ratio & clinical equipoise
Best medical interests of patient
Contact person for research and informed consent

Case C: "Therapeutic Misconception" and Other Distortions in Decision-making
Advising and monitoring roles
Communication with study investigators
Therapeutic misconception
Desperation and frustration of parents
Motivations for participation in research

Case D: Consent, Confidentiality, and Participant Selection
Confidentiality
Requirement of parental permission
Child and adolescent assent
State laws allowing minors to consent to treatment
Capacity determinations
"Rule of 7s"
Therapeutic misconception

Case E: Genetic Research and Information Sharing
Value of genetic results
Clinical usefulness
Incidental findings
Informed decision-making
Genetic discrimination
Separation of medical and research records

CASE A: DECIDING WHETHER TO CONDUCT RESEARCH

Case A

A psychiatrist hears from her pediatrician colleague that his clinic has recently started conducting clinical trials. The pediatrician finds that for some of his patients, enrollment in clinical research offers attractive alternatives to standard medical treatment. He also reports that participation in research offers his clinic an additional source of revenue, and himself, his colleagues, office staff, and any patients who participate a sense of contributing to medical advancement. He notes that the research network offers education and support for adding research to a practice, and he finds the challenges intellectually rewarding. Hearing this, the psychiatrist thinks about several of her patients for whom standard medical treatment is not effective. They have asked her whether she would consider joining a national clinical trial so that they could participate. Until now, she has rejected that suggestion because she has been uncomfortable with the idea, in part because of a vague notion that "doctors ought not experiment on their patients" and in part because she questions whether her medical training is sufficient to allow her to undertake an activity as seemingly foreign as medical research. Now, however, after talking with her colleague, she wonders whether she should reconsider.

Soon after, she contacts a psychiatric colleague across town who has joined the trial she is considering. He tells her that the trial is somewhat complicated and it may not be worth it for her to enroll her own patients because of the resources required. However, he offers to pay her for every patient she refers who enrolls in the trial with him.

What are the issues this psychiatrist should consider in deciding whether and how she wants to participate in research?

Although adding research to one's practice can be rewarding and can be done ethically, it is important that the psychiatrist recognize that research participation inevitably creates tension with the professional obligations she owes to her patients.[17] Adding research to one's clinical practice creates conflicts of interest.[17,25] Although a conflict of interest is not—in and of itself—unethical, it can create pressures or incentives to deviate from acceptable conduct. Even when a conflict of interest does not jeopardize professional judgment, the perception by others of a conflict of interest has the potential to significantly undermine patient or community trust, which are critical features of medical practice and clinical research.

Conflicts of interest occur when a physician's own personal interests or obligations to others conflict with obligations to patients. Examples of nonfinancial personal interests include the gratification, intellectual reward, and prestige that might come from serving as an investigator. Examples of financial conflicts include financial compensation offered for enrolling and monitoring patients in studies or for referring patients to research, or a physician's financial interest in the outcome of research through stock ownership in the company whose product is being studied. Financial conflicts of interest, particularly those engendered by industry-sponsored research, have received a great deal of attention generally, as well as for the field of child and adolescent psychiatry specifically.[26–29]

Although physicians can ethically accept reasonable compensation for the amount of time and energy spent on a research study, as well as actual costs associated with research, amounts above and beyond that are ethically suspect. Payments for simply referring patients to research, so-called "finder's fees," are considered unethical, and the American Medical Association deems them unacceptable.[30] Thus, no matter what her decision with regard to her own future participation in research, the psychiatrist in our case example ought not to accept the finder's fee offered by her colleague. Although other kinds of financial interests are not per se unethical, they may also have the potential to compromise patient care and/or research integrity.

Consistent with the professional obligation to put patients' interests above personal interests, recommendations regarding conflicts of interest start with avoiding such conflicts when possible. When unavoidable, accepted ways to manage them exist, both in clinical care and in research.[31,32] For example, transparency and disclosure gives patients, potential research participants, and their families an opportunity to take potential conflicts of interest into account during their own decision-making. The American Academy of Child and Adolescent Psychiatrists provides an example of a "Statement for Parents" that could be adapted to inform parents about potential conflict of interest situations.[31]

Certain types of nonfinancial conflicts of interest are sometimes referred to as conflicts of commitment.[33] Rather than involving a physician's own self-interest, conflicts of commitment "involve sets of role expectations where competing obligations prevent honoring both commitments or honoring them both adequately."(p. 61)[33] For example, all psychiatrists can recall a situation during residency in which their commitments as physician, teacher, and learner conflicted. For physicians also conducting research, a conflict of commitment may occur, for example, when faced with the choice between enrolling patients in a study that does not allow adjuvant care and providing patients with the best available care. When this occurs, physicians experience a conflict of commitment between their professional obligations to provide or recommend the best available treatments to their patients and the professional commitment they make to contribute to the research enterprise, including to enroll research participants and conduct good science. Conflicts of commitment arising between professional obligations of clinical care and of research exist to some extent in all clinical research conducted by physician-investigators, but research conducted in real-world settings heighten these conflicts, in part because of the purposeful effort to blend research with routine clinical practice.

Although the ultimate goals of clinical practice and clinical research are similar (ie, to prevent and treat illness to the best of one's ability), there are important differences between these two activities. Medical care provided in clinical practice is individualized. Even when following practice guidelines, the medical care that the psychiatrist currently provides her patients is individualized, and the recommendations and treatments she offers are meant to advance their best interests. In contrast, clinical research employs protocol-driven interventions aimed at developing generalizable knowledge to help theoretical future patients who might benefit from the research findings. Although improvement in the medical condition of research participants is hoped for, it is a secondary effect ("side effect") and is not the primary intention of research. It is critically important that patients enrolled in research understand this distinction. If they do not understand it, they may later experience confusion, misunderstanding, and feelings of betrayal.

Justifications for personal risks are also fundamentally different between clinical practice and research. In clinical practice, risk is justified by potential for and expectation of direct personal diagnostic, therapeutic, or preventive benefit. Even when clinical care is innovative, and thus potentially riskier than evidence-based care, the physician's intention is to provide what she thinks is best for her patient, all things considered. The associated risks should be justifiable by the patient's potential to benefit. By contrast, risks incurred by research activities are justified primarily by the potential of the research to benefit future individuals, not necessarily the research participant.

Before deciding to participate in research generally or in a particular research project, the psychiatrist in this example needs to determine whether she will be able to appropriately manage the tensions that will exist between her commitment to care for her patients and her commitment to participate in research. This set of concerns will mean, at a minimum, careful selection of research protocols that she might consider, allocation of sufficient time to ethically enroll and monitor participants, and development of a keen sense of alertness to situations that might arise which would compromise her ability to fulfill her primary obligation, which is as doctor to patient.

Careful attention to ethical issues as one considers whether and how to introduce clinical research into one's practice goes a long way in preparing to manage the ethical dimensions of commingling clinical research and clinical practice. There are also many practical questions to consider before deciding to participate in research. Whether these can be answered satisfactorily will also affect whether the research can be conducted in an ethical manner.[17]

Some of these questions focus on the psychiatrist's relationship with her patients and wider community. How will the addition of research affect the degree of trust the practice has earned and continues to enjoy? Will the effect be positive, because the psychiatrist is seen as particularly current with respect to new treatments, or might it be negative, because patients or the community suspect that the psychiatrist's motivations are financial? Decisions about what kinds of research to undertake, the types of payments to accept, and how to communicate about research opportunities, should all be made with an eye on the potential effects to the psychiatrist's relationship with patients and the community as well as to her own professional identity and sense of integrity.[34]

Other questions focus on the workings of the psychiatrist's office. In addition to having a commitment to her patients and the community, and to a successful practice for her own benefit, a psychiatrist has a commitment to her staff. Will her staff be able to perform the additional obligations of research without diminishing the quality of medical care provided to patients? What will the staff's attitude be toward the addition of research? Will they embrace the opportunity or resent it? Will there be sufficient resources to ensure that appropriate training and continuing education are available?

Before deciding to engage in research, the psychiatrist will need to understand what additional operational matters will have to be undertaken by herself and her staff, at what cost, and with what adjustments to the workings of the office. For example, the practice will need to physically separate clinical and research records. Only in this way can it achieve accurate case reporting for the research protocol and protect research records while also preserving confidentiality of patient information. Similarly, many practices will also find it necessary to hire a research coordinator, even if all existing staff help conduct the research. Before the psychiatrist decides to conduct clinical research in her practice, she should confirm that she will get adequate support for these practical and ethical matters from the PBRN or the CRO soliciting her participation, as described in further detail below.

CASE B: DECIDING WHICH STUDIES TO CONDUCT AND COMMUNICATING WITH PATIENTS ABOUT THEM

Case B

Several psychiatrists in a clinic join a practice-based research network and create a patient advisory board that meets periodically to discuss issues related to choosing particular studies, best practices related to parental permission and participant assent, advertising, confidentiality, and other issues related to conducting research in the practice. The practice is contacted by a CRO asking it to serve as a site for several pharmaceutical trials. By what criteria should these psychiatrists determine whether to participate in particular trials?

After a practice or individual psychiatrist has decided to more actively participate in research, determining which studies to conduct is not always straightforward. Psychiatrists should only consider studies that they believe have scientific, social, or clinical value.[7,35,36] For example, a psychiatrist may find it worthwhile to participate in a study sponsored by a PBRN in which she has the opportunity to help craft the research questions being asked or to conduct an industry-sponsored clinical trial of a truly novel treatment, yet decide to turn down a trial of a "me-too" medication aimed primarily to capture market share from already successful medications.

Because the risks to patient–participants from research are justified by the prospect of contributing important knowledge, psychiatrists should not only feel confident about the value of the knowledge to be gained but also about the protocol's scientific validity. If the study has advanced to the stage of soliciting sites, it should have already undergone several stages of scientific review. Nevertheless, some determination about scientific validity should also be made by the individual psychiatrist, even if she satisfies this requirement in significant part by examining how comprehensive the prior independent reviews have been. Ensuring a study's scientific validity will also require close adherence to the protocol; if some of the protocol's requirements are considered objectionable by the practice or will be difficult to adhere to, then it should decline to participate.[18]

Ethical research requires independent review not only of the scientific merit of the study but also to ensure protection of human participants.[36] Research protocols presented to practicing psychiatrists should already have been reviewed for these purposes by independent bodies (eg, scientific review committees; research ethics committees, which in the United States are called institutional review boards), and at times governmental agencies (eg, FDA).[19,20,22] However, sometimes additional research ethics review committee approval will be required before an individual psychiatrist can participate in a study, which is a question that the sponsors of the research or the PBRN should be able to help answer. Even if additional research ethics review is not required, a psychiatrist will want to know who has reviewed and approved the research, and will also want to critically inquire for herself whether the protocol meets ethical standards. Review by others does not relieve the individual psychiatrist from responsibility, both ethical and legal, for ensuring that the research in which she participates meets ethical standards.[37]

A substantial component of this review asks whether the risk–benefit ratio is favorable. In general, the risks to the research participant are weighed against the benefits of the knowledge to be gained from the research and the prospect of benefit to the participant, if any. For studies involving children and adolescents, there are specific federal regulations that stipulate allowable risk and appropriate safeguards, as described in Case D below. It is important not to overestimate the potential benefit to research participants. For example, although tests performed in research might lead to the discovery of an undiagnosed illness, if the results do not provide clinically useful information or are not made available in a clinically appropriate time-frame, they will not yield actual benefits to the patient–participants.

The concept of "clinical equipoise" is frequently used to determine the reasonableness of risk–benefit ratios in randomized controlled trials.[38] Under this principle, a trial is considered ethically reasonable when there is genuine uncertainty and a lack of consensus within the relevant clinical community as to which treatment is better or, when one of the study arms includes a placebo, whether any effective treatment is available.

Even the existence of clinical equipoise, however, may not lead all psychiatrists to feel sufficiently comfortable with the risk–benefit ratio to conduct a study in their practices or to enroll a specific patient. Although there may be disagreement among the clinical community about the effectiveness of two treatments, the psychiatrist herself may have good reasons for preferring one treatment over the other for a particular patient. In addition, even with equipoise, a trial might still have features, such as standardized dosages or medication washout periods, that set it apart from clinical practice.

How should psychiatrists who consider conducting a study handle these concerns? Should psychiatrists enrolling their own patients in a study view risk–benefit ratios differently than researchers who do not have a doctor–patient relationship with participants? It is not clear that they are required to apply heightened scrutiny with respect to this issue, but it is certainly allowed and perhaps even expected. A psychiatrist–investigator has a duty to look out for her patient's best medical interests even when the patient has voluntarily consented to research with an understanding of the risks involved. Although participation in research will necessarily alter the clinical care that the patient is receiving, any deviation from the patient's best medical interests must be reasonable.[39]

Case B, continued

Suppose after reviewing the protocols of these trials, the psychiatry practice decides to participate in several of them. The CRO gives the practice brochures and posters to let patients know of the opportunity to participate in the trials. How should this information be displayed? The brochures and posters have a space left blank for the practice to fill in to inform patients whom to contact if they might be interested in learning more about the research. What contact should it name?

There is no single right way to inform patients and families about research studies that might interest them. Each method carries ethical advantages and pitfalls. In the case example, the practice may decide not to advertise the research protocols at all if the psychiatrists believe advertising would be viewed negatively by a significant portion of their patient base and undermine patient trust. However, this would mean instead that individual psychiatrists would have to identify and approach patients and families that they think would be appropriate participants for the study. This manner of communication carries its own risks. Patients and families so approached might misunderstand the psychiatrist's inquiry to be a recommendation for joining the study to benefit the patient rather than a call for volunteers to advance scientific knowledge. (Case C discusses this concept of "therapeutic misconception" in more detail.)

Suppose on the other hand that the practice decides to place study brochures in the waiting room and allow patients and families to approach the practice about potential participation. Should the brochures say to contact "your psychiatrist" or instead give the name of the research coordinator (assuming there is one)? Even a decision at this level of detail has ethical implications. If the patient or family speaks with the research coordinator, they may be less likely to misunderstand the patient's enrollment in research as being for her benefit. In addition, the patient and her parents are less likely to agree to participate in research to please the psychiatrist. The more distance created between the treating psychiatrist and the recruitment and informed consent process, the less potential for undue influence by the treating psychiatrist over the decisions made by patients and families about research. Indeed, some consider it essential that someone other than the treating physician obtain informed consent when the physician is also the investigator.[32,40] Of course, if the patient or parents ask the psychiatrist directly for her advice about research participation, the psychiatrist should give her recommendation as well as her rationale for, or against, participation, as discussed in more detail in Case C below.

CASE C: "THERAPEUTIC MISCONCEPTION" AND OTHER DISTORTIONS IN DECISION-MAKING

Case C

A private-practice psychiatrist receives a phone call from the mother of one of his patients to cancel her son's next appointment. The psychiatrist has been treating the 8-year-old boy for ADHD for about a year with appointments every month or every week, depending on how he is doing. His symptoms have been very difficult to manage and over the last 3 months the psychiatrist has started to suspect that the child might have comorbid bipolar disorder. The mother of the patient has expressed dismay at this possibility because her husband's father, whom she disliked, had bipolar disorder. She remains convinced that her son just has a very difficult case of ADHD.

> *In explaining why she is cancelling her appointment, the mother reports with excitement that she has found a new pediatrician for her son who has invited her to enroll him in a 12-week study of a new and promising drug for ADHD. She is convinced that this pediatrician would not have suggested enrolling her son if he did not think that it would help him. She feels somewhat vindicated that his sugges- tion means that he also believes her son has a complicated case of ADHD. She is also excited that her son is contributing to research about this difficult condition.*
>
> *The psychiatrist is concerned that it might be dangerous for the patient to be enrolled in this study because of his possible bipolar disorder. Further, the psychia- trist knows of a practical clinical trial that provides good diagnostic testing and monitoring for patients with suspected comorbid ADHD and childhood bipolar disorder. If the patient and his mother really wish to participate in research, this might be a more appropriate study. The psychiatrist might be able to facilitate his enrollment in this alternative study.*
>
> *The psychiatrist suggests to the mother that it would be a good idea to keep the scheduled appointment so that he can learn more about the study and offer his advice about her son's participation. What should he do now?*

Treating psychiatrists have important roles to play as advisors, monitors, and potential referral sources for patients and their families considering research participation.[6] In this case, the psychiatrist has an opportunity to meaningfully fulfill each of these roles. He made the right decision in convincing the mother to keep the scheduled appointment.

First, he can offer advice to the mother about the risks and benefits of her son's partic- ipation in the ADHD study, and in doing so, attempt to reduce the mother's misunder- standing about the potential benefits to her son from participation. Because of his long-term therapeutic relationship with this patient and family, the psychiatrist is uniquely positioned to recognize whether the mother is misconstruing important aspects of the study so that her assessment of risks and potential benefits is distorted. The mother's own description of the ADHD study reveals that she has confused the pediatrician's invi- tation to volunteer for research as an individualized recommendation made in the best interests of her child. The potential for this sort of confusion between research and medical care, which is termed "the therapeutic misconception",[41–44] is heightened in practice-based studies such as this one because the mother is looking to the pediatrician specifically to provide medical care for her son. Although desperation does not always lead to therapeutic misconception or compromised informed consent,[45] the desperation this mother seems to be experiencing can further feed therapeutic misconception and motivate her to enroll her son in research on the basis of unrealistic hopes about novel interventions, even though the prospect for benefit is both small and uncertain.

In addition to giving general advice about the purposes and conduct of research, this psychiatrist appears well-positioned, by virtue of his established relationship with the patient and his mother and his unique insight regarding the boy's condition, to offer more specific advice about participation in the ADHD study. The psychiatrist should ask the mother to bring the consent form for the study to her son's appoint- ment. In addition to the consent form, the psychiatrist may feel it necessary to contact the pediatrician for more information, to review a copy of the protocol, or to consult the relevant literature. If the psychiatrist believes that the child should not be enrolled in the study, the reasons for this recommendation should be communicated clearly to the patient's mother and the pediatrician.

Even if the patient's mother and pediatrician decide to enroll the child in the study against the psychiatrist's advice, communication by the psychiatrist to the pediatri- cian–investigator will alert him that the child may be at a higher risk for a poor outcome, prompting closer monitoring by the investigators. Ongoing communication between this patient's psychiatrist and the investigator also facilitates the resumption of clinical management after a patient's participation in a trial is complete. Professional standards for such communication are similar to those that govern relationships when treating physicians consult specialists.[46,47]

A second role that the psychiatrist might play in regards to the patient's enrollment in the ADHD study is that of monitoring the patient. This role seems especially important in this case because the investigator is a pediatrician, rather than a psychiatrist, and will not be providing psychiatric care. Here the psychiatrist might suggest to the patient's mother that continuing to see her son on a regular basis will enable him to monitor the boy's symptoms while he is in the study and to watch for early signs of potential worsening. If withdrawal from the study is advisable for the child's health, the psychiatrist will be able to advise it when timely. Further, regular appointments will allow for a smooth resumption of treatment once participation in the study is complete.

In a case like this, some psychiatrists may be tempted to use this opportunity to end their own professional relationship with this patient. Especially when treating very complicated patients whom other clinicians have abandoned, the psychiatrist may share the feelings of desperation and frustration experienced by the patient's family. However, it is important to remember that this patient still needs a doctor—a psychiatrist, in fact—perhaps even more so now.

An opposite reaction might ensue: rather than easing out of a relationship with this patient and family, the psychiatrist in this example appears interested in maintaining that relationship and in fact enrolling the patient in an alternative study that he feels is more appropriate. The psychiatrist should similarly assess the motivations driving him toward suggesting the alternative study. Some physicians express concern that patients who participate in clinical research with another physician might end up transferring all of their care to that physician. The authors are not aware of any study documenting whether this is a common occurrence. Nevertheless, it is easy to see how this concern might tempt some psychiatrists to consider conducting clinical research in their practice when they are not otherwise prepared for the responsibilities entailed in taking this important step. Although the possibility of offering more types of opportunities to their patients is a reasonable motivating factor for psychiatrists to consider conducting studies in their own practice, they still need to ensure that they can do so in an ethically responsible manner, as discussed in Cases A and B.

CASE D: CONSENT, CONFIDENTIALITY, AND PARTICIPANT SELECTION

Case D

A psychiatrist has been providing psychotherapy for a 16-year-old patient with depression for a year without the knowledge of her parents because of her concern that they would disapprove. Her parents do not believe in depression and think that prayer will solve her problems. She does well in school and has been elected student body president for next year. She plans to become a physician, potentially a psychiatrist, because she is so pleased with the help she has received. She recently read about a practical clinical trial about depression in children and adolescents which looks at differences in those who choose psychotherapy versus pharmacotherapy and their clinical courses. She discovered that her psychiatrist is helping to conduct the study. She requests to enroll in the study because she feels strongly that participating in this type of research will allow her to contribute to society and to a treatment community that has helped her. Can this patient be enrolled in the study?

This case raises the unresolved question of whether an unemancipated but mature adolescent, who can legally and ethically consent for her own mental health treatment, is also able to provide her own consent for research without parental involvement.

Informed consent requirements for research are quite formalized and explicitly stipulated in the federal regulations governing research with human participants.[48] With respect to research involving children and adolescents, these regulations follow the spirit of child assent and parental permission requirements as applied in clinical practice.[49,50] There are nevertheless important differences that stem from the differences between clinical practice and clinical research.

As a general rule, the regulations governing federally funded research require that parents or guardians give written permission before minors can participate in research.[7,51] (See **Box 2** for key definitions from the regulations and **Table 1** for a summary of regulations about allowable risk, parental permission and child assent.) Whether permission is required from one or both parents depends on the level of risk presented in the study and whether the study provides a prospect of medical benefit to the participant, as determined by the research ethics committee reviewing the study.[51,52] In addition, depending on the maturity of the minor, he or she must provide assent to participate in the research.[52] Ideally, the parental permission and assent forms, operations manual, and educational instructions that the psychiatrist receives from the study designers have been reviewed by an independent ethics review committee, and will walk investigators through these requirements.

Because requirements for assent of children and, as discussed below, the potential for enrolling adolescents in research without parental involvement, hinge on individual decision-making capacity, significant clinical judgment is required before enrolling children and adolescents in research. Although a specific age cut-off might be stipulated by the study designers and/or the ethics review committee with regard to these issues, the clinical judgments of the individuals enrolling participants are still important.[53] In general, the "rule of 7s" developed for assent in the treatment context applies to the development of capacity for, and thus necessity of, assent in the research context.[7,50] The "rule of 7s" assumes that normally children under the age of 7 years do not have the capacity to assent, that children between the ages of 7 and 14 years can give or refuse assent, and that adolescents age 14 years and up

---

Box 2
Key definitions relating to federally funded research involving child and adolescent participants.

Children are persons who have not attained the legal age for consent to treatments or procedures involved in the research, under the applicable law of the jurisdiction in which the research will be conducted.

Assent means a child's affirmative agreement to participate in research. Mere failure to object should not, absent affirmative agreement, be construed as assent.

Permission means the agreement of parent(s) or guardian to the participation of their child or ward in research.

Minimal risk means that the probability and magnitude of harm or discomfort anticipated in the research are not greater in and of themselves than those ordinarily encountered in daily life or during the performance of routine physical or psychological examinations or tests.

Data from U.S. Department of Health and Human Services: 45 C.F.R. §46.102(i) & 45 C.F.R. §46.402(a)-(d). Available at: http://www.hhs.gov/ohrp/humansubjects/guidance/45cfr46.htm#subpartd. Accessed February 26, 2009.

Table 1
Summary of key U.S. regulations applicable to federally funded research involving child and adolescent participants[a,b]

Amount of risk in protocol	Research with prospect of direct benefit for participants	Research without prospect of direct benefit for participants
No greater than minimal risk	Permissible **Parental permission:** Required of at least one parent **Child assent (if capable):** Not required if prospect of direct benefit important to the health or well-being of the child and is available only in the context of research	Permissible **Parental permission:** Required of at least one parent **Child assent (if capable):** Required
Minor increase over minimal risk	**Permissible if:** • The risk is justified by the anticipated benefit to the participant; *and* • the relation of the anticipated benefit to the risk is at least as favorable to the participants as that presented by available alternative approaches **Parental permission:** Required of at least one parent **Child assent (if capable):** Not required if prospect of direct benefit important to the health or well-being of the child and is available only in the context of the research	**Permissible if:** The intervention or procedure • presents experiences to participants that are reasonably commensurate with those inherent in their actual or expected medical, dental, psychological, social, or educational situations; *and* • is likely to yield generalizable knowledge about the participant's disorder or condition which is of vital importance for the understanding or amelioration of the disorder or condition **Parental permission:** Required of both parents **Child assent (if capable):** Required
Greater than minor increase over minimal risk		**Permissible if:** Approved by the Secretary of the U.S. Department of Health and Human Services **Parental permission:** Required of both parents **Child assent (if capable):** Required

[a] Research subject to FDA regulation must comply with a similar but different set of rules (Food and Drug Administration, Department of Health and Human Services: 21 C.F.R. §§50.50-50.56, Subpart D—Additional Safeguards for Children in Clinical Investigations. Available at: http://www.access.gpo.gov/nara/cfr/waisidx_02/21cfr50_02.html. Accessed April 8, 2009).

[b] For research subject to regulations governing federally funded research, waivers of parental permission are permitted when the research could not practically be carried out without a waiver (Department of Health and Human Services: 45 C.F.R. §§46.116(c) & (d)), or when parental permission is not a reasonable requirement to protect the subjects (for example, neglected or abused children) and an appropriate mechanism for protecting the children is substituted (Department of Health and Human Services: 45 C.F.R. §46.408(c)). Waivers are not permitted for research subject to FDA regulation (Food and Drug Administration, Department of Health and Human Services: 21 C.F.R. §50.55).

Data from Department of Health and Human Services: 45 C.F.R. §§46.401-46.408, Subpart D—Additional Protections for Children Involved as Subjects in Research. Available at: http://www.hhs.gov/ohrp/humansubjects/guidance/45cfr46.htm#subpartd. Accessed February 26, 2009.

have the cognitive capacity to participate in informed consent processes.[7] Although it is likely that many of the illnesses studied in practice-based research will not significantly affect this developmental trajectory, psychiatrists should remain aware that their patient–subject may not follow this trajectory.[8]

The ultimate question posed by this case is whether an adolescent who can legally consent to her own mental health treatment can likewise provide her own consent for related research without parental permission. The study described in the case would not require different treatment for this patient–participant than she is currently receiving; the research component primarily adds periodic structured assessments. Most ethics review committees would consider the research component of this study to involve only minimal risk, and therefore be acceptable for children. However, minimal risk alone is not enough under the federal regulations to justify a waiver of parental permission.

Unfortunately, the regulations governing federally funded research are not clear on this matter, and commentators may disagree about whether this patient may participate without parental permission. The regulations governing federally funded research do delineate certain situations in which it might be reasonable for an ethics review committee to consider waiving (under specific regulatory "waiver" provisions) the requirement for parental permission, but these provisions are quite narrow and would not apply in the case described. Further, if the study were subject to federal FDA research regulations, as are most industry-sponsored trials, waiver of parental permission is not an option.[54–56]

Some clinicians and researchers who are concerned about adolescent health have suggested another route to avoiding the requirement of parental permission: when adolescents are, under applicable state law, able to consent to treatment without parental involvement, ethics review committees should approve research without parental permission on the grounds that these adolescents are not considered children under the regulatory definition.[56–58] In particular, they suggest that ethics review committees should not require parental permission when such studies carry low risk and involve subjects about which adolescents are likely to be reluctant to share information with their parents, especially when the adolescents themselves are generally mature.[56] These suggestions are motivated by concerns that strict requirements for parental permission have hindered research aimed at improving adolescent health.[59,60] This case example is illustrative of the types of studies for which the Society for Adolescent Medicine urges more explicit federal approval for adolescent research without parental permission.[60]

In the absence of such explicit federal approval, however, and because the regulations are fairly strict, it is unclear whether an ethics review committee would, or should, approve the research participation of the 16-year-old in this case without parental permission. Simply because this patient can consent to psychotherapy under applicable state law does not mean that she is able to consent to any kind of research related to her treatment. State laws allowing unemancipated minors to receive certain forms of medical treatment without parental permission are not predicated solely on their maturity but are motivated by concerns over their health and well-being.[61] Because the research component in this study does not carry a prospect of benefit to the patient, reliance on state laws allowing adolescents to consent to mental health treatment carries some risk.

The federal Office of Human Research Protection offers some guidance on this question: "If research on a specific treatment involves solely treatments or procedures for which minors can give consent outside the research context (under applicable state and local laws, for example, research on sexually transmitted diseases or pregnancy), such individuals would not meet the definition of children. . . ."[62] Accordingly, the more that the research protocol varies from or adds to the treatment that would take place in the absence of research, the more likely adolescents would be unable to consent to the research absent parental permission. For example, periodic assessments conducted as part of the research protocol that are not much different from periodic assessments that would otherwise take place in a purely treatment relationship would be less problematic than a genetic study that is merely related to the research.

In another potential wrinkle, although this patient is currently only receiving psychotherapy and would continue to do so under the research protocol, the study also includes an arm of adolescents receiving medication. If state law allows minors to consent only to mental health treatment involving counseling and therapy, and requires parental permission for medication,[63,64] this restriction would likely factor into the ethics review committee's decision whether to approve or disapprove the enrollment of any adolescents without parental permission. Because adolescents in such jurisdictions who did not wish to involve their parents in treatment decisions could only be legally assigned to one arm of the study, a bias sufficient to diminish the study's scientific merit might be introduced.

A treating psychiatrist considering whether to enroll adolescents in research without parental permission should first consider whether the protocol design has already accounted for situations like this. The ethics review committee reviewing the protocol may have already determined that a waiver of parental permission for all research participants in the study is appropriate or have approved a process whereby an individual subject's eligibility to participate (based on qualifications of maturity relevant to applicable state law) can be assessed. Treating psychiatrists who consider enrolling their adolescent patients in research should be alert for these types of situations and, when their clinical judgment suggests that it might be appropriate, should know when to inquire whether such waivers are possible. However, even when an ethics review committee approves a certain protocol for adolescent consent without parental permission this does not mean the psychiatrist–investigator's ethical duties are complete. Before proceeding, the psychiatrist will want to make sure that the review contains a reasoned explanation for its determination that parental permission is not required under the regulations. Secondly, she still must evaluate the appropriateness of receiving consent from this particular patient–participant, considering capacity to understand, voluntariness, and possibility of therapeutic misconception.

CASE E: GENETIC RESEARCH AND INFORMATION SHARING

Case E

A psychiatrist has enrolled a 12-year-old patient in a longitudinal cohort study of the development and progression of childhood obsessive-compulsive disorder (OCD). This study allows medications to be prescribed as needed and collects data on symptoms and functional status every six months. DNA samples are collected and stored in a repository for genetic substudies for which separate parental permission and assent, when appropriate, are obtained.

A substudy assessing the association between the serotonin transporter gene and symptoms of OCD is proposed. The protocol stipulates that genetic results will not routinely be reported back to families or treating psychiatrists; however, specific requests for genetic information will be considered and handled through the treating psychiatrist. As the psychiatrist explains this part of the protocol to the child's parents, they suggest that they would like to receive any information that might be interesting or useful to them. How should the psychiatrist respond?

Clarification of the genetic bases of psychiatric disorders and treatment responses promises to improve diagnosis and treatment and launch important preventive efforts. Thus, genetic research proceeds apace, sometimes in practice-based studies. The pharmaceutical industry is very interested in learning how genes responsible for drug metabolism might affect drug safety in certain individuals, and indeed, so are we all. Identification of individuals for whom prevention or early intervention might avert disease promises to revolutionize what is considered medical care. Personalized medicine always seems to be just around the corner.

The addition of genetic components to almost every type of clinical research from observational, epidemiological studies to randomized controlled trials makes urgent the need for psychiatrists to become fluent in the relevant scientific, clinical, and ethical dimensions of genetic research, and to learn how to help their patients navigate through the promise and potential perils of participating in genetic research. The authors are not able to provide a comprehensive review of these issues in the space here; however, good overviews are available.[65–67] Here, just one specific issue is discussed: how psychiatrists should respond when patients or families ask for genetic research results.

In this case, the protocol provides that the investigators will not share genetic results unless a specific request comes from the patient or family, through the psychiatrist. On the face of it, the request by these parents seems relatively benign: after all, anyone can obtain a full genetic profile through 23andMe for less than $500.[68] In reality, however, this request should prompt a careful and thorough discussion about the kinds of information that might be obtained, what might be appropriate to provide to the parents, and whether the parents would really want any of it.

Ethicists and geneticists generally agree that genetic results should not be given to patients unless they provide clinically meaningful information, the results reveal a risk of disease or disorder that is considerable, and intervention is possible.[67,69,70] Yet, even sharing results that have some predictive power can be ethically problematic— carrying risks of labeling or damage to self-image, guilt on the part of parents, or unnecessary stress through misunderstanding. The serotonin transporter gene is a promising area for genetic research in OCD[71] and it is also implicated in other psychiatric and nonpsychiatric areas.[72–75] However, although this research may lead to potentially interesting findings, many reported genetic risk factors for psychiatric disorders have been subsequently disproved, as have genetic associations in many areas. Under this analysis, participants in psychiatric genetic studies should rarely be given back research findings, even ones as seemingly useful as these.[67]

Ravitsky and Wilfond propose that a research participant's genetic results should be revealed only if they are clinically useful (ie, they can be used to improve a person's well-being).[70] Clinical utility requires consideration of: the clinical validity of the results (to determine if sufficient proof of an association between a genotype and particular clinical outcome exists); the likelihood that the expected clinical outcome of disclosure of the results will be safe and effective (is there treatment available or prevention strategies?); and the value of that outcome to the individual (in making reproductive decisions, for example, or life plans).[70] Lavieri and Garner emphasize that the best person to assess the value of the outcome for the individual is the individual him- or herself.[76]

The fact that the participant in this genetic study is an adolescent makes it even less likely that an ethical analysis would support returning his genetic information.[77–79] This conclusion is true for both research results and for so-called incidental findings.[67,70,80] Incidental findings could be as far-ranging as misattributed paternity or the genetic marker for Huntington's disease. Sharing such findings could have enormous implications for this entire family. Determining an ethically defensible manner in which to proceed is a staple in the ethics literature related to genetic testing and counseling.[67,81–83]

How might the psychiatrist in Case E handle this discussion? First, she should not agree to provide genetic results that are merely interesting. The conveyance of interesting news (eg, a gene for athleticism) is not really a part of her professional role. It would be more appropriate to suggest that if she disclosed any information to them, she would limit disclosure to information that could affect the health or well-being of their child or the family. She would want to discuss the risks and benefits of obtaining even this information. For example, receiving genetic results places one at risk of needing to disclose this information on insurance forms. Loss of insurance benefits or loss of employment are risks if the results become known. State laws have, for a number of years, provided various protections against genetic discrimination, but that protection is often less than comprehensive.[67] The new federal Genetic Information Nondiscrimination Act of 2008 prohibits the use of genetic information to discriminate in health insurance and employment, but it does not address life insurance, disability insurance, or long-term care insurance.[84] Moreover, although legal protection against genetic discrimination may reduce the risk that it will take place, it does not eliminate it. If the psychiatrist in this case is not confident of her ability to discuss these types of issues, she should seek the help of a genetic counselor.

Some research protocols address, in more detail, what kinds of expected or unexpected results it may disclose to participants and how. The psychiatrist may wish to contact the investigators and determine if that is the case in this protocol. Many investigators, however, leave these decisions to the patient and psychiatrist. If this family and psychiatrist choose to go forward, care must be taken in the psychiatrist's office that this research information does not inadvertently get placed into the medical record and passed onto insurers and others who may have a legitimate request for access to medical records.

SUMMARY

Changes in the clinical research enterprise to involve practicing psychiatrists in gathering evidence in real-world settings are truly exciting. The CAPTN breaks important ground as a PBRN in psychiatry. The authors anticipate that more practical clinical trials will come. These changes challenge psychiatrists to reach an entirely new level of understanding and appreciation of the ethical and practical challenges of commingling clinical practice and research. It is time that all practicing psychiatrists prepare to meet these challenges.

ACKNOWLEDGMENTS

Dr. Chen's work in research ethics is supported in part by a grant from the National Institutes of Health (NIH) to the University of Virginia General Clinical Research Center, M01-RR000847. The opinions expressed are the authors' own. They do not reflect any position or policy of the University of Virginia or the NIH.

REFERENCES

1. Geddes J, Carney S. Recent advances in evidence-based psychiatry. Can J Psychiatry 2001;46(5):403–6.
2. Essock SM, Goldman HH, Van Tosh L, et al. Evidence-based practices: setting the context and responding to concerns. Psychiatr Clin North Am 2003;26(4):919–38.
3. March JS, Silva SG, Compton S, et al. The case for practical clinical trials in psychiatry. Am J Psychother 2005;162:836–46.

4. March JS, Silva SG, Compton S, et al. The Child and Adolescent Psychiatry Trials Network (CAPTN). J Am Acad Child Adolesc Psychiatry 2004;43(5):515–8.
5. On December 5, 2008, ClinicalTrials.gov has 65,543 trials listed with locations in 161 countries. Listed studies include phases I- IV as well as observational studies. A search on the term "child AND mental health" finds 865 studies of which 360 studies are open to recruitment. 23 of these open studies are sponsored by industry, 213 are sponsored by NIH, 17 are sponsored by other federal agencies, and 152 studies are sponsored by universities/organizations/other. Two of these studies are part of the Child and Adolescent Psychiatry Trials Network (CAPTN). Available at: http://www.cliwwwnicaltrials.gov. Accessed December 5, 2008.
6. Chen DT, Miller FG, Rosenstein DL. Clinical research and the physician-patient relationship. Ann Intern Med 2003;138(8):669–72.
7. Hoop JG, Smyth AC, Roberts LW. Ethical issues in psychiatric research on children and adolescents. Child Adolesc Psychiatr Clin N Am 2008;17(1):127–48.
8. Arnold LE. Turn-of-the-century ethical issues in child psychiatric research. Curr Psychiatry Rep 2001;3(2):109–14.
9. Hotopf M, Churchill R, Lewis G. Pragmatic randomised controlled trials in psychiatry. Br J Psychiatry 1999;175:217–23.
10. Wasserman RC, Slora EJ, Bocian AB, et al. Pediatric research in office settings (PROS): a national practice-based research network to improve children's health care. Pediatrics 1998;102(6):1350–7.
11. Green LA, Wood M, Becker L, et al. The Ambulatory Sentinel Practice Network: purpose, methods, and policies. J Fam Pract 1984;18(2):275–80.
12. For up-to-date information and examples, see homepage of AHRQ Practice-Based Research Networks. Available at: http://pbrn.ahrq.gov/portal/server.pt. Accessed December 10, 2008.
13. For up-to-date information about contract/clinical research organizations, see the website for the Association of Clinical Research Organizations. Available at: http://www.acrohealth.org/. Accessed December 10, 2008.
14. Rettig RA. The industrialization of clinical research. Health Aff (Millwood). 2000; 19(2):129–46.
15. Wadman M. The quiet rise of the clinical contractor. Nature 2006;441(7089):22–3.
16. Shuchman M. Commercializing clinical trials–risks and benefits of the CRO boom. N Engl J Med 2007;357(14):1365–8.
17. Chen DT, Worrall BB. Practice-based clinical research and ethical decision making–Part I: deciding whether to incorporate practice-based research into your clinical practice. Semin Neurol 2006;26(1):131–9.
18. Chen DT, Worrall BB. Practice-based clinical research and ethical decision making–Part II: deciding whether to host a particular research study in your practice. Semin Neurol 2006;26(1):140–7.
19. Wolf LE, Walden JF, Lo B. Human subjects issues and IRB review in practice-based research. Ann Fam Med 2005;3(Suppl 1):S30–7.
20. Graham DG, Spano MS, Manning B. The IRB challenge for practice-based research: strategies of the American Academy of Family Physicians National Research Network (AAFP NRN). J Am Board Fam Med 2007;20(2):181–7.
21. Excellent overviews and educational materials are available at the Clinical Trials Networks Best Practices website. Available at: https://www.ctnbestpractices.org/. Accessed December 10, 2008.
22. Beach JE. Clinical trials integrity: a CRO perspective. Account Res 2001;8(3):245–60.
23. Snyder L, Mueller PS. Research in the physician's office: navigating the ethical minefield. Hastings Cent Rep 2008;38(2):23–5.

24. Gray T. Getting the most out of community-based research. ACP Observer 2004. Available at: http://www.acpinternist.org/archives/2004/04/cbr.htm. Accessed December 10, 2008.

25. Klein JE, Fleischman AR. The private practicing physician-investigator: ethical implications of clinical research in the office setting. Hastings Cent Rep 2002;32:22–6.

26. Eichenwald K, Kolata G. Drug trials hide conflicts for doctors. New York Times (print) 1999;1:34. Available at: http://www.nytimes.com/1999/05/16/business/drug-trials-hide-conflicts-for-doctors.html%sec=health. Accessed February 24, 2009.

27. Zuckerman G. Biovail is paying physicians prescribing new heart drug. Wall St J July 21, 2003. Available at: http://wsj.com/article/SB105874152264f463400.html?med=americas_business_whats_news. Accessed February 24, 2009.

28. Harris G, Carey B, Roberts J. Psychiatrists, children, and drug industry's role. New York Times May 10, 2007. Available at: http://www.nytimes.com/2007/05/10psyche.html. Accessed February 24, 2009.

29. Harris G, Carey B. Researchers fail to reveal full drug pay. New York Times. June 8 2008. Available at: http://www.nytimes.com. Accessed February 24, 2009.

30. CEJA Report 2 – I-94, Finder's fees: payment for the referral of patients to clinical research Studies. Available at: http://www.ama-assn.org/ama1/pub/upload/mm/369/ceja_2i94.pdf. Accessed December 10, 2008.

31. American Academy of Child and Adolescent Psychiatry. AACAP guidelines on conflict of interest for child and adolescent psychiatrists. Available at: http://www.aacap.org/galleries/transparency-portal/Council%20Approved%20COI%20Guidelines%20for%20Practitioners%201-30-2009.pdf. Accessed February 24, 2009.

32. Morin K, Rakatansky H, Riddick FA Jr, et al. Managing conflicts of interest in the conduct of clinical trials. JAMA 2002;287(1):78–84.

33. Werhane P, Doering J. Conflicts of interest and conflicts of commitment. Prof Ethics 1995;4:47–81.

34. Miller FG, Rosenstein DL, DeRenzo EG. Professional integrity in clinical research. JAMA 1998;280(16):1449–54.

35. Roberts LW, Geppert CM, Brody JL. A framework for considering the ethical aspects of psychiatric research protocols. Compr Psychiatry 2001;42(5):351–63.

36. Emanuel EJ, Wendler D, Grady C. What makes clinical research ethical? JAMA 2000;283(20):2701–11.

37. Noah BA. Bioethical malpractice: risk and responsibility in human research. J Health Care Law Pol 2004;7(2):175–241.

38. Joffe S, Truog RD. Equipoise and randomization. In: Emanuel EJ, Grady C, Crouch RA, et al, editors. The Oxford textbook of clinical research ethics. New York: Oxford University Press; 2008. p. 245–52.

39. Coleman CH. Duties to subjects in clinical research. Vanderbilt Law Rev 2005;58: 387–449.

40. World Medical Association. Declaration of Helsinki. 2008. Available at: http://www.wma.net/e/policy/b3.htm. Accessed December 10, 2008.

41. Kimmelman J. The therapeutic misconception at 25: treatment, research, and confusion. Hastings Cent Rep 2007;37(6):36–42.

42. Dresser R. The ubiquity and utility of the therapeutic misconception. Soc Philos Policy 2002;19(2):271–94.

43. Henderson GE, Churchill LR, Davis AM, et al. Clinical trials and medical care: defining the therapeutic misconception. PLoS Med 2007;4(11):e324.

44. Appelbaum PS, Roth LH, Lidz CW, et al. False hopes and best data: consent to research and the therapeutic misconception. Hastings Cent Rep 1987;17(2):20–4.

45. Miller FG, Joffe S. Benefit in phase 1 oncology trials: therapeutic misconception or reasonable treatment option? Clin Trials 2008;5(6):617–23.
46. Emanuel LL, Richter J. The consultant and the patient–physician relationship. A trilateral deliberative model. Arch Intern Med 1994;154:1785–90.
47. Stoeckle JD, Ronan LJ, Emanuel LL, et al. A manual on manners and courtesies for the shared care of patients. J Clin Ethics 1997;8:22–33.
48. Department of Health and Human Services. 45 CFR §46.116 and 45 CFR §46.117. Available at: http://www.hhs.gov/ohrp/humansubjects/guidance/45cfr46.htm. Accessed April 9, 2009.
49. Department of Health and Human Services. 45 CFR §46.408 (2008). Available at: http://www.hhs.gov/ohrp/humansubjects/guidance/45cfr46.htm. Accessed April 9, 2009.
50. Committee on Bioethics, American Academy of Pediatrics. Informed consent, parental permission, and assent in pediatric practice. Pediatrics 1995;95(2):314–7.
51. Department of Health and Human Services. 45 CFR §46.408(b) and (d) (2008). Available at: http://www.hhs.gov/ohrp/humansubjects/guidance/45cfr46.htm. Accessed April 9, 2009.
52. Department of Health and Human Services. 45 CFR §46.408(a). Available at: http://www.hhs.gov/ohrp/humansubjects/guidance/45cfr46.htm. Accessed April 9, 2009.
53. Kuther TL, Posada M. Children and adolescents' capacity to provide informed consent for participation in research. Adv Psychol Res 2004;32:163–73.
54. Food and Drug Administration, Department of Health and Human Services, 21 C.F.R. §50.55.
55. In brief, waivers are only permitted when the research could not practically be carried out without a waiver (45 C.F.R. §46.116(c) & (d)), or when parental permission is not a reasonable requirement to protect the subjects (for example, neglected or abused children) and an appropriate mechanism for protecting the children is substituted (45 C.F.R. §46.408(c)).
56. Collagan LK, Fleischman AR. Adolescent research and parental permission. In: Kodish E, editor. Ethics and research with children. New York: Oxford University Press; 2005. p. 77–99.
57. Campbell AT. State regulations of medical research with children and adolescents: an overview and analysis. In: Field MJ, Behrman RE, editors. Ethical conduct of clinical research involving children. a report of the Institute of Medicine. Washington, DC: National Academies Press; 2004. p. 320–87.
58. Children are defined in the regulations as "persons who have not attained the legal age for consent to treatments or procedures involved in the research, under the applicable law of the jurisdiction in which the research will be conducted." 45 CFR §46.402(a) (2008).
59. Katzman DK. Guidelines for adolescent health research. J Adolesc Health 2003; 33(5):410–5.
60. Santelli JS, Rogers AS, Rosenfeld WD, et al. Guidelines for adolescent health research: a position paper of the Society for Adolescent Medicine. J Adolesc Health 2003;33(5):396–409.
61. Glantz LH. Research with children. Am J Law Med 1998;24:213–44.
62. Department of Health and Human Services, Office for Human Research Protections, OHRP Research Involving Children Frequently Asked Questions, Question 17. Available at: http://www.hhs.gov/ohrp/researchfaq.html. Accessed April 9, 2009.
63. Campbell AT. Consent, competence, and confidentiality related to psychiatric conditions in adolescent medicine practice. Adolesc Med Clin 2006;17(1):25–47.

64. See, e.g., Cal Fam Code §6924 (2008) (psychotropic drugs); Florida Stat §394.4784 (2008) (any medication); Ohio Rev Code Ann (2008) §5122.04 (any medication). See generally Vukadinovich DM. Minors' rights to consent to treatment: navigating the complexity of state laws. J Health Law 2004;37(4):667–91.
65. Nuffield Council on Bioethics. Mental disorders and genetics: the ethical context. London: Nuffield Council on Bioethics; 1998.
66. Farmer AE, Owen MJ, McGuffin P. Bioethics and genetic research in psychiatry. Br J Psychiatry 2000;176:105–8.
67. Appelbaum PS. Ethical issues in psychiatric genetics. J Psychiatr Pract 2004; 10(6):343–51.
68. 23andMe Home Page. Available at: https://www.23andme/.com. Accessed on December 12, 2008 when the cost was $399, and a "family special" was being offered with a savings of $200.
69. Burke W, Pinsky LE, Press NA. Categorizing genetic tests to identify their ethical, legal, and social implications. Am J Med Genet 2001;106(3):233–40.
70. Ravitsky V, Wilfond BS. Disclosing individual genetic results to research participants. Am J Bioeth 2006;6(6):8–17.
71. Bloch MH, Landeros-Weisenberger A, Sen S, et al. Association of the serotonin transporter polymorphism and obsessive-compulsive disorder: systematic review. Am J Med Genet B Neuropsychiatr Genet 2008;147B(6):850–8.
72. Caspi A, Sugden K, Moffitt TE, et al. Influence of life stress on depression: moderation by a polymorphism in the 5-HTT gene. Science 2003;301(5631):386–9.
73. Prasad HC, Steiner JA, Sutcliffe JS, et al. Enhanced activity of human serotonin transporter variants associated with autism. Philos Trans R Soc Lond B Biol Sci 2009;364(1514):163–73.
74. Camilleri M, Busciglio I, Carlson P, et al. Candidate genes and sensory functions in health and irritable bowel syndrome. Am J Physiol Gastrointest Liver Physiol 2008;295(2):G219–25.
75. Kronenberg S, Frisch A, Rotberg B, et al. Pharmacogenetics of selective serotonin reuptake inhibitors in pediatric depression and anxiety. Pharmacogenomics 2008;9(11):1725–36.
76. Lavieri RR, Garner SA. Ethical considerations in the communication of unexpected information with clinical implications. Am J Bioeth 2006;6(6):46–8.
77. American Society of Human Genetics Board of Directors, American College of Medical Genetics Board of Directors. Points to consider: ethical, legal, and psychosocial implications of genetic testing in children and adolescents. Am J Hum Genet 1995;57(5):1233–41.
78. Nelson RM, Botkjin JR, Kodish ED, et al. Committee on Bioethics. Ethical issues with genetic testing in pediatrics. Pediatrics 2001;107(6):1451–5.
79. Stevenson DA, Strasburger VC. Advise or consent? Issues in genetic testing of adolescents. Adolesc Med 2002;13(2):213–21.
80. Cho MK. Understanding incidental findings in the context of genetics and genomics. J Law Med Ethics 2008;36(2):280–5.
81. Ensenauer RE, Michels VV, Reinke SS. Genetic testing: practical, ethical, and counseling considerations. Mayo Clin Proc 2005;80(1):63–73.
82. Lucassen A, Parker M. Revealing false paternity: some ethical considerations. Lancet 2001;357(9261):1033–5.
83. Lilani A. Ethical issues and policy analysis for genetic testing: Huntington's disease as a paradigm for diseases with a late onset. Hum Reprod Genet Ethics 2005;11(2):28–34.
84. Public Law 110–233 (2008).

Ethical Issues in Psychiatric Research

Liliana Kalogjera Barry, JD[a,b],*

KEYWORDS

- Ethics • Psychiatric research • Informed consent
- Human subjects • Mental illness research

BACKGROUND: THE NEED FOR RESEARCH

Many individuals suffer from mental illness. The National Institutes of Mental Health Web site highlights the following statistics pertaining to the prevalence of mental disorders in the United States[1]:

- Approximately 26% of adult Americans—or approximately 57.7 million people, based on the 2004 U.S. census—experience a mental disorder annually.
- Approximately 1 in 17 of adult Americans who suffer from a mental disorder suffers from a serious mental illness.
- Mental disorders are the leading cause of disability in the United States and Canada for persons age 15 to 44 years.
- Major depressive disorder is the leading cause of disability in the United States for ages persons age 15 to 44 years.
- In 2004, 32,439 people (approximately 11 per 100,000 population) died by suicide in the United States.
- More than 90% of people who commit suicide have a diagnosable mental disorder.
- Approximately 3.5% of adult Americans experience posttraumatic stress disorder per year.

These statistics provide just a few examples of the impact of mental illness in the United States. Individuals who suffer from mental illness experience this impact both in terms of their own health and in terms of their relationships with others, whether

The content of this article is the responsibility of the author alone and does not reflect the views or policies of the United States Department of Veterans Affairs, nor does mention of trade names, commercial products, or organizations imply endorsement by the United States.

[a] Department of Psychiatry and Behavioral Medicine, Medical College of Wisconsin, 8701 Watertown Plank Road, Milwaukee, WI 53226, USA

[b] United States Department of Veterans Affairs, Office of Regional Counsel, Regional Office, 5400 W. National Avenue, Milwaukee, WI 53214, USA

* Corresponding author. United States Department of Veterans Affairs, Office of Regional Counsel, Regional Office, 5400 W. National Avenue, Milwaukee, WI 53214.
E-mail address: liliana.kalogjera@va.gov

Psychiatr Clin N Am 32 (2009) 381–394
doi:10.1016/j.psc.2009.02.003
0193-953X/09/$ – see front matter. Published by Elsevier Inc.

through the direct and indirect effects of a general social stigma or through the more immediate challenges that mental illness creates for interpersonal relationships with friends and family. In addition, mental disorders are associated with substantial socio-economic costs, which have been estimated to exceed $150 billion annually.[2]

INTRODUCTION TO RESEARCH ETHICS

Because mental illness touches so many lives and with various adverse effects—emotional, physical, economic—there remains a great need for increased under-standing of mental illness through psychiatric research. Ethical conduct of this research, however, must incorporate both the general framework for research involving human subjects and a unique understanding of the ethical issues specific to psychiatric research.

General Research Ethics

The ethical foundation for the conduct of research involving human subjects arose, in part, as a reaction to research abuses that spanned the twentieth century. The Nazis, for example, conducted abhorrent experiments on Jewish people, mentally ill individ-uals, and member of other targeted groups, under the guise of scientific research.[3] This "research," utterly disregarded for the humanity of participants and exploited both the participants involved and the institution of scientific research. As a result, the Nuremberg Code emerged in 1947 from the trial of war criminals who conducted these studies.[4] The Nuremberg Code sets forth various ethical principles that helped form the foundation for the field of research ethics. These principles include the following requirements: (1) the participant's voluntary informed consent; (2) the likeli-hood that the study will produce fruitful results; (3) minimization of the physical and mental suffering and risk to the participant, (4) the proportionality of the study's risk to the importance of the problem examined by the research; (5) the requirement that scientifically qualified individuals conduct the research; (6) the participant's freedom to terminate his or her participation during the study; and (7) the investigator's willingness to terminate the study if he or she has reason to believe that continuation is likely to lead to great harm to the participant(s).[4] In the Declaration of Helsinki, first published in 1964 and amended numerous times since, the World Medical Association echoed these principles and expanded on their meaning in terms of the ethical duties of physicians to patients.[5]

The United States has its own unfortunate history of research abuses, which came to light largely through a groundbreaking article published by Beecher in the *New England Journal of Medicine* in 1966.[6] Beecher's article exposed various research studies conducted at academic and other major medical centers in the United States that exemplified unethical treatment of human participants, including the performance of studies that lacked therapeutic value. For example, some studies involved deliber-ately attempting to "give" participants a disease, such as by inducing hepatitis in patients at an "institution for mentally defective children." Other studies involved with-holding treatment and observing the natural progression of disease, such as rheu-matic fever and typhoid fever. Beecher noted that only 2 of the 50 studies he reviewed in connection with the article discussed informed consent. He identified investigator responsibility as being a "more dependable" safeguard than informed consent, however.

Despite Beecher's call for reform in research practices, abuses continued in the United States, with the Tuskegee Syphilis Study representing decades of unethical treatment of research participants.[7] This study's formal title was the "Tuskegee Study of Untreated Syphilis in the Negro Male," and it lasted from 1932 to 1972. As its name suggests, the primary purpose of the study was to observe untreated syphilis among black, male participants; researchers withheld treatment when it became widely available in 1947, and participants were not informed of the full nature of their participation or of the possibility of treatment. The egregiousness of this study was so great that President Clinton formally apologized on behalf of the United States in 1997, prompting some concerns that the apology may result in the unintended consequence of further decline in trust and research participation by African Americans.[8]

The United States Government conducted its own ethically flawed research, using human subjects in studies examining the effects of ionizing radiation.[9] Like the Tuskegee Syphilis Study, these experiments spanned decades, from 1944 to 1974.

These research abuses contributed to the United States' development of regulatory responses and ethical pronouncements. In 1974, the predecessor to the US Department of Health and Human Services (DHHS) published a federal regulatory framework for the protection of human participants in research.[10] These regulations included the requirement that every federally funded research entity have an Institutional Review Board (IRB) to oversee the conduct of research at the local level.[11] Following the promulgation of these and other agency-specific regulations, 16 federal agencies adopted the Common Rule, which essentially applies the DHHS regulations codified at 45 CFR §46 as federal policy.[12] Currently, the Office of Human Research Protections of the DHHS, which serves to protect the rights and well-being of research participants, maintains oversight of IRBs to ensure that federally funded research is ethical and safe.[13]

Complementing the United States' regulatory framework for research is its own body of ethical commentary. In1979, the National Commission for the Protection of Human Subjects of Biomedical and Behavioral Research published the Belmont Report, an articulation of the key ethical principles for conducting research with human participants.[14] These principles, which continue to serve as the foundation of research ethics, consist of: (1) respect for persons, (2) beneficence, and (3) justice. Respect for persons involves honoring the autonomy of an individual to deliberate upon and act according to his/her goals and protecting the autonomy of each individual who lacks complete autonomy. In the case of psychiatric research, this principle involves special efforts to ensure that participants who have impaired decision-making capacity consent to participate in the research in a manner that is truly informed and voluntary. Beneficence involves acting to "do good" for participants or to act for their well-being while also taking steps to avoid and minimize harm (ie, nonmaleficence). These concepts of beneficence and nonmaleficence commonly are understood as expressed in the Hippocratic oath and, thus, extend a physician's duties from the typical doctor–patient relationship to the context of clinical research. Justice involves fairness in the distribution of the burdens (eg, risks) of research and in access to its fruits. The Tuskegee Syphilis Study is an example in which one group, black males, bore a disproportionate burden of the risks of research.

In the spirit of the Belmont Report, various national commissions have addressed particular ethical issues in research. Some of these issues have been associated with specific scientific advances in areas such as genetics and reproduction. Others address vulnerable research populations, such as prisoners and children.[15]

Ethics of Psychiatric Research

Although psychiatric research involves the ethical considerations common to biomedical research, psychiatric research also has its own set of ethical concerns. Initial discussions about ethical issues in psychiatric research focused on the threshold issue of whether research involving persons who have mental illness ever could be performed in an ethical manner. The existence and continued development of the field of psychiatric research ethics, however, represents a paradigm shift from the question of whether to conduct psychiatric research to how to conduct it in an ethical manner.

The President's Commission for the Protection of Human Subjects of Biomedical and Behavioral Research provided some guidance in its 1981 report.[16] Unlike the Commission's recommendations regarding pregnant women, prisoners, and children, however, its guidance pertaining to people who have mental illness did not lead promptly to corresponding federal regulation.[17] Pursuant to an executive order by President Clinton, the National Bioethics Advisory Commission (NBAC) issued its report on "Research Involving Persons with Mental Disorders that May Affect Decision-Making Capacity" in 1998.[15,18] This comprehensive report identified key ethical issues pertaining to research involving this population, ranging from the planning phase (eg, which values should guide such research and how researchers should design such studies) to clarification of the informed consent process for this population and the role of surrogate decision-makers. In addition, to further the dual goals of facilitating such research and protecting participants, the report outlined 21 robust recommendations for the conduct and oversight of such research. This report was controversial because of concerns about its potential to stigmatize this population and either hamper research unduly or protect participants inadequately.[19]

The continued need for understanding and guidance in this area led the psychiatric profession to examine these issues and to issue its own recommendations through the formation of the American Psychiatric Association's (APA's) Task Force on Research Ethics ("Task Force") in 2001.[2] This entity illustrates the recognition of the unique nature of ethical issues in psychiatric research (ie, in contrast to biomedical research generally) and the psychiatric profession's commitment to addressing these issues adequately.

KEY CONCEPTS AND SAFEGUARDS

As a result of efforts of the NBAC, the APA, and others, there is greater clarity regarding the ethical issues associated with psychiatric research and the necessary safeguards for conducting such research in an appropriate manner.

Psychiatric research raises unique ethical concerns because of two key characteristics of mental illness. First, people who have mental illness are, in general, a uniquely vulnerable population.[17] In addition to the immediate effects of mental illness on an individual's physical and mental health and well-being, mental illness has the inherent potential to interfere with an individual's ability to make truly informed, voluntary decisions with regard to participation.[11] Because informed consent is a fundamental aspect of the ethical conduct of research, this potential disability creates profound challenges for researchers and the need for more robust safeguards. Second, mental illness carries its own unique stigma, which affects the ethical requirements for research in a variety of ways. By definition, stigma marginalizes individuals. In the case of people who have mental illness, this marginalization may translate into reduced social support and resources for accessing the political system.[2] The stigma surrounding mental illness also may raise concerns regarding the principle of justice, because stigma may (1) lead to unwarranted, discriminatory exclusion from study participation,[2] and (2) exert an improper influence on research priorities and funding. In addition, because of its potential to cause harm, stigma can create heightened obligations for researchers in terms of confidentiality and the protection of participants' privacy.

Because of these ethical issues, the field of psychiatric research warrants the emphasis on a distinct set of safeguards, in addition to those common to research generally, to protect participants. These safeguards represent pragmatic efforts to honor the principles set forth in the Belmont Report—respect for persons, beneficence, and justice—when conducting research involving persons who have mental illness. These safeguards aim to protect participants at all stages of the research process, ranging from the prestudy phase (eg, initial study design), to the study itself (eg, the informed consent process), to the poststudy phase (eg, publication of research results). **Table 1** illustrates the role of these safeguards in case examples.

Study Design and Recruitment

As an initial matter, safeguards include ethical requirements for study design and recruitment. Each study should investigate a valuable question, about which there exists genuine uncertainty or equipoise,[20] in a scientifically valid manner (ie, in a manner reasonably likely to produce useful results).[21,22] Upholding these standards honors the principle of respect for persons, by avoiding exploitation of individuals though unnecessary exposure to risks of research that is unlikely to benefit those individuals and/or society as a whole. Attempting to benefit persons who have mental illness also furthers the interests of beneficence by striving to improve the condition of this population.[2] Beneficence also requires that a study design minimize risks, both to particular participants and generally, through the use of the least risky design among viable alternatives.[2,22] In the interest of justice, a psychiatric research study should examine a question that is relevant to people who have mental illness, that can benefit that population, and that involves the least vulnerable participants possible within that population.[2,22] In addition, an investigator's duties to participants do not end upon receipt of a signed informed consent form; rather, study design should incorporate adequate monitoring of participants and, when indicated, treatment of symptoms, mechanisms for appropriate withdrawal from the study, and follow-up care.[2]

After selecting the participant population, investigators should strive to recruit individual participants in an ethically sound manner. Ethically sound recruitment includes examination of the potential participant's motivations (eg, altruism) and understanding (eg, an accurate view of the potential for benefit from the study).[23] Investigators should take specific care to ensure that the recruitment process is free of coercion (eg, through disproportionately large financial incentives).[22,24]

Scientific and Ethical Expertise of Research Team

A comprehensive set of safeguards also should address the research team.[21] Investigators should have the expertise and willingness to carry out the study properly from scientific, regulatory (eg, within the IRB framework), and ethics perspectives.[17] The Task Force articulates these standards as both an ethical obligation of the individual researchers and as a general obligation for the psychiatric profession to educate its investigators.[2] A critical aspect of an investigator's ethical duties is a commitment to integrity through appropriate identification and management of potential and actual conflicts of interest.[21,25] These conflicts include challenges posed by the dual roles of treating physician and investigatory physician[17] and challenges stemming from financial incentives, such as those from the pharmaceutical industry, which are discussed in greater detail later in this article.

Informed Consent

The informed consent process is one of the most prominent safeguards for the ethical conduct of research, because it is a component of the foundational ethics documents,

Table 1
Case Scenarios

Scenario	Ethical Issues	Possible Approaches for Prevention/Resolution
Potential study participant lacks decision-making capacity and has an activated durable power of attorney for health care, which, under applicable state law, permits the health care agent to consent to research participation. The health care agent, who also is the potential participant's spouse, has indicated that she would like her husband to participate in the study, which includes a generous financial reward for participation and which may provide treatment benefits to the participant. Investigator is unsure whether the health care agent herself has the capacity to understand the risks, benefits, and alternatives of her husband's participation in the study.	Vulnerability of potential participant because of decisional incapacity Health care agent's potential conflict of interest between desire for financial reward and duty to act according to her husband's previously expressed wishes or in his best interests Investigator's potential conflict of interest between desire to enroll participants and the duties to recruit participants in a nonexploitative manner and to obtain informed consent of participants or their agents	Research advance directive to clarify what potential participant would have wanted IRB or other review of incentive for participation to determine whether it is excessive (ie, potentially coercive) Enhanced focus on the informed consent process involving (1) examination of whether health care agent has the ability to provide informed consent, and (2) pursuant to confidentiality requirements, consultation with others who have knowledge of potential participant's prior express wishes
Initial data collected during study reveal a rare but significant side effect of a psychiatric clinical intervention. Investigator, a resident, does not realize that this data may warrant notification of current participants and the IRB of this potential risk and revision of informed consent forms.	Lack of scientific and ethical expertise of investigator Inadequate informed consent process (ie, failure to identify and disclose potential risks) Duty to warn current participants of potential harm	Improved scientific and ethics training IRB or other oversight Notification and appropriate treatment and monitoring of current participants Revision of informed consent forms to include the recently discovered side effect
Investigator, who is working from home for the day, decides to analyze participant data, including various personal identifiers (eg, name and Social Security Number) and psychiatric diagnosis, on his/her personal computer via a non-password-protected WiFi network. The investigator's neighbor is able to hack into the network and access sensitive participant information.	Investigator's duty of due care to protect the confidentiality of participants' information Lack of technical expertise of investigator Vulnerability of participants to social stigma and emotional harm through improper disclosure of their personal information	Improved training regarding protection of confidential information and physical and technical safeguards Disclosure of potential privacy breaches as part of informed consent process Disclosure of breach and provision of counseling to participants whose privacy may have been compromised

including the Nuremberg Code, Declaration of Helsinki, Belmont Report, and Common Rule. The Belmont Report distills the concept of informed consent into three elements: information, comprehension (which is referred to here in the broader sense as "decisional capacity"), and voluntariness.[14] Fulfilling the requirements of the informed consent process can prove particularly challenging in the context of psychiatric research because of the inherent nature of mental illness.

Albeit obvious, the type and quality of information that investigators provide to participants is of paramount importance to the informed consent process. The information provided to participants should include information regarding the nature and purpose of the study, reasonably anticipated risks and benefits, alternatives to participating in the study along with the anticipated outcomes of each alterative, conflicts of interest, and any other information that a "reasonable volunteer" would like to know to decide whether to participate in a study.[14,17]

Information alone is insufficient, however, and decisional capacity is critical for processing the information in a meaningful way.[14,17] Decisional capacity consists of the the ability to communicate a preference, the ability to understand or comprehend the information that is relevant to the decision, the ability to think rationally or to reason about the decision, and the ability to understand or appreciate the decision and its impact in the context of the individual's life.[26] The determination of decisional capacity is highly particularized and potentially dynamic and may require reassessment of the individual's participation at a subsequent point in the study. The required level of decision-making capacity depends on the nature of the decision to be made, and a participant may be capable of making a simple treatment decision but lack the capacity to process the risks, benefits, alternatives, and other information necessary to make the decision to participate in a research study.[17]

Individuals who lack decision-making capacity still may participate in psychiatric research in an ethical manner through appropriate alternatives, including the use of surrogate decision-makers and advance directives for psychiatric research.[17] Although such alternatives may be particularly important in the case of an individual whom a court has declared legally incompetent, it may be appropriate for investigators to explore consent through a surrogate decision-maker, consistent with legal requirements and additional safeguards, in the case of any individual who lacks decision-making capacity.

The two primary standards for surrogate decision-making consist of either "substituted judgment"—that is, the choice that the individual would have wanted if he/she could express his/her wishes—or the individual's "best interests"—that is, the choice that the surrogate believes would further the well-being of the individual[17] Because the substituted judgment approach aims to make the decision in a manner consistent with the potential participant's preferences and beliefs and thus attempts to promotes the patient's autonomy, this approach is preferable to the "best interests" standard (provided that the surrogate's estimation of the individual's preferences is possible). The Task Force has endorsed states' facilitation of the use of surrogate decision-makers for adults who lack full decision-making capacity, provided that the surrogate decision-makers act according to standards that parallel United States federal regulations restricting research involving children.[2]

Another alternative is to honor an individual's advance directive for psychiatric research, if a valid one exists. Like all advance directives, these documents express an individual's preferences about specific decisions, such as whether a person would ever wish to receive ventilator support or artificial nutrition and hydration, in anticipation of a time when these decisions must be made and the individual is unable to express his/her preferences. An individual also may use an advance directive to express his/her preferences regarding participation in research, either by incorporating language addressing these preferences in a general advance directive or by executing a specific advance directive for research purposes. For psychiatric research in particular, a psychiatric research advance directive also may address specific aspects of the study, such as the acceptability of rescue medication or involuntary hospitalization.[17] State policies and laws pertaining to research advance directives vary widely, however. For example, Wisconsin law prohibits a health care agent from consenting to experimental mental health research,[27] and Maryland and New York have promoted a requirement that, to participate in research, adults who have cognitive impairment have completed a research advance directive while competent.[28,29] In addition to interstate variation, another significant issue involving research advance directives is the concern that a general statement regarding consent to research participation may not be sufficient evidence for consent to participate in research involving a higher degree of risk.[28]

In its simplest interpretation, voluntarism, the third element of the informed consent process, means that participation in research occurs without coercion.[22] The absence of voluntarism may be obvious in the examples of participants who lack physical and or legal liberties, such as individuals who are institutionalized or prisoners.[30] In the context of current psychiatric research in the United States, however, voluntarism requires a more nuanced understanding, such as "the individual's ability to act in accordance with one's authentic sense of what is good, right and best in light of one's situation, values, and prior history."[30] To assess this more expansive concept of voluntarism, one model uses a four-pronged approach, which considers the following types of factors: developmental considerations (eg, children's cognitive inability to make complex decisions); illness-related considerations (eg, impaired judgment caused by psychotic or substance abuse disorders); psychological, cultural, and religious considerations (eg, refusal of treatment because of beliefs, as by a Christian Scientist); and external considerations (eg, financial incentives).[30] This framework provides some guidance in determining whether participants who have mental illness have the capacity to participate voluntarily in research, a determination that may involve a inquiry distinct from the determination of an individual's ability to make a decision about participation.

Confidentiality

The concept of confidentiality has deep roots in the medical profession, as seen in its expression in the Hippocratic oath.[31] Confidentiality is a privilege (eg, between a treating physician and patient) in which at least one party agrees to uphold the other's right to privacy by not disclosing his/her information without that individual's permission. Confidentiality is both an ethical and a legal concept,[22] and legal requirements exist at the state and federal levels. Perhaps the most prominent and widely applicable of these requirements are the Privacy Rule regulations issued by the DHHS pursuant to the Health Insurance Portability and Accountability Act of 1996, which apply specific privacy protections to the research context.[32] From an ethical perspective, confidentiality promotes an individual's autonomy and illustrates respect for that person, by allowing the individual the freedom to decide who may access his/her private information and, consequently, how that information will affect his/her life.[33] The duty of confidentiality also comports with the paired principles of beneficence and nonmaleficence, in that breaches of confidentiality can cause harm (eg, social, psychological, and economic) to the individual who is the subject of the information disclosure.[33] In addition to ethical obligations, the stigma associated with mental illness highlights the importance of safeguards to protect the confidentiality of participants in psychiatric research, in that they serve the pragmatic function of encouraging individuals to seek treatment.

Investigators must uphold the confidentiality of participants' personal information throughout the research process, including data collection, analysis, presentation, and publication.[2,21] This duty involves taking appropriate steps to provide physical protection of participant information (eg, storing paper records in locked cabinet), to implement technical safeguards (eg, firewalls and passwords for electronically stored information), to de-identify or aggregate information when possible, and to train and monitor study personnel for compliance with these requirements.[2,21] In addition, the informed consent process should inform participants fully about the risks of privacy breaches, which are particularly relevant in light of the prevalence of electronic health information and the potential risks of improper access and dissemination (eg, computer hackers). The informed consent process also should discuss potential exceptions to the duty of confidentiality, such as when the law requires disclosure of information to prevent an imminent risk of serious bodily harm or regulatory disclosures to oversight bodies.

Under the authority of Congress and the Secretary of Health and Human Services, the National Institutes of Health (NIH) issues Certificates of Confidentiality to augment the confidentiality protections for research participants.[34] Certificates of Confidentiality give investigators and institutions the legal right to withhold certain sensitive information in civil, criminal, administrative, legislative, and other proceedings at the state and federal levels. To qualify for protection, this information must identify an individual participant. The information also must be sensitive in nature, which the NIH describes as potentially damaging to a person's "financial standing, employability, insurability, or reputation," if disclosed. According to the NIH, examples of potentially sensitive research activities include collection of the following: genetic information; information regarding an individual's psychological well-being; information regarding an individual's sexual attitudes, preferences, or practices; and substance abuse or other illegal risk-taking behaviors. Although Certificates of Confidentiality have limits and exceptions (eg, researchers may voluntarily disclose child abuse if the informed consent form allows that type of disclosure), they represent an important federal policy decision to promote potentially sensitive research, such as psychiatric research, through the protection of participants' privacy.

Oversight

Finally, psychiatric research should take place within a regulatory framework, such as the one set forth by the Common Rule, which provides oversight and enforces the implementation of safeguards.[17] Intraprofessional efforts also may prove valuable for achieving progress in the ethical conduct of research. Examples include the Task Force's standards and recommendations, the peer review process for publication, and the use of Data Safety Monitoring Boards to examine study data as it accrues during the course of the study, reassess the potential risks to participants, and identify when study revision or cessation may be necessary.[21,22]

CURRENT ISSUES
Emerging Evidence

As the theoretical discourse of psychiatric research ethics has developed, empirical research in this area has expanded the understanding of its practical implications.[35] This research has provided insight into the attitudes and clinical factors that influence psychiatric research, and, because it influences ethics discourse, may represent the evolution of evidence-based ethics as a field.[25]

Studies of psychiatrists and of persons who have mental illness indicate that appropriate use of safeguards is the key means of promoting knowledge of mental illness through research in an ethical manner. A 2004 study by Roberts and colleagues[36] of psychiatrists and of people who had schizophrenia suggests that ethical safeguards for research participation may positively influence patients' willingness to participate in research. A previous study by Roberts and colleagues[37] reports that both the psychiatry faculty and residents at one institution viewed safeguards and scientific merit as holding paramount importance to the conduct of clinical research. These findings, in light of the Task Force's report, illustrate the continuing trend of viewing psychiatric research through a positive lens, provided that appropriate safeguards are in place.

The general public, however, seems to be more conservative than psychiatrists or people who have mental illness in terms of openness to psychiatric research. A survey of the general public by Muroff and colleagues[38] revealed that the public is stricter about permitting research involving participants who have psychiatric illnesses than research involving participants who have nonpsychiatric medical illnesses. Perhaps this difference arises from the stigma of mental illness, which, as the Task Force highlighted, "can lead people to exaggerate the deficits and vulnerabilities of individuals with mental illness and to overlook or discount their strengths."[2] This study, however, suggests that substantial education may be necessary before the general public will understand that sufficient protections exist for persons who have mental illness to participate in psychiatric research in an ethically sound manner.

Empirical evidence also has augmented the insight regarding the capacity of persons who have mental illness to participate in psychiatric research, and, overall, this understanding is promising for the continued growth of psychiatric research. It suggests that persons who have mental illnesses such as schizophrenia tend to have the ability to provide informed consent for research participation, particularly through improved informed consent processes, and that their motivations for participating in research are similar to those of individuals who have other types of illnesses.[2,24,39] This research also helps clarify the potential vulnerabilities of participant populations. For example, a study by Misra and colleagues[40] of individuals who had bipolar disorder revealed that, although mania had no significant impact on the appreciation of the risks of a particular study, individuals in both the euthymic and manic states exhibited diminished ability to distinguish treatment from research participation and had an overly optimistic view of research participation.

Through increased empirically based knowledge about ethical issues in psychiatric research, the understanding of the relevant concerns and responses should continue to grow.

Emerging Technology: Genetics

Technological advancements also can raise novel ethical issues, as is the case with psychiatric genetic research, which represents another pressing topic for psychiatric research ethics.[41]

Extensive literature exists regarding the ethics of genetics. This body of literature includes substantial discussion of what, if anything, distinguishes genetic information from other types of information.[42,43] Genetic information may be "exceptional" or have particular significance because of its potential predictive value of an individual's future health, its potential to reveal information about an individual's relatives, its potential for stigma, and its potential to cause an individual psychological harm.[41,43]

Although a full discussion of the debate about genetic exceptionalism is beyond the scope of this discussion, recent developments in psychiatric genetic research, such as initial findings of potential genetic links to schizophrenia, bipolar disorder, and major depression, suggest that this field is ripe for increased ethics discourse.[41,44] As highlighted herein, the ethics discourse regarding psychiatric research continues to grow. Perhaps not surprisingly, the field of psychiatric genetic research, as a subset of psychiatric research, is relatively underdeveloped.[41] Accordingly, continued examination of the ethical issues in this area might help clarify relevant considerations, safeguards, and objectives for research.

Emerging Threat: Conflicts of Interest

Conflicts of interest involving research and the pharmaceutical industry have become a particularly important issue in the field of psychiatric research.[22] Generally, a conflict of interest arises when a physician has "competing roles, relationships, or interests"[24] that have the potential to hamper the physician's ability to fulfill the moral obligations attendant to his/her roles.[22] For example, any physician who is a clinician and an investigator faces a potential conflict of interest when he/she invites a patient to participate in the physician's research study; the physician may face tensions between clinical duties to act in the best interests of the patient and the desire to promote the physician's research interests. In psychiatric research, in particular, the participants' potential vulnerability because of their mental illness may call for heightened scrutiny of conflicts of interest.

As in other areas of medicine, the use of pharmaceuticals in psychiatry continues to grow and brings with it concerns about a particular type of conflict of interest: the influence of the pharmaceutical industry on the integrity of the psychiatric research endeavor.[45] This influence may occur at various phases throughout the research process; examples include investigators who positively skew data analysis or who fail to disclose financial arrangements in the publication of results.[45] The Task Force acknowledged this concern through its recommendations for avoiding, disclosing, and mitigating conflicts of interest (eg, though the use of independent monitors of research involving a significant conflict).[2] Continued scrutiny of conflicts of interest and implementation of safeguards should help reduce harm to participants and uphold the integrity of psychiatric research; increased empirical data regarding best practices and outcome measures will further these efforts.[46]

Emerging Population: Veterans of Operations Enduring Freedom and Iraqi Freedom

The recent deployment of United States military personnel in Iraq and Afghanistan under Operations Enduring Freedom and Iraqi Freedom (OEF/OIF) also raises a novel set of issues for psychiatric research ethics. The most recent report of the Mental Health Advisory Team of the United States Army Surgeon General found that OIF soldiers who reported high combat experiences and poor leadership also reported very high levels of mental health problems, and suicide rates among OEF/OIF soldiers were higher than historic Army rates.[47] Studies of this population thus far suggest that OEF/OIF veterans who return to the United States have a distinct risk of certain mental health problems and use mental health services at higher rates.[48] These mental health disorders include increased risk of posttraumatic stress disorder, depression, and substance abuse.[48–52]

Because of their heightened level of mental health risks and unique needs, additional psychiatric research of returning OEF/OIF veterans seems necessary to improve the ability to help this population. In addition to furthering the principle of beneficence, such research furthers the interests of justice by helping care appropriately for individuals who voluntarily have put their lives at risk to serve their country. As with other potentially vulnerable populations, however, such research should proceed only with appropriate safeguards that are tailored to address the vulnerabilities of this population.

SUMMARY

The field of psychiatric research ethics has evolved in recent years. This evolution seems to stem from the efforts of various groups (eg, medical ethicists, regulatory bodies, and the profession's own association, the APA) and from increased understanding of the endeavor of psychiatric empirical research. Current data regarding mental illness highlight the need for the continued expansion of psychiatric research to help relieve the suffering of the many individuals whom mental illness affects. The ethics for psychiatric research should parallel this expansion of psychiatric research to ensure that studies sufficiently address ethical considerations and thus foster the proper, delicate balance between progress and protection (see **Table 1**).

ACKNOWLEDGMENTS

The author gratefully acknowledges Laura Weiss Roberts, M.D., M.A., for her guidance and review of this paper, Ann Tennier, B.S., for her assistance in the preparation of this article, Jinger G. Hoop, M.D., M.F.A, for her support, and Ikar J. Kalogjera, M.D., for his inspiration.

REFERENCES

1. National Institutes of Mental Health. The numbers count: mental disorders in America. Available at: http://www.nimh.nih.gov/health/publications/the-numbers-count-mental-disorders-in-america.shtml. Last Accessed November 12, 2008.
2. American Psychiatric Association's Task Force on Research Ethics. Ethical principles and practices for research involving human participants with mental illness. Psychiatr Serv 2006;57(4):552–7.
3. Wolpe PR, Moreno J, Caplan A. Ethical principles and history. In: Pincus HA, Lieberman JA, Ferris S, editors. Ethics in psychiatric research. Washington, DC: American Psychiatric Association; 1999. p. 1–22.
4. Trials of war criminals before the Nuremberg Military Tribunals under Control Council Law No. 10, vol. 2, Nuremberg, October 1946-April 1949 (Washington, DC: US Government Printing Office, 1949), 181–2. Available at: http://ohsr.od.nih.gov/guidelines/nuremberg.html. Accessed November 12, 2008.
5. The World Medical Association, Ethics Unit, Declaration of Helsinki. Available at: http://www.wma.net/e/ethicsunit/helsinki.htm. Accessed March 27, 2009.
6. Beecher HK. Ethics and clinical research. N Engl J Med 1966;274(24):1354–60.
7. Available at: http://www.cdc.gov/tuskegee/timeline.htm. Accessed November 12, 2008.
8. White RM. Unraveling the Tuskegee Study of untreated syphilis. Arch Intern Med 2000;160:585–98.
9. The Human Radiation Experiments. Final Report of the President's Advisory Committee. New York: Oxford University Press; 1996.
10. 45 CFR Part 46 (2008).
11. Brody B. The ethics of biomedical research: an international perspective. New York: Oxford University Press; 1966. p. 31–53, 129–35.
12. Department of Health and Human Services. National Institutes of Health. Office of Protection from Research Risks: in Code of Federal Regulations, Title 45. public welfare. Part 46: Protection of Human Subjects. Available at: http://ori.dhhs.gov/

education/products/ucla/chapter2/page04b.htm. Last Accessed November 12, 2008.

13. United States Department of Health and Human Services, Office for Human Research Protections (OHRP). Available at: http://www.hhs.gov/ohrp/. Accessed November 12, 2008.

14. National Commission for the Protection of Human Subjects of Biomedical and Behavioral Research. The Belmont report: ethical principles and guidelines for the protection of human subjects of research. Washington, DC: U.S. Government Printing Office; 1979.

15. The President's Council on Bioethics, Former Bioethics Commissions. Available at: http://www.bioethics.gov/reports/past_commissions/index.html. Accessed November 12, 2008.

16. President's Commission for the Protection of Human Subjects of Biomedical and Behavioral Research. Protecting human subjects. Washington, DC: US Government Printing Office; 1981.

17. Roberts LW. Ethics and mental illness research. Psychiatr Clin North Am 2002;25: 525–45.

18. National Bioethics Advisory Commission, Research Involving Persons with Mental Disorders That May Affect Decisionmaking Capacity. Available at: http://bioethics. georgetown.edu/nbac/capacity/TOC.htm. Accessed November 12, 2008.

19. Project Muse, Kennedy Institute of Ethics Journal. Available at: http://muse.jhu.edu/ journals/kennedy_institute_of_ethics_journal/v012/12.1meslin.html. Accessed November 12, 2008.

20. Freedman B. Equipoise and the ethics of clinical research. N Engl J Med 1987; 317(3):141–5.

21. Roberts LW, Geppert CMA, Brody JL. A framework for considering the ethical aspects of psychiatric research protocols. Compr Psychiatry 2001;42(5):351–63.

22. Roberts LW, Dyer AR. Ethics in mental health care. Washington, DC: American Psychiatric Publishing, Inc.; 2004. p. 261–92.

23. Lieberman JA, Stroup S, Laska E, et al. Issues in clinical research design: principles, practices, and controversies. In: Pincus HA, Lieberman JA, Ferris S, editors. Ethics in psychiatric research. Washington, DC: American Psychiatric Association; 1999. p. 23–60.

24. Roberts LW, Hoop JG, Dunn LB, et al. An overview for mental health clinicians, researchers, and learners. In: Roberts LW, Hoop JG, editors. Professionalism and ethics: Q & A self-study guide for mental health professionals. Washington, DC: American Psychiatric Publishing, Inc.; 2008. p. 3–72.

25. Roberts LW, Heinrich TH. Walking a tightrope: ethics and neuropsychiatric research. Psychiatric Times October 2005;XXII:24–26.

26. Hoop JG, Smith AC, Roberts LW. Ethical issues in psychiatric research on children and adolescents. Child Adolesc Psychiatr Clin N Am 2008;17:127–48.

27. Wis. Stats. § 155.20(3) (2007–08).

28. Wendler D, Prasad K. Core safeguards for clinical research with adults who are unable to consent. Ann Intern Med 2001;135(7):514–23. .

29. Mutthapan P, Forster H, Wendler D. Research advance directives: protection or obstacle. Am J Psychiatry 2005;162:2389–91.

30. Roberts LW. Informed consent and the capacity for voluntarism. Am J Psychiatry 2002;159:705–12.

31. History of Medicine Division, National Library of Medicine, National Institutes of Health. Available at: http://www.nlm.nih.gov/hmd/greek/greek_oath.html. Accessed November 12, 2008.

32. Health Insurance Portability and Accountability Act of 1996, Pub. L. 104-191 (Aug. 21, 1996); 45 CFR Parts 160 and 164 (2008).
33. Dubois JM. Ethics in mental health research: principles, guidance, and cases. New York: Oxford University Press; 2008. p. 179.
34. United States Department of Health and Human Services, Office of Extramural Research, National Institutes of Health. Available at: http://grants.nih.gov/grants/policy/coc/background.htm. Accessed November 12, 2008.
35. Tsao CI, Layde JB, Roberts LW. A review of ethics in psychiatric research. Curr Opin Psychiatry 2008;21:572–7.
36. Roberts LW, Green Hammond KA, Warner TD, et al. Influence of ethical safeguards on research participation: comparison of perspectives of people with schizophrenia and psychiatrists. Am J Psychiatry 2004;162(12):2309–11.
37. Roberts LW, Warner TD, Brody JL, et al. What is ethically important in clinical research? A preliminary study of attitudes of 73 psychiatric faculty and residents. Schizophr Bull 2003;29(3):607–13.
38. Muroff JR, Hoerauf SL, Kim SYH. Is psychiatric research stigmatized? An experimental survey of the public. Schizophr Bull 2006;32:129–36.
39. Carpenter WT, Gold JM, Lahti AC, et al. Decisional capacity for informed consent in schizophrenia research. Arch Gen Psychiatry 2000;57:533–8.
40. Misra S, Socherman R, Hauser P, et al. Appreciation of research information in patient with bipolar disorder. Bipolar Disord 2008;1:635–46.
41. Hoop JG. Ethical considerations in psychiatric genetics. Harv Rev Psychiatry 2008;16(6):322–38.
42. Ross LF. Genetic exceptionalism vs. paradigm shift: lessons from HIV. J Law Med Ethics 2001;29(2):141–8.
43. Green MJ, Botkin JR. "Genetic exceptionalism" in medicine: clarifying the differences between genetic and nongenetic tests. Ann Intern Med 2003;138(7):571–5.
44. Hoop JG, Roberts LW, Hammond KAG, et al. Psychiatrists' attitudes regarding genetic testing and patient safeguards: a preliminary study. Genet Test 2008; 12(2):245–52.
45. Schowalter JE. How to manage conflicts of interest with industry? Int Rev Psychiatry 2008;20(2):127–33.
46. Warner TD, Roberts LW. Scientific integrity fidelity and conflicts of interest. Curr Opin Psychiatry 2004;17:381–5.
47. United States Army Surgeon General. Mental Health Advisory Team (MHAT-V): report. Washington, DC: Dept of the Army, Office of the Surgeon General. 5. Available at: http://www.armymedicine.army.mil/reports/mhat/mhat_v/MHAT_V_OIFandOEF-Redacted.pdf. Accessed November 12, 2008.
48. Hoge CW, Auchterlonie JL, Milliken CS. Mental health problems, use of mental health services, and attrition from military service after returning from deployment to Iraq or Afghanistan. JAMA 2006;295(9):1023–32.
49. Seal KH, Bertenthal D, Miner CR, et al. Bringing the war back home: mental health disorders among 103 788 US veterans returning from Iraq and Afghanistan seen at Department of Veterans Affairs facilities. Arch Intern Med 2007;167:476–82.
50. Hoge CW, Castro CA, Messer SC, et al. Combat duty in Iraq and Afghanistan, mental health problems and barriers to care. N Engl J Med 2004;351:13–22.
51. United States Army Surgeon General. Mental Health Advisory Team (MHAT-11): report. Washington, DC: Dept of the Army, Office of the Surgeon General; 2005. p. 1–30.
52. Kang HK, Hyamns KC. Mental health care needs among recent war veterans. N Engl J Med 2005;352:1289.

Research Ethics Issues in Geriatric Psychiatry

Laura B. Dunn, MD[a],*, Sahana Misra, MD[b]

KEYWORDS

- Research ethics • Decision making capacity
- Surrogate consent • Geriatric psychiatry
- Advanced directives • Research participation

Geriatric psychiatry research seeks to elucidate the etiology, course, and modifying factors of mental disorders affecting older people and to develop treatment options with greater safety, tolerability, and effectiveness than those currently available. Despite many advances, further research is urgently needed on mood, anxiety, psychotic, and cognitive disorders, and disorders that are commonly seen in older medically ill patients, such as delirium. Alzheimer's disease (AD) is a looming public health crisis; in the United States alone, the prevalence is estimated to rise to 13 million people by the year 2050.[1] A host of other neurologic and medical conditions that are often accompanied by behavioral sequelae and/or psychiatric comorbidity, including other forms of dementia, Parkinson's Disease and stroke, will also increase in prevalence as the population ages. Given these predictions and the need for improved treatment options for older adults suffering from these illnesses, much work toward the development of improved treatment options remains to be done.[2]

Clinical research relies on the participation of volunteers with (or at risk for) the disorder being studied. Ethical issues in the design, conduct, and monitoring of research involving older adults overlap substantially with those issues relevant to human subjects research in general (for an excellent summary, see[3]). There are, however, issues unique to research involving older adults that warrant further discussion. This paper reviews pressing ethical issues in geriatric psychiatric research, including capacity and cognition, the role of surrogates, and research involving suicidal individuals.

INFORMED CONSENT AND CAPACITY ASSESSMENT
Conceptual Issues

Three principles—respect for persons, beneficence and justice—guide the ethical conduct of human subject research.[4] The principle of "respect for persons" articulates

[a] Department of Psychiatry, University of California, San Francisco, 401 Parnassus Avenue, Box GPP-0984, San Francisco, CA 94143-0984, USA
[b] Mental Health Division, Portland VA Medical Center; Department of Psychiatry, Oregon Health & Science University, 3710 SW U.S. Veterans Hospital Road, Portland, OR 97239, USA
* Corresponding author.
E-mail address: laura.dunn@ucsf.edu (L.B. Dunn).

Psychiatr Clin N Am 32 (2009) 395–411
doi:10.1016/j.psc.2009.03.007
0193-953X/09/$ – see front matter © 2009 Elsevier Inc. All rights reserved.

that researchers endeavor to support individual autonomy and the right to self-determination, while protecting those with diminished autonomy. "Beneficence" ensures that researchers maximize benefits, minimize risks, and do not harm individuals. "Justice" requires that researchers equitably distribute the benefits and burdens of research. For example, subject selection consists of an appropriate sampling of participants based on the problem being studied rather than individuals that are readily accessible or easily manipulated.

"Respect for persons" provides the foundation for the doctrine of informed consent. The informed consent process is comprised of three unique components: (1) disclosure of pertinent information including risks, benefits and alternatives; (2) decision-making capacity; and (3) voluntariness (a free and genuine choice made without coercion).[5]

Decision-making capacity is most commonly conceptualized as involving four decisional abilities (often equated with legal standards of competence, but actually legal standards vary according to jurisdiction). These four abilities or domains are to: (1) understand relevant information (re: research, the specific research protocol, and the research enterprise, including risks and benefits) (2) appreciate the information by applying it to one's personal situation, (3) reason through the information in a rational manner (the "reasoning" standard), and; (4) communicate a clear and consistent choice (re: research, whether or not to participate).[6] A second, similar model incorporates a fifth legal standard of "reasonableness of choice."[7] In clinical and legal contexts, the stringency with which each of these decisional abilities (or some combination) is demonstrated should vary according to the risk-to-benefit ratio of the decision in question. This sliding-scale concept sees the threshold for sufficient capacity as resting on a continuum based on the risk to benefit ratio of the specific decision: a lower threshold for capacity is adequate for decisions with minimal risks, while decisions that involve greater risk necessitate a greater level of capacity. Of interest, some legal jurisdictions do not require demonstration of all four legal standards for an individual to be judged competent, thus having a lower threshold of sufficient demonstration of competence compared with other jurisdictions.

The research setting is inherently different than clinical or legal settings, as participation is voluntary and the risk-to-benefit ratio is typically skewed toward more direct risk with less direct benefit. Nevertheless, the sliding-scale concept of decisional capacity is the most useful guide for investigators in determining how stringent to be when evaluating capacity for research participation.[8]

Capacity assessments begin with the informed consent process, ideally occurring as an information sharing process. For potential research participants, full disclosure of relevant information pertaining to a study is required to make knowledgeable decisions that reflect personal values. A capacity assessment should be performed only after relevant information, including the purpose of the study, risks and benefits of participation, the alternatives to study participation, is disclosed, and questions are elicited and answered. Capacity assessments are focused on the specific decision in question (eg, whether to undergo a surgical procedure, a desire to leave the hospital against medical advice, or whether to participate in research participation). Through examination of the four decisional abilities mentioned above, the process of how someone ultimately arrives at their choice becomes clear. Whether the final decision or choice is considered ideal or preferred by the examiner is not a focus of the examination. In the clinical setting, if an individual demonstrates diminished capacity for a pressing medical decision, consent is generally sought from an appropriate proxy or surrogate decision maker who is typically a close family member.[6] The use of proxies for research decisions is discussed later in this paper.

Methods of Assessing Research Consent Capacity

In recent years, various instruments have been developed to assist clinicians and researchers in conducting decision-making capacity assessments. These tools are designed to allow the interviewer to systematically evaluate the decisional abilities outlined above. Yet, variation exists among these instruments; as a result, when selecting an instrument, it is important to understand the purpose of the evaluation and the specific characteristics of the tool chosen. In a review of studies published from 1980 to 2004 that included 23 instruments designed to assess decisional capacity in both research and treatment contexts, substantial variation in format, degree of standardization, flexibility of content, and scoring, as well as widely varying reliability and validity was found.[9]

Of the instruments identified, the MacArthur Competence Assessment Tools for Clinical Research (MacCAT-CR)[10] and Treatment (MacCAT-T)[11] were considered the most well-studied and well-validated.[12] They were developed from substantially lengthier instruments used in a hallmark study of competence, the MacArthur Treatment Competence Study, which included psychiatric and medical patients, as well as healthy controls.[12] The MacCAT-T and MacCAT-CR take between 15 and 20 minutes to administer and, given the content-specific nature of capacity assessments, must be adapted to the treatment or research protocol in question. The Competency to Consent to Treatment Inventory (CCTI) is another tool that has been validated in patients with dementia for treatment decisions.[7] In this tool, two hypothetical treatment vignettes are presented and followed by standardized questions to evaluate decision-making capacity based on five legal standards (including the "reasonable-ness of choice" standard described above).

One of the limitations of existing instruments, including the MacCAT-T and MacCAT-CR, is the lack of a final determination of whether someone has or lacks sufficient capacity to provide informed consent.[9] In the MacCAT-CR, for example, subscores for each decisional ability are obtained, but there is no predetermined cut-point above which sufficient capacity can be said to exist. The rationale for this aspect of the instrument lies in the previously mentioned notion that the desired threshold for "adequate capacity" should be considered a continuum, or sliding scale, depending on the risk–benefit ratio of the decision at hand. As a result, there continues to be an element of subjectivity in capacity assessment. Nevertheless, using a systematic and structured method for assessing decisional abilities can enable researchers to gain a more complete picture of individuals' decision-making abilities, as well as to highlight where there may be common and specific difficulties with understanding the specific protocol (which can lead, in turn, to adjustment of the consent process to facilitate better understanding).

Cognitive tests or screens, such as the Mini-Mental State Examination (MMSE)[13] — although not substitutes for a systematic assessment of decisional abilities — can provide useful complementary information for decision-making capacity assessments. The MMSE has been shown in several studies to correlate with performance on measures of decision-making capacity;[14–17] however, it does not have adequate predictive validity to be used as a stand-alone or surrogate marker for decisional impairment.[15,17] Also, some screens, such as the MMSE, may be less sensitive to higher order executive deficits seen in patients with frontal-focused neuropathology.[18] Thus, if specific cognitive test or tests are used as an adjunct to a capacity assessment, they should be selected with the target population and a clear rationale for the cognitive test in mind.

To underscore a main point of this review: when deficits in understanding (or other domains of capacity) are detected, the deficits do not necessarily justify excluding the participant from research participation. Rather, such deficits in performance indicate the need for enhanced methods of consent, such as by providing consent information in an interactive and iterative format that facilitates information sharing and, for many, may improve decisional abilities.[19] The use of enhanced methods of consent is discussed further in a later section.

DECISION-MAKING CAPACITY AND THE OLDER RESEARCH PARTICIPANT

Although age has been demonstrated to be associated with lower scores on assessments of capacity in a number of studies,[15,20,21] these findings have sometimes been confounded by other factors (eg, education, verbal reasoning, reading skills) that also affect performance on decision-making assessments. It is clear, however, that cognitive impairment seen in disorders associated with aging places patients at risk for impaired decision-making capacity.

AD, the most common form of dementia, affects the very cognitive abilities (eg, memory, language, judgment, abstraction, conceptualization) necessary for informed decision making.[7,14,16,22,23] Although a diagnosis of AD is not equivalent to impaired capacity to consent, a number of studies conducted over the last decade indicate that AD patients inevitably lose decisional capacity: some patients in the mild stages, most patients probably somewhere in the transition from mild to moderate disease.[7,16,17,24,25] Moreover, as shown by several research groups, executive functioning and verbal recall are closely associated with clinical assessments of decision-making abilities.[26–28] These types of impairments are not always readily apparent to the medical professional, researcher, or research staff. For instance, among medical inpatients who were tested for treatment-related decisional capacity by Raymont and colleagues,[15] nearly one-third of them were found to lack capacity, based on a consensus among the researchers who used the MacCAT-T. However, only one quarter of these patients had been identified by their treating physicians or their relatives as having impaired capacity; cognitive impairment and age were the only independent predictors of incapacity. Such findings suggest that older individuals who are medically ill or who have cognitive impairment are at increased risk for impaired capacity, but they cannot be assumed to lack capacity without assessment.

Although psychiatric diagnoses have been a focus of intense scrutiny with respect to capacity to consent to research, capacity studies specifically focusing on older adults with specific psychiatric diagnoses are relatively few. Studies of decision-making capacity in depressed patients, either for treatment or research decisions, have overall reported good performance on measures of capacity, and little-to-no association with depression severity. Among the depressed inpatients studied in the original MacArthur Treatment Competence Study (who scored primarily in the high moderate to low severe range on the Beck Depression Inventory),[29,30] treatment-related capacity performance was lower than that of controls, but the majority of the depressed patients were not impaired. Studies of decisional capacity in patients with schizophrenia, including older patients, have demonstrated mean scores worse than control or depressed comparison populations. Factors associated with poor performance include cognitive symptoms, conceptual disorganization, negative symptoms, and acute psychosis. Of importance, significant heterogeneity in performance was apparent with a substantial proportion of subjects (in some studies a majority of subjects) meeting thresholds for adequate capacity, stressing that the diagnosis of schizophrenia itself is not sufficient to establish lack of capacity.[31]

Studies of consent capacity in patients with bipolar disorder are sparse. Misra and colleagues examined research consent capacity in manic (n = 26) and euthymic subjects (n = 25). Compared to euthymic subjects, those with mania demonstrated poorer understanding of relevant research information.[32] Palmer and colleagues[33] similarly assessed research consent capacity in patients with bipolar disorder and compared them to patients with schizophrenia and normal controls. The patients with bipolar disorder had worse understanding than the healthy controls and did not differ from the patients with schizophrenia. For the entire sample, poor performance on the MacCAT-CR was associated with neurocognitive deficits and negative symptoms. Importantly, in both studies, patients with bipolar disorder, including manic patients, demonstrated improvement in understanding when relevant research information was re-reviewed.

To summarize, consent capacity studies have not found an association between decision-making capacity and specific diagnoses. Certain diagnoses may have higher rates of diminished capacity than others, but on an individual basis, many patients with psychiatric illnesses are able to provide informed consent. Impairments in cognitive abilities, on the other hand, particularly memory and frontal lobe-mediated executive functioning, do seem to affect decisional abilities.

Methods of Enhancing the Research Consent Process

Intrapersonal factors, the sociocultural context, and factors related to the study itself all influence the consent and decision-making process.[34] Some intrapersonal factors (eg, level of arousal, anxiety, distraction, pain) may be transitory and are potentially modifiable. Other intrapersonal factors may be more stable and thus difficult to modify (eg, prior experience with research, educational level, vocabulary/reading abilities). These factors nevertheless must be taken into account in tailoring the enrollment, consent, and overall research experience for individual participants, to ensure that the process is respectful of these individual differences and enhances autonomy whenever possible. External to the individual, factors including complexity of the information presented and the quality of the consent discussion will directly impact the decision-making process. Researchers and their staffs should endeavor to assess whether potential subjects are alert, attentive, and comfortable during the informed consent process and that relevant information is discussed in a quiet environment.

Growing concerns about capacity to consent, particularly in people with psychiatric illnesses, have led to increased interest in identifying educational interventions that will improve the overall decision-making process and consent-related abilities in people at risk for decisional impairments. Although the inherent complexity of pertinent research information may not be easily modified, the nature in which the information is communicated by the researcher can be improved. To this end, educational interventions ("enhanced consent" procedures) have been increasingly examined.

Tested interventions have ranged from multiple repetitions of consent information (reiterative review) to using different modalities of providing information (eg, presentation software, DVDs, group discussions).[35–37] Iterative review of pertinent information has been demonstrated to improve patients' understanding of relevant information in multiple populations, including populations with cognitive, affective and psychotic disorders.[31,36–38]

SPECIAL ISSUES IN GERIATRIC PSYCHIATRY RESEARCH
Surrogate Consent for Research: Current Context and Ethical Issues

Informed consent raises ethical challenges in geriatric research protocols (particularly in studies of AD or other cognitive disorders) because many potential participants will have impaired decision-making capacity.[16,23,24,39] Investigators most commonly address the consent dilemma through "double consent," ie, obtaining consent from the proxy, as well as assent from the subject,[39] making proxy consent central to the ethical integrity of clinical AD research.[40] Reliance on proxy consent for research on adults who lack capacity is done either formally or informally, depending on specific state law and institutional review board (IRB) requirements.[41,42] In part, this variability is because there is no unified accepted approach, and no federal regulations that speak directly to this issue. Ethics codes, organizational and governmental guidelines, legislative efforts, and commentators' proposals vary widely in their approach to proxy consent (see **Table 1**), representing what Appelbaum called a "gray zone of law and ethics."[41] For instance, although California and Virginia have laws specifically allowing proxy consent for research, the two laws differ in degree of detail regarding protocols to which proxies can consent.[43] It is unclear how differences would be reconciled, for instance, in a multisite protocol. In the absence of clear guidance, individual IRBs may adopt more restrictive or cautious stances. In addition, although a great deal of discussion of proxy consent centers on risks and benefits, some believe that further definition of levels and types of risks and benefits is needed.[44]

Proxy consent also raises ethical questions, because proxies must decide on behalf of another person, which may involve accepting potential risks and unknown benefits for someone whose research-related preferences are unknown.[45,46] Karlawish and colleagues[47] studied the views of competent older adults (n = 538, all 65 years or older) toward delegating decisions about AD research to proxies. Interview questions included items about how much power subjects would grant their proxy to enroll them (even against their wishes) in studies that presented more than minimal risk (ie, a study involving a lumbar puncture) but no potential for direct benefit. Two hypothetical research scenarios were used to explore these attitudes. Presumably these scenarios were provided in less detail (ie, shorter vignettes) than typical, lengthy consent forms given for actual research studies. However, only those participants who demonstrated sufficient understanding of core research concepts relevant to proxy consent were interviewed regarding the hypothetical research protocols. The majority of subjects endorsed willingness to be enrolled by their proxy, even against their advance consent, in the blood draw study (81% willing) and the blood draw plus lumbar puncture study (70%). Interview items also examined subject views on providing advanced consent for future studies. Advanced research directives have been proposed as another strategy to complement surrogate decision making for conditions anticipated to result in lack of research consent capacity in the future. Most adults (83%) said they would be willing, in advance, to consent to a study involving a blood draw, while approximately half (48%) would be willing to give consent in advance to a blood draw plus a lumbar puncture. Challenges to advanced directives include being able to discuss in detail key elements about specific studies to be conducted in the future as well as the genuineness of desire to participate for a situation that is yet to happen. Overall, general positive attitudes toward biomedical research predicted willingness to be enrolled, although, for the greater-than-minimal risk vignette, ethnic minorities were less willing to be enrolled.

Kim and colleagues,[48] using 10 briefly described research studies, varying in objectively-defined (by expert consultants) level of risk, looked at views of people at risk for AD regarding the acceptability of surrogate consent for research either for themselves or for their loved ones. Overall, subjects viewed surrogate consent for themselves favorably yet were more cautious when considering decisions for others versus themselves. The results suggested greater acceptability of lower risk/lower benefit studies and lower acceptability of higher risk/higher benefit studies.

Although proxy consent seems to be viewed favorably by patients with dementia, evidence suggests this cannot be assumed to be true for other populations. Misra and colleagues[49] demonstrated that patients with bipolar disorder rejected a role for family in decision-making about research participation Roberts and colleagues[50] similarly reported in patients with schizophrenia that family have a weak influence on patients' decisions whether to participate in research. These results raise concern about the acceptability of proxy consent for research in these populations and populations yet to be studied.

Influences on Proxies' Willingness to Enroll Relatives in Research

A number of studies suggest that proxies cite motivations for participation similar to those reported in the broader literature on research participation: altruism, trust in researchers and institutions, desperation, and hope for direct benefit.[14,51,52] The roles of perceived risk and benefit have received moderate attention in the literature on proxy decision making in the research context.[53,54] Several studies suggest that proxies' willingness to enroll their relative decreases in relation to increased risk, and that proxies cite both risk and benefit in their considerations about whether to participate.[14,51] Sugarman and colleagues[54] found that, although informed of risks, proxies seldom seemed to weigh these risks; they seemed to assume that if the institution was doing the study, it must be safe. In several studies, many proxies hoped for direct benefits, even from nondirect benefit research or those with very low probabilities of benefit[52,54]—even when explicitly told the study did not carry potential for direct benefit.[14]

Decision-making Abilities and Processes of Proxies

The importance of studying proxies' own decisional abilities is twofold. First, in any research involving vulnerable populations, ensuring protection of those with diminished autonomy is paramount. Second, if some proportion of proxies (even if relatively small) has poor understanding of key aspects of research, it would be important for IRBs, investigators, and safety monitoring boards to be aware of this possibility and to enact appropriate safeguards. It is also worth noting that some proportion of AD caregivers may themselves be suffering from cognitive impairment.[55]

One study found that some proxies did not adequately understand research-specific procedures;[56] another found that proxies described understanding the methods and risks as relatively unimportant to them.[54] In two studies of proxy decision making for AD research, gaps in understanding of research were identified.[14,57] Such findings should not come as a surprise, given the literature documenting suboptimal understanding of informed consent in numerous study populations.[21,56] Other factors potentially relevant to proxy consent include the role of caregiver burden or depression[52] on decision making, as well as the possibility of proxies feeling burdened by the research decision itself.[54] Such findings are relevant, not only for ensuring that recruitment, consent, monitoring, and debriefing procedures are sensitive to these possibilities, but also for the generalizability of AD trials' findings. Patient illness severity, proxies' perception of patient quality of life, and the nature/quality of the relationship may also affect proxy decision making. For example, Sugarman and colleagues[54] reported that severe illness was associated with less decision burden experienced by proxies than mild or moderate illness. In another study, adult children were more likely than spouses to decline enrollment in a placebo-controlled medication trial.[57]

Two models of proxy decision-making include the "best interests" standard and the "substituted judgment" standard. Several researchers have examined the modes proxy decision-makers use in the research setting to make decisions for their relative. Muncie and colleagues[58] and Sachs and colleagues[51] found that proxies' decisions more

Table 1
Codes, statements, and proposed guidelines relevant to research with cognitively impaired

Organization/Author	Proxy Consent Allowable	Proxy Consent Not Allowable	Gaps Remaining
A) ETHICS CODES, FEDERAL REGULATIONS, AND STATE LAWS			
Nuremberg Code[69]	• Never		• Does not address issue of proxy consent for research in cognitively impaired (and was not intended to)
Declaration of Helsinki[70] (most recent amendment 2000; two clarifications in 2002 & 2004)	• When condition impairing capacity is focus of research; consent from legally authorized representative; research with some risk if it has potential to benefit population from which incompetent subjects are drawn	• If research could be performed on competent persons	• Lack of clarity regarding levels of risk and benefit; refers to legally authorized representative but definition is left to legal bodies (which have failed to address this for the most part)
Belmont Report[4]	• Possible, but unclear under what circumstances. • Subject's wishes should be taken into account when possible	• Unclear	• Numerous gaps, eg, who can serve, for what types of research; unclear course when subject's wishes unknown
The Common Rule (Code of Federal Regulations 45CFR46)[71]	• Legally authorized representative (LAR)	• Unclear: if no "LAR"?	• "Exceedingly vague" [44]: LARs not clearly defined (left up to the states), making research vulnerable to inconsistencies
California Amendment[72]	• Research related to cognitive impairment, lack of capacity, or serious or life threatening diseases and conditions; hierarchical list of surrogates;	• Research participant is inpatient on a psychiatric unit or in mental health facility or on psychiatric hold	• Unclear status of research unrelated to cognitive impairment but important to quality of life • Does not distinguish among protocols of different levels of risk or potential for direct benefit

Virginia Code[73]	• Minimal risk research • Minor increase over minimal risk research (as determined by human research committee), regardless of potential for therapeutic effect	• Major increase over minimal risk research if no potential for therapeutic effect	• How are risk levels operationalized? (variation in how IRBs evaluate risks and benefits).
B) ORGANIZATIONAL POSITION STATEMENTS/PROPOSED GUIDELINES (EXAMPLES)			
American College of Physicians[74]	• Legally authorized surrogate consent permissible if no advance consent document, and if in subject's best interests		• Proxies should use mixed substituted judgment/best interests standard—but how is this operationalized? • IRBs should establish "special protections" (consisting of what?)
Alzheimer's Association[75]	• Minimal risk research • Research with potential therapeutic effect • No more than minor increase over minimal risk research if no potential for therapeutic effect	• Greater than minor increase over minimal risk research if no potential for therapeutic effect (with two exceptions: condition causing cognitive impairment is object of the study; or individual has given a research advance directive	• Variation in how IRBs assess risk and benefit is not addressed. • Suggests that proxies be instructed to use a substituted judgment standard when possible; if impossible, then best interests standard—suggesting need for study of actual practices

(continued on next page)

Table 1
(continued)

Organization/Author	Proxy Consent Allowable	Proxy Consent Not Allowable	Gaps Remaining
NIH ("Points to Consider")[76]	• "Where permitted by law"	• Subject indicates a wish to withdraw from study	• Safeguards should be commensurate with severity of capacity impairment or magnitude of experimental risk—but how to operationalize risk levels?
C) ETHICIST POSITIONS (selected examples)			
"Proposed Guidelines" for consent with cognitively impaired research subjects (Berg)[77]	• Minimal risk research • Research with potential therapeutic effect • Additional protections as risks increase	• Most restrictions in studies with high degree of risk with no potential for therapeutic benefit	• Proposes hierarchy of protections with increasing level of risk, eg, surrogate consent monitor—operationalization and stakeholders' views of such protections in need of study
"Full Spectrum Proxy Consent" (Post, 2003)[44]	• Research at or below maximum potential risk, regardless of potential for therapeutic effect	• Research above maximum potential risk	• Argues need for consensus regarding risk threshold for dementia research, eg, through a consensus conference—yet, empirical work should also inform such discussions

closely reflected wishes for themselves than what patients reported as their wishes, suggesting a dominance of a "best interests" versus "substituted judgment" mode of decision-making.[52] Karlawish and colleagues[57] reported that disagreement between proxy and patient about whether to enroll was more common among those who declined enrollment in a trial. Taken together, these findings highlight how difficult it is to generalize regarding how proxies actually use the "best interests" versus "substituted judgment" standards when asked to decide about research for their relative.

DEPRESSION AND SUICIDE RESEARCH

In 2004, adults 65 years of age or older comprised 12% of the United States population yet accounted for 16% of suicide deaths. In addition, 14.3 of every 100,000 adults that were 65 and older died from suicide compared with 11 of every 100,000 in the general population.[59] Older United States adults, white males in particular, are at increased risk for completed suicide compared with other age groups.[60] Research on suicide in older adults is clearly an area in need of further study, including identifying those at greatest risk and developing effective interventions. Suicide research, however, has been challenging to conduct, in part because of real, as well as perceived, ethical issues. In most mental health research, as a result, an endorsement of suicidality frequently results in exclusion or, if detected during the study, withdrawal. Moreover, institutional review boards and grant reviewers will ask for detailed plans on how researchers will handle potentially suicidal individuals.

Because of these challenges, an NIH and American Foundation for Suicide Prevention sponsored meeting was convened in 2001 entitled "Ethical Issues in Including Suicidal Individuals in Clinical Research." An outgrowth of this meeting, a discussion by Fisher and colleagues[61] of these issues should be required reading for investigators (and reviewers) involved in any depression or suicide research. One question central to designing an ethical research design is whether suicide research is analogous to research enrolling people with terminal illnesses. As argued by these experienced researchers and ethicists, IRBs have not "assessed equitably" the risk-to-benefit ratio of research involving suicidal individuals. The authors argue "for scientifically sound research on suicide prevention to move forward, and eventually benefit those at risk, death by suicide needs to be understood as an expectable event."

In addition, the authors challenge widely held assumptions (ie, those held by researchers, institutional review boards and the public) that attribute responsibility for suicide to the individual and/or the health care provider, and that oversimplify the liability. In contrast, again using the authors' own words, "…preliminary evidence would suggest that psychosocial, pharmacologic, and community-based efforts require systematic, multipronged, and sustained efforts to provide real protection against suicide." A second question that remains unclear is whether suicidal patients have diminished capacity to consent to research, given that this is the same population who clinically may meet criteria for involuntary hospitalization. This area is in need of systematic research. Finally, there are challenges around determining the presence of sufficient clinical equipoise with existing treatments for suicide prevention to justify randomized clinical trials and, if equipoise is thought to be present, there are many difficulties in designing an adequate control arm, such as the "treatment as usual" (TAU) model.[61]

Reynolds (one of the lead investigators for the multisite NIMH-funded PROSPECT Study [Prevention of Suicide in Primary Care Elderly]) and colleagues[62] further elaborated on the tensions between research design and ethics that occur when using TAU designs in suicide research, using the PROSPECT study as an example. The

Table 2
Special issues in geriatric psychiatry research

Concept	Ethical and Practical Challenges	Future Research Directions
Decision-making Capacity	• Impairment in cognitive abilities, such as memory and executive function, are associated with decision-making capacity deficits, including ability to consent to research participation	• Further examination of interventions aimed at improving decision-making capacity • Enhance the informed consent process (different modalities of presenting pertinent information, improving intra and extra personal factors that influence the decision-making process)
Surrogate/Proxy Consent	• Variations in patients' desire for surrogate consent • Variations in extent of knowledge about impaired relative's wishes • Different models of proxy making –"best interest" (what I would do) versus "substituted judgment" (what my relative would want) • Lack of uniform federal regulations – different states vary regarding types of studies that qualify for surrogate consent (problematic for multi-site studies)	• Examination of state laws on research in cognitively impaired individuals and the impact on conduct of research • Examination of how various stakeholders (public, patients, IRBs)define and weigh risks and benefits in research involving proxy consent • Examination of factors associated with patients' desire for or against surrogate consent, ie, demo graphics, primary illness, risk:benefit ratio of study in question • Interventions aimed at improving concordance rates between patients and potential surrogates
Advanced Directives for Research Participation	• Inability to address specific information about a future study that is required for an informed consent process • Questions about the genuineness of consent for future studies –based on hypothetical considerations	• Design of an advanced directive for research participation and examination of its utility, feasibility and applicability • Usefulness of an advanced directive for research participation for a surrogate when faced with con senting for a study for their loved one
Suicide Research	• Inclusion of suicidal subjects in studies • Can suicide be viewed as an expected event in a study including suicidal subjects • Do suicidal patients have diminished capacity to consent to research • Strong scientific design plus clinical equipoise for all arms including control arms	• Examination of how various stakeholders (public, patients, researchers, IRBs) define and weigh risks and benefits in research involving suicidal patients • Development of procedures for conduct of research that maintain the highest ethical and scientifically sound standards.

PROSPECT study sought to determine whether depression health specialists, placed in primary care clinics (intervention arm), would prevent or reduce suicidal ideation, hopelessness and depressive symptoms in elderly primary patients. To determine the effectiveness of the intervention, the design included a TAU comparison arm. "Treatment as usual," however, when incorporated into a study design becomes altered for both research design and ethical reasons. In PROSPECT, all subjects including the TAU control group needed to be initially screened for depression (eligibility criteria), and the control group also needed to be monitored over time for any adverse effects of study participation (in this case worsening depression or suicidal ideation). The authors noted that this enhanced TAU design, although confounding their ability to detect the true effect of the addition of depression health specialists in the primary care clinics, was a necessary and important part of meeting the ethical standard of beneficence.[62] Despite limitations, PROSPECT demonstrates that careful research can be conducted—and should be conducted— in populations potentially at risk for suicidal ideation or suicide to provide the critical information needed on how best to identify and address their unmet needs.

SUMMARY

Progress in geriatric psychiatric research may be impeded by lack of attention to collecting evidence relevant to ethical issues. As has been noted for some time, unless proactive work is done to identify, clarify, and remediate ethical challenges (see **Table 2** for research directions), deleterious effects on research can result, including research bans, unduly overprotective stances, or inaccurate weighing of risks and benefits of research by review boards.[41,63–67] With regard to proxy consent, a number of issues require further study. These include: how state laws address (or fail to address) research involving cognitively impaired individuals and what effects this has on research conduct;[41–43] how IRBs define and weigh risks and benefits in considering research involving proxy consent;[68] how various stakeholders, including the general public, people with disorders that may impair decision-making capacity, and proxies themselves view proxy consent for research;[47,48] and to what degree proxies' research decisions reflect what patients themselves would decide. The use of advanced directives as a stand alone method for future consent is fraught with difficulties around adequate informed consent for a particular study; however, future study may clarify if such directives provide surrogates with improved understanding of their relative's overall views of the research enterprise and possibly the types of studies they would be willing to participate in even if they are no longer able to provide their own consent. In depression and suicide research, further work is needed to develop standard procedures for meeting the ethical demands of research while conducting rigorous, crucial research.

REFERENCES

1. Arch Neurol – Alzheimer Disease in the US Population, Hebert LE, Scherr PA, Bienias JL, et al. Prevalence estimates using the 2000 census, August 2003. Available at: http://archneur.ama-assn.org/cgi/content/full/60/8/1119. 2008;60(8):1119. Accessed December 12, 2008.
2. Jeste DV, Alexopoulos GS, Bartels SJ, et al. Consensus statement on the upcoming crisis in geriatric mental health: Research agenda for the next 2 decades. Arch Gen Psychiatry 1999;56(9):848–53.
3. Emanuel EJ, Wendler D, Grady C. What makes clinical research ethical? JAMA 2000;283(20):2701–11.

4. National Commission for the Protection of Human Subjects of Biomedical and Behavioral Research. The belmont report: ethical principles and guidelines for the protection of human subjects of research. Washington, DC: Government Printing Office; 1979.

5. Faden R, Beauchamp T, King N. A history and theory of informed consent. New York: Oxford University Press; 1986.

6. Grisso T, Appelbaum P. Assessing competence to consent to treatment: a guide for physicians and other health professionals. New York: Oxford University Press; 1998.

7. Marson DC, Ingram KK, Cody HA, et al. Assessing the competency of patients with Alzheimer's disease under different legal standards. A prototype instrument. Arch Neurol 1995;52(10):949–54.

8. Drane JF. Competency to give an informed consent. A model for making clinical assessments. JAMA 1984;252(7):925–7.

9. Dunn LB, Nowrangi MA, Palmer BW, et al. Assessing decisional capacity for clinical research or treatment: a review of instruments. Am J Psychiatry 2006;163(8):1323–34.

10. Appelbaum PS, Grisso T. MacCAT-CR: MacArthur competence assessment tool for clinical research. Sarasota (FL): Professional Resource Press; 2001.

11. Grisso T, Appelbaum PS, Hill-Fotouhi C. The MacCAT-T: a clinical tool to assess patients' capacities to make treatment decisions. Psychiatr Serv 1997;48(11): 1415–9.

12. Grisso T, Appelbaum PS. The MacArthur treatment competence study. III: abilities of patients to consent to psychiatric and medical treatments. Law Hum Behav 1995;19(2):149–74.

13. Folstein MF, Folstein SE, McHugh PR. "Mini-mental state". A practical method for grading the cognitive state of patients for the clinician. J Psychiatr Res 1975; 12(3):189–98.

14. Karlawish JH, Casarett DJ, James BD. Alzheimer's disease patients' and caregivers' capacity, competency, and reasons to enroll in an early-phase Alzheimer's disease clinical trial. J Am Geriatr Soc 2002;50(12):2019–24.

15. Raymont V, Bingley W, Buchanan A, et al. Prevalence of mental incapacity in medical inpatients and associated risk factors: cross-sectional study. Lancet 2004;364(9443):1421–7.

16. Kim SY, Caine ED, Currier GW, et al. Assessing the competence of persons with Alzheimer's disease in providing informed consent for participation in research. Am J Psychiatry 2001;158(5):712–7.

17. Kim SY, Caine ED. Utility and limits of the mini mental state examination in evaluating consent capacity in Alzheimer's disease. Psychiatr Serv 2002;53(10):1322–4.

18. Malloy PF, Cummings JL, Coffey CE, et al. Cognitive screening instruments in neuropsychiatry: a report of the committee on research of the American Neuropsychiatric Association. J Neuropsychiatry Clin Neurosci 1997;9(2):189–97.

19. Kim SY, Karlawish JH, Caine ED. Current state of research on decision-making competence of cognitively impaired elderly persons. Am J Geriatr Psychiatry 2002;10(2):151–65.

20. Dunn LB, Jeste DV. Enhancing informed consent for research and treatment. Neuropsychopharmacology 2001;24(6):595–607.

21. Sugarman J, McCrory DC, Hubal RC. Getting meaningful informed consent from older adults: a structured literature review of empirical research. J Am Geriatr Soc 1998;46(4):517–24.

22. Marson D, Dymek M, Harrell L. Neuropsychological correlates of the factor structure of competency to consent in Alzheimer's disease. J Int Neuropsychol Soc 1995;2(1):60.

23. Palmer BW, Dunn LB, Appelbaum PS, et al. Assessment of capacity to consent to research among older persons with schizophrenia, Alzheimer's disease, or diabetes mellitus: comparison of a 3-item questionnaire with a comprehensive standardized capacity instrument. Arch Gen Psychiatry 2005;62(7):726–33.
24. Buckles VD, Powlishta KK, Palmer JL, et al. Understanding of informed consent by demented individuals. Neurology 2003;61(12):1662–6.
25. Kim SY, Karlawish JH. Ethics and politics of research involving subjects with impaired decision-making abilities. Neurology 2003;61(12):1645–6.
26. Marson DC, Hawkins L, McInturff B, et al. Cognitive models that predict physician judgments of capacity to consent in mild Alzheimer's disease. J Am Geriatr Soc 1997;45(4):458–64.
27. Holzer JC, Gansler DA, Moczynski NP, et al. Cognitive functions in the informed consent evaluation process: a pilot study. J Am Acad Psychiatry Law 1997;25(4):531–40.
28. Royall DR, Mahurin RK, Gray KF. Bedside assessment of executive cognitive impairment: the executive interview. J Am Geriatr Soc 1992;40(12):1221–6.
29. Appelbaum PS, Grisso T. The MacArthur competence study I, II, III. Law Hum Behav 1995;19(2):105–74.
30. Grisso T, Appelbaum PS, Mulvey EP, et al. The MacArthur treatment competence study. II: measures of abilities related to competence to consent to treatment. Law Hum Behav 1995;19(2):127–48.
31. Dunn LB, Candilis PJ, Roberts LW. Emerging empirical evidence on the ethics of schizophrenia research. Schizophr Bull 2006;32(1):47–68.
32. Misra S, Socherman R, Park BS, et al. Influence of mood state on capacity to consent to research in patients with bipolar disorder. Bipolar Disord 2008;10(2):303–9.
33. Palmer BW, Dunn LB, Depp CA, et al. Decisional capacity to consent to research among patients with bipolar disorder: comparison with schizophrenia patients and healthy subjects. J Clin Psychiatry 2007;68(5):689–96.
34. Dunn LB, Palmer BW, Karlawish JH. Frontal dysfunction and capacity to consent to treatment or research: conceptual considerations and empirical evidence. In: Miller BL, Cummings JL, editors. The human frontal lobes. 2nd edition. New York: Guilford Press; 2007.
35. Carpenter WT, Gold JM, Lahti AC, et al. Decisional capacity for informed consent in schizophrenia research. Arch Gen Psychiatry 2000;57(6):533–8.
36. Moser DJ, Reese RL, Hey CT, et al. Using a brief intervention to improve decisional capacity in schizophrenia research. Schizophr Bull 2006;32(1):116–20.
37. Jeste DV, Palmer BW, Golshan S, et al. Multimedia consent for research in people with schizophrenia and normal subjects: a randomized controlled trial. Schizophr Bull 2008 Jan 31 [Epub ahead of print].
38. Palmer BW, Cassidy EL, Dunn LB, et al. Effective use of consent forms and interactive questions in the consent process. IRB 2008;30(2):8–12.
39. Karlawish JH, Knopman D, Clark CM, et al. Informed consent for Alzheimer's disease clinical trials: a survey of clinical investigators. IRB 2002;24(5):1–5.
40. Stocking CB, Hougham GW, Baron AR, et al. Are the rules for research with subjects with dementia changing? views from the field. Neurology 2003;61(12):1649–51.
41. Appelbaum PS. Involving decisionally impaired subjects in research: the need for legislation. Am J Geriatr Psychiatry 2002;10(2):120–4.
42. Kim SY, Appelbaum PS, Jeste DV, et al. Proxy and surrogate consent in geriatric neuropsychiatric research: update and recommendations. Am J Psychiatry 2004;161(5):797–806.

43. Saks ER, Dunn LB, Wimer J, et al. Proxy consent to research: the legal landscape. Yale J Health Policy Law Ethics 2008;8:37–92.

44. Post SG. Full-spectrum proxy consent for research participation when persons with Alzheimer's disease lose decisional capacities: research ethics and the common good. Alzheimer Dis Assoc Disord 2003;17(Suppl 1):S3–11.

45. Wendler D, Martinez RA, Fairclough D, et al. Views of potential subjects toward proposed regulations for clinical research with adults unable to consent. Am J Psychiatry 2002;159(4):585–91.

46. Bravo G, Paquet M, Dubois MF. Knowledge of the legislation governing proxy consent to treatment and research. J Med Ethics 2003;29(1):44–50.

47. Karlawish J, Rubright J, Casarett D, et al. Older adults' attitudes toward enrollment of non-competent subjects participating in Alzheimer's research. Am J Psychiatry 2008. Accessed December 12, 2008. 10.1176/appi.ajp.2008.08050645.

48. Kim SYH, Kim HM, McCallum C, et al. What do people at risk for Alzheimer's disease think about surrogate consent for research? Neurology 2005;65:1395–401.

49. Misra S, Socherman R, Hauser P, et al. Appreciation of research information in patients with bipolar disorder. Bipolar Disord 2008;10(5):635–46.

50. Roberts LW, Warner TD, Brody JL, et al. Patient and psychiatrist ratings of hypothetical schizophrenia research protocols: assessment of harm potential and factors influencing participation decisions. Am J Psychiatry 2002;159(4):573–84.

51. Sachs GA, Stocking CB, Stern R, et al. Ethical aspects of dementia research: informed consent and proxy consent. Clin Res 1994;42(3):403–12.

52. Hougham GW, Sachs GA, Danner D, et al. Empirical research on informed consent with the cognitively impaired. IRB 2003;Suppl 25(5):S26–32.

53. Elad P, Treves TA, Drory M, et al. Demented patients' participation in a clinical trial: factors affecting the caregivers' decision. Int J Geriatr Psychiatry 2000;15(4):325–30.

54. Sugarman J, Cain C, Wallace R, et al. How proxies make decisions about research for patients with Alzheimer's disease. J Am Geriatr Soc 2001;49(8):1110–9.

55. Beach SR, Schulz R, Williamson GM, et al. Risk factors for potentially harmful informal caregiver behavior. J Am Geriatr Soc 2005;53(2):255–61.

56. Pucci E, Belardinelli N, Borsetti G, et al. Information and competency for consent to pharmacologic clinical trials in Alzheimer's disease: an empirical analysis in patients and family caregivers. Alzheimer Dis Assoc Disord 2001;15(3):146–54.

57. Karlawish JH, Casarett D, Klocinski J, et al. How do AD patients and their caregivers decide whether to enroll in a clinical trial? Neurology 2001;56(6):789–92.

58. Muncie HL Jr, Magaziner J, Hebel JR, et al. Proxies' decisions about clinical research participation for their charges. J Am Geriatr Soc 1997;45(8):929–33.

59. National Institute of Mental Health. Older adults: depression and suicide facts. Available at: http://www.nimh.nih.gov/health/publications/older-adults-depression-and-suicide-facts.shtml. Accessed December 18, 2008.

60. Conwell Y, Duberstein PR, Caine ED. Risk factors for suicide in later life. Biol Psychiatry 2002;52(3):193–204.

61. Fisher CB, Pearson JL, Kim S, et al. Ethical issues in including suicidal individuals in clinical research. IRB 2002;24(5):9–14.

62. Reynolds CF, Degenholtz H, Parker LS, et al. Treatment as usual (TAU) control practices in the PROSPECT study: managing the interaction and tension between research design and ethics. Int J Geriatr Psychiatry 2001;16(6):602–8.

63. Bonnie RJ. Research with cognitively impaired subjects. unfinished business In the regulation of human research. Arch Gen Psychiatry 1997;54(2):105–11.

64. National Bioethics Advisory Commission. Research involving persons with mental disorders that may affect decisionmaking capacity. Rockville (MD): National Bioethics Advisory Commission; 1998.
65. Oldham JM, Haimowitz S, Delano SJ. Protection of persons with mental disorders from research risk: a response to the report of the National Bioethics Advisory Commission. Arch Gen Psychiatry 1999;56(8):688–93.
66. Charney DS. The National Bioethics Advisory Commission report: the response of the psychiatric research community is critical to restoring public trust. Arch Gen Psychiatry 1999;56(8):699–700.
67. Roberts LW. Ethics and mental illness research. Psychiatr Clin North Am 2002; 25(3):525–45.
68. Silverman H, Hull SC, Sugarman J. Variability among institutional review boards' decisions within the context of a multicenter trial. Crit Care Med 2001;29(2): 235–41.
69. Katz J. World medical association declaration of Helsinki. In: Thomas CC, editor. Experimentation with human beings. New York: Russel Sage Foundation; 1972.
70. World Medical Association Declaration of Helsinki: Ethical Principles for Medical Research Involving Human Subjects: Adopted by the 18th WMA General Assembly, Helsinki, Finland, June 1964, and amended by the 29th WMA General Assembly, Tokyo, Japan, October 1975; the 35th WMA General Assembly, Venice, Italy, October 1983; the 41st WMA General Assembly, Hong Kong, September 1989; the 48th WMA General Assembly, Somerset West, Republic of South Africa, October 1996; and the 52nd WMA General Assembly, Edinburgh, Scotland, October 2000. Ferney-Voltaire, France, WMA.
71. Department of Health and Human Services. Code of Federal Regulations, Title 45: Public Welfare. Part 46, Subpart A: Protection of Human Subjects, 1991.
72. Amendment to section 24178 of the California Health and Safety Code, 2002.
73. Health - human research - informed consent. Code of Virginia: 32.1, 162.18. 2002.
74. Cognitively impaired subjects. American College of Physicians. Ann Intern Med 1989;111(10):843–8.
75. Alzheimer's Association. Position statement: ethical issues in dementia research (with Special Emphasis on "informed Consent"). Vol. 2005; 1997. Available at: http://www.alz.org/national/documents/statements_ethicalissues.pdf.
76. National Institutes of Health Office of Extramural Research. In: Research involving individuals with questionable capacity to consent: points to consider, Vol. 2007. National Institutes of Health; 1999. Available at: http://grants.nih.gov/grants/policy/questionablecapacity.htm.
77. Berg JW. Legal and ethical complexities of consent with cognitively impaired research subjects: proposed guidelines. J Law Med Ethics 1996;24(1):18–35.

The Ethics of Psychiatric Education

John Coverdale, MD, MEd, FRANZCP[a,b,*], Laurence B. McCullough, PhD[b],
Laura Weiss Roberts, MD, MA[c,d]

KEYWORDS

- Ethics • Education • Psychiatry • John Gregory
- Sexual boundaries • Conflicts of interest • Suicidal patients

Ethical issues pervade all of psychiatric clinical practice. These issues range from managing suicidal patients to obtaining assent for care from a young adolescent and from dealing with complicated sexualized issues that may arise in performing psychotherapy to introducing "cutting edge" clinical approaches such as somatic therapies and genetic testing in the care of patients. In addition, the behavior of some psychiatrists causes concern when their interests are promoted over and above those of patients. Such situations can occur when psychiatrists violate social and sexual boundaries with patients, when financial gain becomes an influential consideration in decision-making about the admission of a patient, or when conflicts of interest arise in relationships with pharmaceutical companies or the health care industry. Although these issues pertain to all medical professionals, one early national survey of program training directors in psychiatry asking what topics should be taught in psychiatric ethics found that physician–patient sexual contact and financial considerations in practice were deemed the most important.[1] In a second survey of residents at 10 training programs, the majority of trainees requested that additional curricular attention be given to 19 of 26 ethics topics encompassing issues related to withholding information from patients, informed consent and decisional capacity, responsibilities in terminating with therapy, allocation of health care resources, and colleague impairment.[2]

Psychiatric educators must attend to learners' ability to address constructively the ethical concerns inherent in both routine and challenging clinical problems and to prevent ethical conflicts that arise in everyday practice, particularly when their own

[a] Menninger Department of Psychiatry and Behavioral Sciences, Baylor College of Medicine, Houston, TX, USA
[b] Center for Medical Ethics and Health Policy, Baylor College of Medicine, Houston, TX, USA
[c] Department of Psychiatry and Behavioral Medicine, Medical College of Wisconsin, Milwaukee, WI, USA
[d] Department of Population Health, Medical College of Wisconsin, Milwaukee, WI, USA
* Corresponding author. Menninger Department of Psychiatry and Behavioral Sciences, Baylor College of Medicine, One Baylor Plaza, BCM 350, Houston, TX 77030.
E-mail address: jhc@bcm.tmc.edu (J. Coverdale).

Psychiatr Clin N Am 32 (2009) 413–421
doi:10.1016/j.psc.2009.02.007
0193-953X/09/$ – see front matter © 2009 Elsevier Inc. All rights reserved.

interests could supersede those of patients. Ethics, in turn, concerns the clinical judgment, decision-making, and behavior of practitioners (and health care organizations) and both the evidence and arguments that support what these should be.[3] Thus, an ethics of psychiatric education must attend not only to promoting competent clinical judgment and clinical practice but also to promoting ethical behaviors.

This article discusses the central elements of an ethics of psychiatric education. This discussion is framed in light of the work of John Gregory, whose medical ethics helped shape medicine as a profession. References to John Gregory's medical ethics are used here to inform the ethics of psychiatric education in three selected areas of importance to the profession: the management of suicidal patients, managing sexual boundaries between psychiatrists and patients, and avoiding conflicts of interest.

JOHN GREGORY'S ETHICS OF MEDICINE

John Gregory (1724–1773) wrote the first professional medical ethics in the English language that was based on the physician's responsibility to promote and protect the interests of patients. Thus, John Gregory introduced the concept of medicine as a profession and heavily influenced Thomas Percival (1740–1804), who in turn was a major influence on the code of ethics promulgated by the American Medical Association in 1847.[4] John Gregory's contribution was truly revolutionary given the circumstances of practice in Scotland during his lifetime.

In eighteenth century Scotland, medicine was practiced as an entrepreneurial and self-interested business, creating a crisis of intellectual and moral trust among the sick that prompted Gregory to write and lecture on medical ethics. A comprehensive account of this history has been provided by one of the present authors (LBM) elsewhere.[4,5] There was no standard medical curriculum, no licensure, no uniform pathway to becoming a physician, or regulation of practice, and there were a number of different concepts of health and disease. Many of the sick did not trust physicians intellectually, in terms of what they said or how they treated their illnesses. Many of the sick also did not trust physicians morally, in terms of putting the interests of the sick individual first and physicians' financial and other interests second. Some physicians assumed the good manners of a gentleman to pry their way into the houses of the sick and to take advantage of them financially. Some also became sexual predators of the sick. Gregory took the view that this behavior toward the vulnerable ill was unacceptable and was concerned by both a lack of scientific competence and unbridled self-interest.

Gregory responded to this crisis in trust by using the tools of ethics and philosophy of medicine to open medicine to public scouting and accountability. Three key components of his response serve to inform the teaching and practice of medicine today. The first addresses the problem of intellectual trust by calling for medicine to be based on scientific principles and evidence. The second component of his response addressed the problems of moral trust by emphasizing that protecting and promoting the interests of patients should be the physician's primary concern or motivation. The third component was the call to physicians to subordinate the pursuit of their own interests in favor of the needs of patients (**Box 1**).

In addressing the lack of intellectual trust in physicians, Gregory looked to Francis Bacon (1561–1626), who had called for medicine to be based on experience or on the rigorously collected results of natural and designed experiments. The first component then requires that physicians become and remain scientifically and clinically competent. Gregory referred to an openness to conviction that enables a physician to

---

Box 1

John Gregory's response to a lack of intellectual and moral trust in physicians

1. Medicine should be based on the rigorously collected results of natural and designed experiments.

2. Physicians should be concerned primarily with protecting and promoting the interests of the patient.

3. Physicians should be concerned only secondarily with protecting their own interests.

---

acknowledge errors and to correct mistakes and not to adhere obstinately to unsuccessful treatment methods.

In addressing the problem of moral trust of physicians, Gregory appealed to David Hume's (1711–1776) principle of sympathy. Sympathy activates feeling in fellow human beings, which, as Gregory described, "incites" physicians to relieve the distress of the sick. The second component of Gregory's response thus directs the physician's attention away from self-interest and toward the interests and needs of patients. The virtues of integrity, compassion, self-effacement, and self-sacrifice give substance to Gregory's responses (**Box 2**) and together constitute a starting point for an ethics of medical and psychiatric education.

Integrity is the highest virtue and relates to the attainment of a high standard of scientific and clinical excellence in all medical pursuits, whether in teaching, administration, clinical practice, or research.

Compassion, similar to the notion of sympathy, motivates physicians to reduce suffering in patients. This virtue should be cultivated by balancing obligations to patients with time spent in the pursuit of personal activities and interests that reinvigorate enthusiasm for clinical work and thus help keep compassion intact.

Self-effacement reduces the possibility that any differences in a physician–patient relationship (eg, ability to pay or differences in social class, manners, hygiene, ethnicity, or religion) do not influence or adversely affect treatment.

Self-sacrifice moves the physician to put aside his or her own interests and to make sacrifices in his or her own life to protect and promote the well-being of patients. Self-sacrifice thus requires educators and learners to direct their attention to the needs and concerns of patients and to promote these interests in teaching settings. Patients should not, for instance, be "used" for educational "purposes" or "gains." Instead, patients should be invited into the care of a physician-in-training who, with supervision and support, can provide care of excellent quality while also

---

Box 2

The four fundamental virtues

Integrity: The lifelong commitment to the practice of medicine in accord with the standards of intellectual and moral excellence.

Compassion: The determination to promote patients' best interests, including relief of their pain and suffering through identification with their distress.

Self-effacement: The putting aside of differences between physicians and patients that should not count as clinically relevant.

Self-sacrifice: The routine willingness of physicians to take risks in their own lives to protect and promote the interests of patients.

helping attain a second aim, a positive "double effect," of helping the early career caregiver to learn.

In aspiring to support the development of physicians whose responses will be governed by these specific virtues, psychiatric educators are obligated to embody and teach to standards of intellectual or academic excellence and to standards of moral excellence. Stated differently, to fulfill the duties inherent to their roles, psychiatric educators are responsible for serving as professional role models and for designing pedagogical approaches with appropriate ethics content and learning methods.[6] An ethics of education uninformed by the virtues of Gregory and the behaviors they inspire will, in the authors' view, lack integrity. Learners at all stages of training, moreover, quickly will perceive the distance between their teachers' actions and their words. If it is a long stretch, all curricular efforts in ethics and professionalism become lost causes. On the other hand, learners have a professional responsibility to engage wholly in their educational tasks: learners are obligated to aim to do their best in educational settings and to make the most of the learning opportunities so that they may serve present and future patients better.

TEACHING EVIDENCE-BASED MEDICINE

John Gregory and Francis Bacon, by calling for medicine to be based on experiments, articulated a nascent concept of the evidence-based medicine of today. The practice of evidence-based medicine is a lifelong directed learning process that is founded on the science of epidemiology and is linked to providing optimal care. It is a systematic, disciplined process for implementing the best evidence into clinical care settings. The major thrust of evidence-based medicine is to reduce the possibility of bias in clinical decision-making.

There are four steps to evidence-based medicine,[7] beginning with a question about what is the evidence for a particular view or decision. Questions can arise from diagnostic, prognostic, ethics, harm, economic, or treatment considerations. The second step involves searching the literature for the best evidence which, when available, normally includes information obtained from systematic reviews or meta-analyses or from randomized, controlled trials.[8] When well conducted, these study designs are less open to the potential for bias.

The third step involves reading the evidence critically to evaluate the reasonableness of the conclusions in relation to the study's goals, adequacy of methods, and results. This step also involves determining the applicability of the study findings to the diagnostic, prognostic, or treatment problem of the individual patient, with regard to specific patient issues including ethnicity, age, gender, and socioeconomic level. Applicability is determined by the inclusion and exclusion criteria of the relevant studies. Attention to these criteria can enable psychiatrists to place the available evidence into the context of individual patients. The fourth critical step in evidence-based medicine is to integrate the results of the previous steps and the clinical recommendations that follow from these steps into routine care, while taking account of the availability of resources and expertise.

The ethical principle of beneficence links directly to these strategies of evidence-based medicine. Obligations of beneficence direct the psychiatrist to apply expertise, rigorously derived, in the service of the patient.[9] Obligations of beneficence further govern the psychiatrist's approach to seek the greater balance of clinical benefits over harms in the care of patients, as understood from a careful, often meticulous, evidence-based perspective.[9] Obligations of beneficence are to be balanced against the ethical principle of respect for autonomy. In respecting a patient's autonomy, the psychiatrist seeks to provide a greater balance of goods over harms in the care of the patient, as understood from the patient's own perspectives of those goods and harms, which in turn are derived in part from that person's experiences and life circumstances.[10] Thus, because evidence alone is insufficient to make clinical decisions, evidence-based medicine is evolving to incorporate the values and preferences of the informed patient into clinical decision-making as fully as possible.[11]

Educators therefore should teach learners to explore patient perspectives and to give weight to patients' preferences, including the option of receiving no treatment, in light of the clinical imperatives of the case. Educators also will help learners understand approaches to managing conflicts between the obligations of beneficence and respect for autonomy when they arise. These approaches constitute important and commonly applied skills in psychiatric practice.

An ethical approach to psychiatric education must seek routinely to minimize the potential for bias to influence clinical decision-making and to find an ethical balance of patients' preferences and the obligations of beneficence. Educational curricular goals routinely should promote the use of evidence-based medicine in clinical settings, promote patterns of lifelong learning, and help learners become familiar with the medical literature and its application to patient care.

CULTIVATING THE VIRTUES

The second and third components of an ethics of psychiatric education, as informed by Gregory, emphasize the importance of protecting and promoting the interests of patients while treating the physician's interests as only secondary to those of patients. These components of an ethics of psychiatric education are illustrated by two commonplace examples in psychiatric practice: managing suicidal patients and managing sexual boundaries with patients.

Managing Suicidal Patients

Psychiatrists routinely manage suicidal patients, and between 32% and 61% of psychiatry residents experience the suicide of at least one patient during training.[12] Prevention of suicide through the provision of appropriate treatment is a central ethical concern,[13] although some neuropsychiatric diseases properly should be understood as potentially terminal illnesses, and not all suicides are preventable. Challenges in managing suicidal patients include that prediction is inherently probabilistic and never certain,[13] and that hospitalization and enforced treatment do not ensure safety.

The ethical issues related to managing suicide relate first to the ethical imperative to act beneficently in helping alleviate the distress and despair experienced by people living with mental illness who believe that ending their lives will solve the problem of their suffering.[9] In such a situation, intervening to safeguard the patient seems to subordinate the preferences of the patient. Helping the learner recognize when disease processes may be distorting the perceptions, ideas, reasons, feelings, and beliefs of the patient will help the learner correctly prioritize beneficently motivated actions to protect the patient and to understand that such actions are not disrespectful of the patient's autonomy when the patient's judgment is significantly impaired by mental illness. Indeed, many of the most difficult ethical issues encountered in the care of suicidal patients arise from the emotional responses of their caregivers.[14] Managing suicidal patients can cause trainees to worry about their reputation and about a malpractice suit should a suicide occur.[15] A sense of frustration can ensue when patients do not follow recommendations about safety. In addition, the suicide of a patient might lead residents to become overly protective of patients.[12,16–18]

Therefore a critical component of the ethics of psychiatric education is to assist residents or trainees in recognizing those strong feelings as a first step in protecting against their distorting clinical judgment. These strong feelings can interfere with clinical judgment when patients are hospitalized unnecessarily or when a discussion with patients or team members about sensitive issues of risk is avoided.

The virtues of self-effacement and self-sacrifice are especially relevant in managing these ethical concerns. Self-effacement obligates psychiatrists to put aside feelings of worry, fear, or frustration when these feelings impair clinical judgment and when they are not relevant to treatment. Self-sacrifice obligates the psychiatrist to de-emphasize self-interest and to tolerate fear and frustration when doing so is necessary to ensure appropriate treatment of a patient. This obligation means that psychiatry should accept some risk on the behalf of the chronically suicidal patient, unless, of course, that risk becomes more acute. Self-effacement and self-sacrifice together focus attention on the needs of the patient, promote thoughtful, reasoned judgment, and support the provision of excellence in clinical care. Educators should teach and model these virtues in clinical practice.

Sexual Boundaries between Patients and Psychiatrists

Almost 5% of psychiatrists[19] and almost 1% of psychiatry residents[20] report having had sexual contact with patients. Although response rates were low in earlier surveys, the prevalence may be similar that in surveys of sexual contact between physicians and patients in other specialties.[21] Medical students also can hold attitudes that conflict with the standards of the profession,[22] even after an educational intervention designed to correct those attitudes.[23] This issue is of considerable importance to the medical profession, which has codified strict prohibitions against sexual contact between doctors and their current patients.[24,25]

The American Psychiatric Association also has classified all sexual activity with either current or former patients as unethical.[26] These prohibitions are driven by several considerations, particularly that sexual contact with patients is almost always harmful,[27–29] and that the doctor may exploit the trust of a patient who is vulnerable because of the patient's emotional state or because of the doctor's knowledge or influence resulting from the professional relationship.[25] Long ago, the Hippocratic writings forbade "mischief making" with patients in addition to stating the imperatives to act beneficently, protect confidentiality, confer optimism, and perform work within the limits of one's clinical competence. Later Gregory also spoke against sexual contact with patients in response to complaints of abuse against the practitioners of his day.[30] Two of the present authors (LBM, JHC) have proposed a virtues-based ethical argument reinforcing previous arguments and demonstrating that sexual relationships between physicians and their current patients are always unethical.[31] In particular self-effacement obligates the psychiatrist to forego acting on personal characteristics that should not count as relevant to the professional relationship. These characteristics include a patient's gender, ethnicity, personal manners, religious views, socioeconomic status, and sexual attractiveness. Self-sacrifice requires psychiatrists to put aside their sexual interest in patients when it occurs. Those two virtues, linked with integrity, form a bulwark against acting on a sexual attraction toward a patient.[31]

Publicized occasions in which physicians engage in sexual contact with patients can be very damaging to the profession, undermining trust in all medical professionals. Psychiatrists, and indeed all physicians, have an obligation to protect the reputation of the profession and thus to preserve the trust of patients by foregoing sexual contact with patients. Psychiatrists also have a responsibility to the profession to protect and foster trust in the institutions and medical organizations of the profession.

As noted previously, sexual contact with a patient is on a par with discriminating against a patient based on other factors that should not count in the physician–patient relationship. Psychiatric educators should work hard to promote a culture of respect for patients as well as for colleagues. They also should be vigilant to identify how the environment of learning might impede or erode respect for patients and to counter any demeaning, sexual, or negative comments directed to patients. They also should promote the understanding that self-observation is a key professional obligation. By recognizing sexual feelings as they arise, students, residents, and all physicians should be better equipped to prevent those feelings from undermining the professional relationship with patients. A rigorous attention to a resident's own attitudes and behaviors should be encouraged throughout the training experience, and efforts also should be undertaken to reveal and deconstruct potentially adverse or contrary lessons taught in the "hidden curriculum." This culture of respect and attention to the needs of patients should pervade all clinical and educational encounters. The curriculum should provide opportunities to reflect on how such a culture of respect can be achieved.

Sexual relationships with patients are unacceptable ethically because of the significant differential in power that exists between the expert who can provide help and resources and the patient who is in need. Similarly, there are constraints, although perhaps less strict, that discourage sexual relationships between educators or supervisors and learners. The relationship between teacher and student is based on a relative empowerment of the teacher, and learners can be vulnerable to exploitation. Relationships that involve people in overlapping and dual roles introduce ethical vulnerability to both individuals. Consequently, such relationships can be harmful both to the learner and to the milieu of the training program. Furthermore, such relationships can impair the educator's objectivity. When feedback about clinical performance is unduly positive or biased or when learners are promoted inappropriately, the standards of the profession are undermined, and the safety of patients is compromised. Intimate relationships between teachers and learners that in time disintegrate also create repercussions that require role separation and active ethical safeguards to prevent damage to the careers of both individuals.

Responsibly Managing Conflicts of Interest

A conflict of interest exists when the psychiatrist has a conflict between obligations to the patient, on the one hand, and self-interest, on the other. Gregory was one of the first to address the ethics of conflicts of interest and did so on the basis of the professional virtue of self-sacrifice. He was very concerned about the bias that economic self-interest can introduce into both clinical practice and research when economic self-interest becomes the physician's primary consideration. He was equally concerned about the ability of patients to be able to trust their physicians to put the patient's interests first and not the physician's acquisition of money, prestige, or power. Gregory called for the systematic sacrifice of economic self-interest. If physicians commit themselves to scientific and ethical excellence in the practice of medicine, they will become professional physicians, and patients will be able to differentiate them from self-interested physicians. Professional physicians can be confident that, in the long run, the market will recognize and reward their commitment to scientific and ethical excellence. This point needs to be emphasized, especially with students and residents who are skeptical.

An essential component of teaching psychiatric ethics is to provide students and residents with the concept of a conflict of interest and the concept of the professional virtue of self-sacrifice as the basis for the responsible management of conflicts of interest. Discussions of actual conflicts of interest (eg, setting one's own fee for psychotherapy, or negotiating rates of payment with insurance companies, or accepting gifts from industry) should focus on the responsible management of these conflicts, especially the requirement to justify giving priority to individual self-interest. This topic has become especially urgent in light of recent exposés of the failure of university psychiatrists to disclose honestly payments from industry.[32]

SUMMARY

Evidence-based medicine and the professional virtues of integrity, compassion, self-effacement, and self-sacrifice constitute the cornerstones of an ethics of psychiatric education. As informed by the pioneering work of John Gregory, psychiatric educators must promote evidence-based and ethically justified behaviors in learners and practicing physicians through example and by formal teaching. These processes together will enable patients to trust the competence of psychiatrists and that psychiatrists will serve the interests of patients first.

REFERENCES

1. Coverdale J, Bayer T, Isbell P, et al. Are we teaching psychiatrists to be ethical? Acad Psychiatry 1992;16:199–205.
2. Roberts LW, McCarty T, Lyketsos C, et al. What and how psychiatry residents at ten training programs wish to learn about ethics. Acad Psychiatry 1996;20(3): 127–39.
3. McCullough L, Coverdale J, Chervenak F. Argument-based medical ethics: a formal tool for critically appraising the normative ethics: literature. Am J Obstet Gynecol 2004;191:1097–102.
4. McCullough LB. John Gregory (1724-1773) and the invention of professional medical ethics and the profession of medicine. Dordrecht, The Netherlands: Kluwer Academic; 1998.
5. McCullough LB. John Gregory (1724-1773) and the invention of professional relationships in medicine. J Clin Ethics 1997;8:11–21.
6. Roberts LW, McCarty T, Roberts BB, et al. Clinical ethics teaching in psychiatric supervision. Acad Psychiatry 1996;20(3):172–84.
7. Rosenberg W, Donald A. Evidence-based medicine: an approach to clinical problem-solving. BMJ 1995;310:1122–6.
8. Grimes DA. An overview of clinical research: the lay of the land. Lancet 2002;359: 57–61.
9. Beauchamp TL, Childress JF. Principles of biomedical ethics. 6th edition. New York: Oxford University Press; 2009.
10. McCullough LB, Chervenak FA. Ethics in obstetrics and gynecology. New York: Oxford University Press; 1994.
11. Montori VM, Guyatt GH. Progress in evidence-based medicine. JAMA 2008;300: 1814–6.
12. Fang F, Kemp J, Jawandha A, et al. Encountering patient suicide: a resident's experience. Acad Psychiatry 2007;31:340–4.
13. Roberts LW, Dyer AR. Concise guide to ethics in mental health care. Washington, DC: American Psychiatric Publishing; 2004.

14. Coverdale J, Roberts LW, Louie AK. Encountering patient suicide: emotional responses, ethics, and implications for training programs. Acad Psychiatry 2007;31:329–32.
15. Shein HM. Suicide care: obstacles in the education of psychiatric residents. Omega 1976;7:75–81.
16. Sacks HS, Kibel HD, Cohen AM. Resident response to patient suicide. J Psychiatr Educ 1987;11:217–26.
17. Pilkington P, Etkin M. Encountering suicide: the experience of psychiatric residents. Acad Psychiatry 2003;27:93–9.
18. Tillman JG. When a patient commits suicide: an empirical study of psychoanalytic clinicians. Int J Psychoanal 2006;87:159–77.
19. Gartrell N, Herman J, Olarte S, et al. Psychiatrist-patient sexual contact: results of a national survey. 1. Prevalance. Am J Psychiatry 1986;143:1126–31.
20. Gartrell N, Herman J, Olarte S, et al. Psychiatric residents' sexual contact with educators and patients: results of a national survey. Am J Psychiatry 1988;145:690–4.
21. Bayer T, Coverdale J, Chiang E. A national survey of physicians' behaviors regarding sexual contact with patients. South Med J 1996;89:977–82.
22. Coverdale J, Bayer T, Chiang E, et al. Medical students' attitudes on specialist physicians' social and sexual contact with patients. Acad Psychiatry 1996;20:35–42.
23. Coverdale J, Turbott SH. Teaching medical students about the appropriateness of social and sexual contact between doctors and their patients: evaluation of a programme. Med Educ 1997;31:335–40.
24. Kay J, Roman B. Prevention of sexual misconduct at the medical school, residency, and practitioner levels. In: Nadelson CL, Notman MT, editors. Physician-sexual misconduct. Washington, DC: American Psychiatric Press; 1999. p. 153–76.
25. Code of Medical Ethics. Current opinion of the Council of Ethical and Judicial Affairs of the American Medical Association. Chicago: American Medical Association; 1992.
26. American Psychiatric Association. The principles of medical ethics with annotations especially applicable to psychiatry. Washington, DC: American Psychiatric Press; 2008.
27. Gartrell NK, Milliken N, Goodson WH, et al. Physician-patient sexual contact: prevalence and problems. West J Med 1992;157:139–43.
28. Pope KS. Therapist-patient sex syndrome: a guide for attorneys and subsequent therapists to assessing damage. In: Gabbard G, editor. Sexual exploitation in professional relationships. Washington, DC: American Psychiatric Press; 1989. p. 39–56.
29. Burgess AW. Physician sexual misconduct and patients' responses. Am J Psychiatry 1981;138:1335–42.
30. Porter R. A touch of danger: the man-midwife as sexual predator. In: Rousseau GS, Porter R, editors. Sexual underworld of the enlightenment. Manchester (England): Manchester University Press; 1987. p. 206–32.
31. McCullough LB, Chervenak F, Coverdale J. Ethically justified guidelines for defining sexual boundaries between obstetrician-gynecologists and their patients. Am J Obstet Gynecol 1996;175:496–500.
32. Harris G. Top psychiatrist didn't report drug makers' pay. New York Times. October 4, 2008. Available at: http://www.nytimes.com/2008/10/04/health/policy/04drug.html?scp=3&sq=psychiatry%20emory&st=cse. Accessed December 3, 2008.

The Revolution in Forensic Ethics: Narrative, Compassion, and a Robust Professionalism

Philip J. Candilis, MD

KEYWORDS

• Forensic ethics • Robust professionalism • Historical narrative

For the past 50 years forensic psychiatry has struggled with the seminal question of which master it serves. Does it answer chiefly to the law or to psychiatry? It is the law, after all, that privileges forensic experts in the courtroom, but it is psychiatry that grounds them in the medical ethics of care and cure. This question is not merely a conceptual one; it has profound implications for practitioners' daily work. It determines which values hold sway, which definitions are applied, and which goals are most important.[1–3]

A LEGAL OR MEDICAL PROFESSION?

Considered on its own, the law can be envisioned as the arbiter of social order, an authority with broad powers and responsibilities. It must have the capacity to command and control individuals and communities while allowing sufficient flexibility to address the full range of human behavior. The law exacts reparation and retribution, enforces or dissolves agreements, and visits serious and intentional harm on some individuals in its purview. In the Unites States, emphasis on the rule-based resolution of disputes—an approach that is adversarial and heavy with procedures and precedents—results in a certain kind of ethical system, one that may serve social order to the detriment of the individual.

Psychiatry, of course, is a different enterprise. Built on values of care and healing, psychiatry is (largely) medical in its approach, focusing on improving an individual's health and optimizing potential. Rather than relying on the justification of social order, psychiatry builds its collaborations on scientific and empirical information that supports its helping mission. Social order is still important, as civil commitment,

Law and Psychiatry Program, University of Massachusetts Medical School, 55 Lake Avenue North, Worcester, MA 01655, USA
E-mail address: philip.candilis@umassmed.edu

Psychiatr Clin N Am 32 (2009) 423–435
doi:10.1016/j.psc.2009.02.005
0193-953X/09/$ – see front matter © 2009 Elsevier Inc. All rights reserved.

psych.theclinics.com

community leverage, and organizational psychiatry attest, but when the care of an individual patient is primary, a different ethical system is formed—one often discussed in reverential terms as covenant, advocacy, or relationship. This is qualitatively different from the law.

The two fields, however, frequently intersect on matters of behavior, perception, thinking, and emotion. In fact, the law counts on psychiatry to perform exculpatory or explanatory functions. Was the defendant acting under compulsion? Was she of sound mind, behaving knowingly and voluntarily? Or was she unable to conform her conduct to the requirements of the law? Competence and mitigation hearings, insanity defenses, commitments, and guardianships all call for the two systems to overlap, causing a serious clash of values and priorities.

How are practitioners to adapt to this clash? Is it a matter of adopting the mantle of the law and being guided by its attorney representatives or of transplanting the values of the clinic or hospital to the legal setting? Is there a third option, one that considers the values of both but caters to neither?

An exploration of the historical narrative of forensic ethics may show that it has developed to the point where it is not enough to apply legal or medical ethics alone.[1,4,5] The intersection of these highly evolved and differing fields calls for more than a passing familiarity with cases and cures. It is only an appreciation of broader perspectives, mixed theories, and sophisticated ethical habits and skills that allows negotiation of the complex meeting of courtroom and clinic.

One can begin by looking at the approaches that set legal priorities first, above psychiatric or medical considerations. It is an approach with a firm foundation in legal and ethical scholarship and championed by careful thinkers in forensic medicine.

THE PRIMACY OF LEGAL ETHICS

Seymour Pollack[6] is the forensic scholar most prominently associated with the primacy of legal values for forensic psychiatrists. A professor and insanity expert at the University of Southern California, Pollack believed that forensic expertise concerns itself "primarily with the ends of the legal system." Forensic psychiatric evaluation, for him, was "directed primarily to the legal issues in which [the patient] is involved." This view accepted the law's social goals and invited psychiatrists to conceive a role outside their usual responsibilities as physicians.

Heavily grounded in role theory, Pollack's approach allowed the context or setting to set the tone for the forensic psychiatrist's work. He accepted the law's ends as legitimate and its procedures as appropriate to the task. It was the work taken in context that determined the role of the professional; and the context was a legal one.

Of course, Pollack did not agree with all the goals of the legal system. He had an almost revelatory experience after his testimony against Sirhan Sirhan, Robert Kennedy's assassin. Deeply troubled that he had contributed to the death sentence meted out at trial, Pollack never again testified in a capital case. His personal opposition to the death penalty ultimately trumped his deference to the law's objectives. So, although legal ends were primary in the forensic context, Pollack exercised personal judgment in applying his expertise. Such personal judgment allowed an opening for other ethical considerations.

Physician-ethicist Paul Appelbaum[7,8] is the most prominent of recent advocates for the primacy of legal values in forensic work. Appelbaum argues forcefully that forensic psychiatry's purpose is legitimate only insofar as it *can* act outside psychiatry's usual role: it must accept a role that can be intentionally harmful to the individual. Indeed forensic psychiatry would be useless otherwise. What purpose would it serve in the courts if psychiatry took only a caring, nurturing stance?

In crafting the first formal theory of forensic practice. Appelbaum[8] argued that principles supporting truth and justice outweigh those supporting care. Underscoring the primacy of truth in forensic psychiatry, Appelbaum nonetheless identified both objective and subjective truth in forensic work—the objective truth found in the medical literature and the subjective truth found in the expert's opinion. Identifying this nuance in the truth sought by forensic work, Appelbaum implicitly recognized the influence of nonlegal values and judgments—both scientific and personal ones.

Because finding truth was more important than caring for the individual, distinguishing the forensic role from the clinical one was a cardinal element of Appelbaum's approach. The separation of roles in forensic work is critical because of the danger that an evaluee will assume the psychiatrist is there to help. The evaluee may believe that the usual rules of the hospital or clinic apply: she may feel free to reveal damning information, to neglect her defense, or ignore her attorney. If roles are not separated cleanly, experts too may fall into this trap. Experts may not recognize the effect their traditional role has on evaluees: they may exercise empathic, clinical strategies to muddy the waters and extract information that takes advantage of the evaluee's misconception.

Lawrence Strasburger,[9] a professor and past president of the American Academy of Psychiatry and the Law (AAPL), and his colleagues at Harvard illustrated the differences between the two roles by describing how each approaches the patient or evaluee. The treating psychiatrist who takes a psychodynamic approach, for example, may focus on the patient's perspective or personal formulation of truth. The patient's perceptions and distortions are the focus of the therapeutic work, with the patient's narrative influenced by internal psychological experiences and the search for meaning.

The forensic expert, by contrast, is interested in more objective versions of the truth, versions that can be agreed upon by social institutions such as police departments and courts. The truth in the forensic role is necessarily more societally based, with a responsibility toward "the fair adjudication of disputes and the determination of innocence and guilt."[9]

For both Strasburger and Appelbaum, the importance of truth and justice is tempered by sensitivity to these differences between roles; both authors endorse separation of the clinical and forensic functions. To bolster this approach, Appelbaum endorses the principle of respect for persons, a principle that protects vulnerable evaluees with confidentiality warnings about the forensic psychiatrist's work. This approach tempers the unimpeded pursuit of truth with a concern for the protection of the vulnerable individual—an individual in the control of the legal system, and facing an uncertain future.

Appelbaum's important framework for forensic psychiatry nonetheless sets legal values above medical ones in a hierarchy of ethical principles. Although clinical techniques are used to interview and explore reasoning, behavior, and emotions, they serve the law first. Protections are included in the framework, as are certain basic medical duties (eg, when an evaluee suffers a medical crisis during an interview). These medical duties, however, fall outside the role of the forensic psychiatrist— a specialist with a specific task outside the traditional function of a physician.

THE PRIMACY OF MEDICAL ETHICS

Bernard Diamond[10] provides the antithesis to this "put-the-law-first" approach. Diamond, a Berkeley professor who had a profound impact on California law, worked only for the defense. He believed strongly that psychiatrists should preserve their physicianly values, using the legal system to attain more therapeutic ends. Diamond[11] notably wrote, "The psychiatrist is no mere technician to be used by the law as the law sees fit."

Diamond used the expert's fiduciary responsibility to define the professional requirements of the role.[12] This relationship of confidence and trust, common to both medicine and law, presaged the grounding of forensic ethics in the moral relationship of evaluator and evaluee. It was an early recognition of parallel ethical values in the two professions.[3]

Through his clinical lens, Diamond saw the partiality and subjectivity of forensic work. Although he practiced an ethic of total honesty in describing his biases in a case, he knew that fraught topics like criminality and litigation could undermine the objectivity of the most seasoned forensic psychiatrist. The adversarial nature of United States law and ongoing controversies in law and psychiatry would see to that.

This paradigm of forensic ethics finds a more recent voice in the writings of Robert Weinstock[13,14] of the University of California, Los Angeles. Weinstock, a forensic psychiatrist and educator, is a strong modern-day proponent of grounding forensic practice in medical ethics. After all, forensic practitioners develop first as physicians, then as psychiatrists, and only after that as forensic experts. In this view, medical ethics can be helpful in finding psychiatric evidence to assist a defendant and in deciding what kinds of cases an expert is competent to accept. Considerations of physical and mental harm, of the strength of clinical evidence, and of clinical skills such as self-reflection and awareness of one's limits and biases all come into play through medical ethics.

Weinstock's classic practitioner surveys identified the broad support for this framework by showing the strong influence of medical ethics on forensic practitioners.[15–17] Respondents to his surveys repeatedly identified the importance of medical values in their work.

At the same time, forensic psychiatrists recognized competing responsibilities to the community. In their surveys, they endorsed statements that identified the conflicting values and multiple duties in forensic work. This balance among the actual practitioners of the craft opened the door to nonmedical influences (eg, community, public safety), much as Pollack's opposition to the death penalty opened the door to considerations of personal, nonlegal values.

THE INADEQUACY OF PURIST APPROACHES

The recognition that purist ethical frameworks are inadequate to address the complexities of forensic practice is evident in the work of all the preceding authors. In fact, each draws on diverse philosophical constructs to enrich his views. Appelbaum, as we have seen, recognized basic human duties between forensic clinician and evaluee and both medical and legal elements of forensic testimony. Diamond and Pollack recognized the personal and professional challenges to pure objectivity, and Weinstock exposed (and endorsed) the balancing approach found among his survey respondents. It is the deficiency of any single ethical framework that underscores the challenge of forensic ethics.

Harvard professor and former AAPL president Thomas Gutheil and his colleagues[18] highlighted precisely this deficiency when they wrote that forensic experts must account for the interactions of individuals, institutions, and society. It is not enough to arrive at specific, scientifically based answers to forensic questions when there is uncertainty in their observation, measurement, and analysis. Neither human behavior nor the behavior of social institutions is a purely objective construct. Consequently, there should be a clear recognition that uncertainties, probabilities, and values confound any pristine approach to forensic thinking.

To address the vicissitudes of working within both the legal and medical systems, the University of Rochester's Richard Ciccone,[19,20] with ethicist Colleen Clements, proposed an elegant approach to forensic work that related the medical and legal systems instead of differentiating them. In his "systems approach," there were far more possibilities for ethical analysis when cases could be decided by "brokering and negotiation between the systems." When practitioners recognized the imperfection of solutions offered by one system alone, a balance of medical and legal values could be achieved.

NARRATIVE ETHICS

It was not, however, until cross-cultural psychiatrist and Yale professor Ezra Griffith[4,21] weighed in, that a sea change was evident in the evolution of forensic ethics. Instead of the usual distinction between legal and medical ethics, Griffith proposed a cultural formulation for forensic ethics. There was no justice, he wrote, in ethical frameworks that did not specifically address how dominant and nondominant groups were treated differently before the bar. Indeed, antiseptic appeals to justice, truth, or objectivity ring hollow when the narratives of oppressed minorities are ignored.

This call for cultural sensitivity was more than a reaction to the usual exercise of cultural dominance in society's institutions. It was the formal introduction of cultural narrative as a tool for forensic practitioners. Forensic ethics to this point had identified roles and principles as the cardinal tools for guiding forensic practice, but the discussion had an unfinished quality. Here finally was a framework—narrative ethics—that could apply roles and principles to specific cases.

Narrative had been evident before in forensic psychiatry, albeit without the stature of a freestanding moral theory. Indeed it provided a touchstone in the organizational history of psychiatry. In 1980 Alan Stone,[22] president of the American Psychiatric Association (APA) and a Harvard law professor, recounted the now widely repeated "Parable of the Black Sergeant."

As an Army psychiatrist, Stone had been asked to evaluate a military officer of color who was accused of stealing government supplies. During his examination of the highly cooperative sergeant, Stone found considerable evidence of racist victimization and personal anger but none of the "kleptomania" proposed by the defense. Without an opportunity in court to describe the cultural context of the black sergeant's behavior, Stone was unable to describe a formal mental condition excusing his actions. This led to the sergeant's conviction and a sentence of 5 years at hard labor. Stone was left with the feeling that justice had not been served.

Stone[23] drew further narrative ammunition from the historical example of Dr. Leo, a Jewish physician in England testifying on behalf of a Jewish defendant accused of stealing four silver spoons. Dr. Leo tried valiantly to defend his fellow citizen in the anti-Semitic court, succeeding only in bringing ethnically charged ridicule and disapprobation upon himself. "Could he say," Dr. Stone asked, "that [given the primitive state of psychiatry in 1801] his purpose in testifying was other than to help a fellow Jew escape what the law of the day considered just punishment...?"

Based on these narratives, Stone[22,23] famously challenged the APA and AAPL to identify anything they really could offer the courts. Stone's challenge was very much based in concerns that psychiatrists could seduce evaluees into revealing too much information, as might have occurred with the black sergeant, or that psychiatrists themselves could be seduced into pretending too much expertise and advocating improperly for one side, as he contended occurred with Dr. Leo.

Griffith, of course, was not surprised by the conviction of the black sergeant or by Dr. Leo's attempt to defend a vulnerable fellow citizen. Griffith nonetheless expressed compassion, rather than disgust, for cases that did not offer sufficient opportunity to explore the full narrative of the forensic encounter. Social context mattered, and assuring that the nondominant perspective was heard represented another step toward a full accounting of forensic morality. In one fell swoop, Griffith had clarified for psychiatry what moral philosophers and ethicists had been trying to explain to their fields for years: that roles and principles do not do enough to explain the moral nuances of professionalism.

Narrative itself had entered medicine through medical ethics, responding to the concern that classic principles such as autonomy, beneficence, and justice did not do enough moral work in complicated cases.[1,3,24] Narrative ethicists, as the new proponents were called, believed more could be done to address the intentions and motives of moral actors. For these new commentators, meaning and nuance could be established only through a more complete understanding of the actor's story.

Narrative was a powerful new tool for exploring the human drama, conflict, and tension of forensic cases. It offered a frame for unfamiliar perspectives, much as the new-found cultural sensitivities of law and medicine called for greater awareness of non-Western and immigrant values.

Resonating deeply with the psychodynamic instincts of psychiatrists like Bernard Diamond and Lawrence Strasburger—psychiatrists who could craft nuanced narratives of their patients' mental lives—narrative nonetheless had some important shortcomings. It was not enough, in a moral or legal sense, for one's story alone to justify right action. The power of individual narratives notwithstanding, there still must be rules for deciding between them when disagreements arose. Ciccone[20] was among those who pointed out the troubling moral relativism that would arise if the individual's perspective were all that mattered in a pluralistic society.

Fortunately modern professional ethics had never relied on a single theoretical approach. Principles still were needed to connect cases to theory;[24] narrative was necessary for providing detail.[1] Indeed even a strong understanding of roles could not define the boundaries of complex cases sufficiently to determine ethical outcomes. Consequently, choosing *from* theories rather than among them remained a compelling option for appreciating the multiple facets of complex forensic interactions.[25]

COMPASSION AT THE CORE OF FORENSIC ETHICS

With social justice now a consideration in forensic ethics, the ethical armamentarium had expanded from legal ethics to medical ethics, from principles and role theory to narrative. There was increasing room for social context and moral values, for the independent moral presence of the practitioner and the narrative of the evaluee.

But for Michael Norko[5] of Yale there was something more than story-telling and truth-telling in Griffith's cultural formulation. In Griffith's writings (and some others that are explored more extensively later in this article), Norko saw an expression of compassion that went beyond the efforts a Dr. Leo might make in a racist setting. Here compassion was a moral foundation for forensic ethics as a whole.

Drawing on widely available constructs in religious and secular traditions, Norko emphasized the themes of fairness and justice (especially "do unto others") found throughout religious and philosophical systems. From before the Bible to Immanuel Kant, these were themes that mattered in basic human interactions. Norko wrote,

"A moral foundation for forensic work that is based on compassion is thus not an argument that can be easily dismissed as a parochial construct. In fact, employing

this construct places our work in a larger context of human endeavor and struggle. And where else should we look to find adequate cultural justification for our involvement in the struggles of the courtroom [p. 388]?"[5]

Norko called for Appelbaum's protective respect for persons to be achieved through the commonality of human experience and compassion for others. The social obligation between citizens required that the law be entrusted to "those who understand the obligation." Otherwise power and influence would be exercised in the ways decried by Griffith, Diamond, and Stone.

With this evolution in forensic ethics, it was possible to consider fairness along with objectivity; to recognize greater nuance in the truth-seeking of the forensic encounter. It was not only context that mattered, but culture and care for one's fellow man. This construct was sorely needed in the political firestorm that followed.

THE FORENSIC ETHICS OF GUANTANAMO BAY

The interrogation of "military detainees" at Guantanamo Bay raised a significant alarm when Behavioral Science Consultation Teams (BSCT or "biscuit" teams) were developed to advise military interrogators.[26] Using both psychiatrists and psychologists, BSCT teams employed mental health professionals outside their traditional roles, famously advising interrogators about one detainee's fear of the dark and about another's close relationship with his mother.[27,28] Based in the Survival, Evasion, Resistance, and Escape training of the United States military, this new brand of interrogation had taken an increasingly aggressive turn in the aftermath of September 11, 2001. Terms such as "stress positions" and "water-boarding" entered the common parlance as media outlets decried the use of medical and psychological professionals in supporting interrogations that could no longer be distinguished from torture.[27–29]

In psychiatry, APA president Steven Sharfstein visited Guantanamo Bay with the president of the American Psychological Association and formally asked that psychiatrists not be involved in the proceedings there. The APA and American Medical Association consequently published strong ethical statements against physicians participating in the new interrogation techniques. Participation was clearly outside the frame of medical ethics. The American Psychological Association, however, was more circumspect, recognizing an overarching legitimacy of social order and the potential for monitoring these aggressive interrogations.

Psychologists were not alone in suggesting that health-related professionals could participate legitimately in controversial activities outside their traditional roles. Forensic psychiatrist and educator Emily Keram,[30] who herself witnessed the effects of interrogation during her involvement as expert to Salim Hamdan, Osama bin-Laden's driver,[31] pointed out that Department of Defense (DOD) regulations clearly left the door open to nontraditional professional activities such as aggressive interrogation. Professionals acting in consultative roles could, in the view of the DOD, legitimately behave in a manner "inconsistent with traditional medical ethics."

Robert Phillips,[32] an officer of the APA and past president of AAPL, also suggested that forensic psychiatrists could justifiably assist in developing and monitoring interrogation techniques. In their forensic work, psychiatrists were acting in a different professional role. When working for law enforcement, he wrote, psychiatrists may function properly outside their traditional obligations, acting legitimately as consultants. Their duty was not to the individual but to the institution that hired them or to society at large.

This form of "exceptionalism," that is, allowing exceptions in which health care professionals could ignore core professional values, provided a context unrecognizable to many ethicists (eg, see Refs.[3,33,34]). Merely declaring certain ethics inapplicable does not make it so, particularly when social expectations, the profession's history, basic human values, and past professional atrocities of the kind perpetrated by the Nazi doctors and Soviet psychiatrists all militate against it. The historical narrative of the profession and its place in the social fabric require that arguments for exceptionalism be viewed with great caution.

The implications for forensic psychiatry were stark. Putting psychiatrists entirely outside their historical narrative severed the moderating influence of medical ethics, of certain social values, of history, and balance—influences that had been recognized in forensic ethics for decades.[1–21]

A ROBUST PROFESSIONALISM

Efforts to describe a unified approach to forensic ethics began as soon as the ink had dried on Griffith's 1998 critique. Originally offered as a presidential address to AAPL the year after Appelbaum's theory was unveiled, Griffith's introduction of narrative and the cultural formulation seemed to provide the missing piece for a robust description of forensic professionalism.

The weaknesses of strict role theory for forensic psychiatry had been exposed first in the inadequacy of purist approaches and later in the cages of Guantanamo Bay, so an approach that went beyond merely defining the limits of professional activity would extend the minimalist obligations to the forensic evaluee. In preparation for a description of a robust professionalism, Candilis and Martinez[1–3,35] joined Weinstock[14] and others[33,34] in exploring the potential damage that could arise from excluding the more recent ethical considerations.

First, the assumption that a separate role for physicians could be constructed for forensic, police, or national security functions created a speculative world where psychiatrists could be free of influences arising from their clinical training, life experiences, and world view. This was the very world of pure objectivity rejected by early theorists. Indeed, psychiatrists were among those professionals who developed tools of self-reflection and self-awareness to identify the blind spots and influences that disrupted their work. The suggestion that they would not be affected by such influences in a purely forensic role, or that they would require extraordinary mindfulness to overcome them, was a risky standard when an evaluee's freedom or life was at stake.

Second, a strict role view of professionalism excluded personal values, the very values most relevant to one's identity as a citizen and moral actor. Forensic practitioners, after all, are professionals who have "many diverse yet particular beginnings."[2] To drive these values underground hid more relevant influences, suggested it was possible to ignore personal values, and relegated the individual professional to a technician's function in forensic work.

Third, excluding historical elements of the parent clinical profession ignored history that could illuminate important moral traps. The dangers of seducing the evaluee into divulging too much information, of testifying beyond one's expertise, and of advocating outright for a certain judicial outcome had already been well described (ie, in the cases of The Black Sergeant and Dr. Leo). The recognition that the historical narrative of forensic psychiatry itself was still evolving allowed more work to be done by those who were still exploring the sociological, cultural, and historical influences on forensic medicine (recall Weinstock, Gutheil, and Griffith). It was too soon to close debate and define the professional role merely as a representation of one institution or another, of one job-specific context or another.

Finally, minimalist obligations to a role or evaluee did not leave room for professional aspirations toward moral ideals.[35] It is only aspirational ethics that allows professionals to advance and improve the standards of their work. These aspirations include the refusal to accept the status quo of unequal treatment, of overstated scientific certainty, and of a single ethical perspective for all cases. A more complex ethic was called for, one that enriched discourse and offered more resources for difficult forensic cases.

Robust Professionalism: Integrity First

Those advocating for a robust professionalism[1-3,35] built on the realization that integrity matters in professional work—not integrity in the sense of honesty or truthfulness, but in the sense of unification or integration of parts. For the complex personal, social, and institutional commitments of forensic work, the qualities of wholeness or intactness yielded the richest model of forensic thinking.[1] In this view, robust forensic professionalism was not found in the artificial splintering of roles or of foundational ethical systems (ie, law versus medicine). Instead, a working definition of professional integrity was found in a model by ethicists Franklin Miller and Howard Brody,[36] who identified three necessary elements: (1) a set of well-regarded personal principles that remain somewhat stable over time and are coherent, (2) verbal expression of those values and principles, and (3) consistency between what one says and what one does.

This model recognized the formative influence of personal values, the salience of personal identity in one's work, and the connection of personal and professional identities. It was the outward expression of one's values in word and deed that made professional integrity a more communitarian venture. Here there was room for publicizing one's ethics and interacting with the community's values. The community then could define limits and expectations, creating in the professional a balance of personal and community values.[1] This was a more realistic, complete, and robust vision of what it meant to be a professional.

A unification or integration of personal, professional, and community values allows improved access to the more unfortunate temptations of forensic work, namely, fame and fortune. The criticism of forensic psychiatrists as "hired guns" had long been a name-calling exercise for experts who disagreed with each other in court. But now, with personal values open to examination, critics could go beyond vague challenges to one another's objectivity. They could examine explicitly their own and each other's biases and predilections. The importance of one's forensic track record, of testifying for both defense and prosecution, of turning down a percentage of cases, and other behavioral markers could be developed to explore heretofore inscrutable influences. Here was a framework for examining the influences on forensic psychiatrists that unified both theory and practice.

The integration of personal and community values consequently joined the profession's historical narrative in filling out the frameworks available for forensic ethics. Alongside legal and medical ethics, principles, narrative, and compassion, the stage was set for a definition of forensic professionalism itself.

Robust Professionalism: Defining Professionalism

It was becoming clear that a robust, textured, and deep professionalism does more than meet minimal standards and expectations of a single role or ethical theory. It is aspirational and strives for moral ideals. It seeks a path that does more than avoid dual roles and conflicts of interest.

A definition of robust professionalism consequently requires more than a list of training characteristics, job qualifications, or role duties. It requires a moral justification that transcends the psychiatric training of its experts or the legal venues of their practice. Wynia and colleagues[37] provided exactly this kind of definition when they wrote of professionalism as "an activity that involves both the distribution of a commodity and the fair allocation of a social good, but that is uniquely defined *according to moral relationships* [emphasis added]. Professionalism is a structurally stabilizing morally protective force in society." This is a professionalism that "protects not only vulnerable persons but also vulnerable social values."

The resonance of this definition with the concerns of Stone, Appelbaum, and Griffith is striking. If the purpose of the work itself includes advancing the concerns of vulnerable persons and values, the vulnerability of evaluees and the seduction of experts are addressed at the outset. Unethical outcomes are not a surprise at the end of a case.

Considering the forensic encounter a moral relationship allows a place for examination of personal values, of the evaluee's narrative, and of a connection to a crime victim or community safety in general. The forensic psychiatrist is a broker of the interplay between individuals and institutions, not simply of the retaining attorney or mentoring physician.

Grounding a profession in moral relationships allows the use of multiple perspectives, of multiple theories, balance, and negotiation. There are more analytic resources for solving ethical dilemmas. There is greater encouragement for pursuing moral aspirations—what the profession ought to be.[2] Because the perspectives of the evaluator, the evaluee, and the community have weight in the relationship, and because theories of law, medicine, and ethics come together in the evaluation, the forensic psychiatrist can transcend the mere technician's responsibility for a case.

How then do practitioners achieve aspirational goals that seem to require recognition of multiple perspectives, theories, and models?

Robust Professionalism: Applying the Model

Robust professionalism is put into practice through the behaviors that operationalize the theory (**Table 1**). In writings on psychiatric and forensic ethics, these behaviors have been called the habits and skills of the ethical practitioner.[3,38,39] Pollack and Diamond, for example, practiced these behaviors by transparently explaining their reasoning and allowing their bias in favor of either prosecution or defense to be apparent. In this way, courts could expand or restrict their judgments based on the approach to the case they found most compelling.

Both Pollack and Diamond therefore practiced openness and transparency as cardinal habits of the ethical practitioner. As they worked to describe the evaluee's condition and its connection to the criminal or civil complaint, they exposed the subjective influences on their thinking. Because they recognized the difficulty of achieving objectivity, they personified another skill now known as "striving for objectivity."[3]

Striving for objectivity recognizes that honest efforts must be made to describe the influences on the professional's work—influences on the evaluation, the evaluator, and the evaluee. This approach, also called "disciplined subjectivity" by ethicist Jay Katz,[40] recognized the illusory nature of objectivity and approximated more closely the messy reality of forensic interactions.

Striving for objectivity seemed to integrate honesty, transparency, self-reflection, self-awareness (especially knowing the limits of one's expertise), and exploration of the various aspects of a case. These qualities and skills would be important both in guiding ethical judgment and in responding to courtroom events. The practicality of

Table 1 Practicing robust professionalism: ethical habits and skills of the forensic practitioner	
Ethical Precepts	**Habits and Skills**
Sensitivity to vulnerable evaluees	Recognizing evaluee's disadvantage (economic, social, cultural, institutional) Recognizing ethical problems within a relationship of unequal power Applying cultural formulation Protecting vulnerable persons
Sensitivity to role problems	Identifying misperceptions of the examiner/examination Offering/crafting confidentiality warnings Separating clinical from forensic functions Recognizing limitations of role theory (avoiding "exceptionalism")
Self-awareness	Identifying/monitoring personal bias
Self-reflection	Practicing internal processing of emotions, behaviors
Honesty	Practicing openness, transparency when explaining one's role and findings Remaining within bounds of the facts and one's training Striving for objectivity
Integrity	Recognizing/integrating values of evaluator, evaluee, and community Recognizing fiduciary values in law and psychiatry Balancing personal and community values
Professionalism	Keeping professional expertise up to date Learning different approaches to ethical problems Choosing among ethical theories/solutions Balancing individual and societal claims Following the profession's historical narrative Protecting vulnerable values Aspiring to improve the profession

applying such skills in actual courtroom procedures (eg, in cross-examination, in which the expert is challenged and alternative explanations are explored) assured that the integrated or unified approach could be reproduced and taught. It was not long before the AAPL included "striving for objectivity" within its own professional guidelines, mirroring movements in other fields such as bioethics and journalism.[3]

These habits and skills of the ethical practitioner now could unify forensic thinking in the trenches. Recognizing multiple aspects of a case meant recognizing the strengths and weaknesses of one's own analysis. Recognizing one's personal values and biases and being transparent about them added to the effectiveness of this analysis. Tying these analyses to the evaluee's and profession's narrative, especially through the recognition of cultural narrative and the dangers of Guantanamo-style exceptionalism, provided a further integration of multiple perspectives. This more robust view of forensic professionalism consequently allowed for better forensic work, not just a deeper appreciation of the field's theoretical approaches.

In the settings in which most forensic psychiatrists practice, these habits and skills have special usefulness. In prisons, jails, and forensic and state hospitals, patients are uniquely vulnerable to the nuances of forensic examination. In these institutions, patients often are mentally ill, economically disadvantaged, and members of nondominant social groups. Without the protection of principles such as respect for persons, of tools such as cultural formulation, of habits such as automatic confidentiality warnings, or skills such as openness and transparency, the confluence of law and psychiatry could become a tragic mockery. Only a robust professionalism folded all these into an aspirational account of forensic ethics.

Forensic psychiatry had consequently evolved from its consideration of either law or medicine as its primary ethical guide. There was new room for personal values and their examination, for appreciation of the evaluee, evaluator, and community within a moral relationship, for recognition of social and institutional forces, and for acknowledgment of the profession's roots and history. It was a richer, more robust, forensic ethic, one that offered more potential solutions to ethical dilemmas and a more coherent approximation of actual forensic practice.

ACKNOWLEDGMENT

The author is grateful to Drs. Richard Martinez and Robert Weinstock for their collaboration in conceptualizing robust professionalism for forensic psychiatry.

REFERENCES

1. Candilis PJ, Martinez R, Dording C. Principles and narrative in forensic psychiatry: toward a robust view of professional role. J Am Acad Psychiatry Law 2001;29:167–73.
2. Martinez R, Candilis PJ. Commentary: toward a unified theory of personal and professional ethics. J Am Acad Psychiatry Law 2005;33:382–5.
3. Candilis PJ, Weinstock R, Martinez R. Forensic ethics and the expert witness. New York: Springer; 2007.
4. Griffith EE. Ethics in forensic psychiatry: a response to Stone and Appelbaum. J Am Acad Psychiatry Law 1998;26:171–84.
5. Norko MA. Commentary: compassion at the core of forensic ethics. J Am Acad Psychiatry Law 2005;33:386–9.
6. Pollack S. Forensic psychiatry in criminal law. Los Angeles (CA): University of Southern California Press; 1974.
7. Appelbaum PS. The parable of the forensic psychiatrist: ethics and the problem of doing harm. Int J Law Psychiatry 1990;13:249–59.
8. Appelbaum PS. A theory of ethics for forensic psychiatry. J Am Acad Psychiatry Law 1997;25:233–47.
9. Strasburger LH, Gutheil TG, Brodsky A. On wearing two hats: role conflict in serving as both psychotherapist and expert witness. Am J Psychiatry 1997; 154:448–56.
10. Diamond BL. The fallacy of the impartial expert. Archives of Criminal Psychodynamics 1959;3:221–36.
11. Diamond BL. The forensic psychiatrist: consultant vs. activist in legal doctrine. Bull Am Acad Psychiatry Law 1992;20:119–32.
12. Diamond BL. The simulation of sanity. Journal of Social Therapy 1956;2:158–65.
13. Weinstock R, Leong GB, Silva JA. The role of traditional medical ethics in forensic psychiatry. In: Rosner R, Weinstock R, editors. Ethical practice in psychiatry and the law. New York: Plenum Press; 1990. p. 31–51.
14. Weinstock R. Commentary: a broadened conception of forensic psychiatric ethics. J Am Acad Psychiatry Law 2001;29:180–5.

15. Weinstock R. Controversial ethical issues in forensic psychiatry: a survey. J Forensic Sci 1988;33:176–86.
16. Weinstock R. Perceptions of ethical problems by forensic psychiatrists. Bull Am Acad Psychiatry Law 1989;17:189–202.
17. Weinstock R, Leong GB, Silva JA. Opinions by AAPL forensic psychiatrists on controversial ethical guidelines. Bull Am Acad Psychiatry Law 1991;19:237–48.
18. Gutheil TG, Bursztajn HJ, Brodsky A, et al. Decision-making in psychiatry and the law. Baltimore (MD): Williams and Wilkins; 1991.
19. Ciccone R, Clements C. The ethical practice of forensic psychiatry. Bull Am Acad Psychiatry Law 1984;12(3):263–77.
20. Ciccone JR, Clements C. Commentary: forensic psychiatry and ethics—the voyage continues. J Am Acad Psychiatry Law 2001;29:174–9.
21. Griffith EE. Personal narrative and an African-American perspective on medical ethics. J Am Acad Psychiatry Law 2005;33:371–81.
22. Stone AA. Presidential address: conceptual ambiguity and morality in modern psychiatry. Am J Psychiatry 1980;137:887–91.
23. Stone AA. The ethical boundaries of forensic psychiatry: a view from the ivory tower. Bull Am Acad Psychiatry Law 1984;12:209–19.
24. Beauchamp TL, Childress JF. Principles of biomedical ethics. 5th edition. New York: Oxford University Press; 2001.
25. Kipnis K. Confessions of an expert witness. J Med Philos 1997;22(4):325–43.
26. Margulies J. Guantanamo and the abuse of presidential power. New York: Simon & Schuster; 2007. p. 123–4.
27. Lewis NA. Interrogators cite doctors' aid at Guantanamo Prison Camp. NY Times June 24, 2005;A1.
28. Levine A. Collective unconscionable. How psychologists, the most liberal of professions, abetted Bush's torture policy. Wash Mon January/February 2007.
29. McKelvey T. First do some harm. Physicians and psychologists are now taking part in interrogations. Am Prospect August 14, 2005.
30. Keram EA. Will medical ethics be a casualty of the war on terror? J Am Acad Psychiatry Law 2006;34:6–8.
31. US v Hamdan 548 US 557, 126 S. Ct. 2749, 165 L. Ed. 2d 723 2006.
32. Phillips RT. Expanding the role of the forensic consultant. Newsl Am Acad Psychiatry Law 2005;30(1):4–5.
33. Pellegrino ED. Societal duty and moral complicity: the physician's dilemma of divided loyalty. Int J Law Psychiatry 1993;16:371–91.
34. Freedman AM, Halpern AL. Response: a crisis in the ethical and moral behavior of psychiatrists. Curr Opin Psychiatry 1998;11:13–5.
35. Candilis PJ, Martinez R. Commentary: the higher standards of aspirational ethics. J Am Acad Psychiatry Law 2006;34:242–4.
36. Miller FG, Brody H. Professional integrity and physician-assisted death. Hastings Cent Rep 1995;25:8–17.
37. Wynia MK, Lathan SR, Kao AC, et al. Medical professionalism in society. N Engl J Med 1999;341:1612–6.
38. Roberts LW, Hoop JG. Professionalism and ethics. Washington, DC: American Psychiatric Publishing, Inc.; 2008.
39. Roberts LW, Dyer AR. Clinical decision-making and ethics skills. In: Concise guide to ethics in mental health care. Washington, DC, American Psychiatric Publishing, Inc. 2004.
40. Katz J. "The fallacy of the impartial expert" revisited. Bull Am Acad Psychiatry Law 1992;20:141–52.

Philosophical and Ethical Issues at the Forefront of Neuroscience and Genetics: An Overview for Psychiatrists

Jinger G. Hoop, MD, MFA[a],*, Ryan Spellecy, PhD[b]

KEYWORDS

- Neuroethics • Medical ethics • Genetics • Neuroscience
- Enhancement • Philosophy of medicine

The twenty-first century holds promise to be an era of great scientific discovery about the workings of the brain from molecular to cellular to anatomic levels. These discoveries have far-reaching implications for future psychiatric practice as well as for our understanding of the biologic basis of normal and abnormal mental functioning. For example, new imaging technologies such as functional MR imaging (fMRI) have enabled researchers to visualize the act of remembering and other mental phenomena.[1,2] Molecular genetics research has begun to identify genetic variants associated with mental disorders, conditions, and traits. Although progress in psychiatric molecular genetics has been slow, there is still great excitement about its potential for achieving greater understanding of the pathophysiology of mental illness.[3] Progress has also been made in developing new brain-based therapies for mental disorders. On the molecular level, psychopharmacology research is exploring relatively uncharted areas such as cognitive enhancers. On the anatomic level, neuromodulation interventions such as deep brain stimulation are exploring new methods

Dr. Hoop and coworkers are funded through the Research for a Healthier Tomorrow Program Development Fund, a component of the Advancing a Healthier Wisconsin endowment at the Medical College of Wisconsin, Milwaukee, Wisconsin.

[a] Department of Psychiatry and Behavioral Medicine, Medical College of Wisconsin, 8701 Watertown Plank Road, Milwaukee, WI 53226, USA
[b] Center for the Study of Bioethics, Medical College of Wisconsin, 8701 Watertown Plank Road, Milwaukee, WI 53226, USA
* Corresponding author.
E-mail address: jhoop@mcw.edu (J.G. Hoop).

Psychiatr Clin N Am 32 (2009) 437–449
doi:10.1016/j.psc.2009.03.004
0193-953X/09/$ – see front matter © 2009 Elsevier Inc. All rights reserved.

psych.theclinics.com

of treating depression, obsessive-compulsive disorder, and other psychiatric conditions.[4]

People with mental illnesses and those who care for them may benefit greatly from these scientific advances. Brain-based technologies could improve diagnosis and treatment, and neuroimaging and genetic screening could potentially identify high-risk individuals to receive preventive services. In addition to these benefits to individuals, there may be social benefits as well in terms of reducing the social burden of mental illness and its stigma. Although this latter point is controversial, at least some experts in mental illness stigma believe that new technologies may help demonstrate that these disorders are "real" (ie, biologically based) and not the result of personal or moral failings of the sufferer.[5]

Brain-based research advances have also raised a great deal of attention among bioethicists and philosophers—so much attention that a new field of "neuroethics" has emerged with its own professional society founded in 2006 (Neuroethics Society), a journal established in 2008 (*Neuroethics*), the publication of numerous books, and several meetings and symposia. For a full discussion of the scope of new technologies, their applications, and the ethical issues surrounding them, we direct the reader to the recently published literature in this area.[1,2,6–8] This article is intended to provide psychiatrists with a sense of the types of philosophical issues provoked by brain-based technologies. It then explores more deeply a major foci of neuroethics scholarship that is especially pertinent to the work of clinical psychiatrists, the issue of "neuroenhancement," that is, using neuromodulation technologies, psychopharmacology, and genetics not only to treat illness but also to improve normal human functioning.[9–12]

PHILOSOPHICAL QUESTIONS RAISED BY NEUROSCIENCE AND GENETIC RESEARCH

The recent leap in our knowledge about the workings of the human brain and about the biologic basis of human behavior has provided an opportunity for science to begin to weigh in on a range of philosophical discussions. Herein we touch on how neuroscience and genetics are beginning to add empiric data to our understanding of three philosophical issues—the mind/body debate, the concept of free will, and the role of emotions in moral decision making.

Is the Human Mind Independent from the Brain?

The brain is by definition a physical organ, consisting of neurons and glial cells organized into structures, whereas the term *mind* encompasses consciousness and intellect, including the phenomena of thinking, feeling, imagining, perceiving, and remembering. Philosophers have long debated whether the mind is an independent, immaterial phenomenon separate from the body, specifically the brain, or whether an immaterial mind cannot exist. Many have maintained that the mind does exist independently of the body for philosophical reasons (ie, the belief that the mind cannot be reduced to just the brain) and religious reasons (ie, the belief in the existence of an eternal, immaterial soul and mind).

The relatively new field of cognitive neuroscience focuses on localizing mental phenomena within the brain. Its methodology includes the study of brain-damaged individuals and imaging techniques such as positron emission tomography, magneto-encephalography, and fMRI.[1] Landmark studies in this exploding field of research have demonstrated the workings of the human brain during a wide and growing range of mental acts, such as perceiving visual and auditory stimuli, processing language, recognizing faces, remembering, feeling, and even lying.[2]

Some argue that eventually neuroscience will be able to link detectable brain activity to all mental phenomena—a person's every thought, emotion, memory, perception, and imagining. Because neuroscience by its very nature is devoted to the study of physical phenomena, it cannot be used to prove that any immaterial concept, including the human mind, does *not* exist; however, it is possible that neuroscience could provide such a full account of brain activity during all mental states that reference to immaterial minds and mental states becomes unnecessary.

Do Human Beings have Free Will?

Traditionally, the concept of free will has been the focus of a debate between those who subscribe to the view that at least some human actions are freely chosen by the individual (ie, they are not controlled by external forces) and those who view the notion of free will as a myth. This latter view, often called "determinism," argues that actions we think are freely chosen can and must be entirely explained by causes other than human volition. For example, although one might think he or she freely chooses to buy a particular soft drink when thirsty, that choice is really entirely a function of past experiences such as exposure to advertising, which have molded current preferences. Proponents of the deterministic view of human action might question what a free action could even be. Because we live in a physical world in which events follow law-like patterns (eg, objects fall downward, not upward, due to gravity), a truly freely chosen human action might seem to be a complete separation from this orderly pattern of cause and effect, and even this may begin to look more like a random event than one that is chosen and controlled by a person.

A middle ground in the free will debate that we find plausible, "compatibilism," holds that although the world and our actions follow orderly cause-and-effect patterns, we may call a human action "free," at least for the purpose of assigning responsibility, as long as the action is not clearly coerced (eg, a robber forcing someone to relinquish a wallet at gunpoint) and as long as it is not the result of some clear pathology (eg, Tourette's disease causing someone to have verbal outbursts).

Neuroimaging and genetic research have provided empiric data relevant to the debate over free will. For example, twin, family, and adoption studies suggest that many mental illnesses, personality disorders, and personality traits such as conscientiousness, impulsivity, and aggressiveness have complex genetic inheritance, that is, each condition or trait is the product of two or more genes (perhaps hundreds), environmental factors, epigenetic factors (such as DNA methylation and histone formation), gene-gene and gene-environment interactions, and random chance.[13–15] Proponents of a deterministic view of human behavior may interpret scientific evidence of the role of genetics in human behavior as a demonstration that individual actions are determined and not the result of free will. Nevertheless, the complex inheritance patterns associated with most behaviors do *not* preclude the influence of personal factors such as "will."

The eventual social and legal ramifications of genetic research in this area are extremely hard to predict. In at least one recent US criminal trial, a defendant has tried to introduce genotyping data to suggest he was predisposed to aggressive behavior.[16] In theory, prosecutors might use the same genetic evidence to argue that an individual should receive harsher sentencing due to an allegedly high likelihood of recidivism.

In a similar fashion, the effect of the "geneticization" of mental illness, substance abuse, or other socially stigmatized behaviors on public attitudes is not yet clear. Knowledge of a biologic basis to illness may lead to reduced stigma because these illnesses are no longer seen as solely an individual's fault,[17] or it may worsen stigma because the illnesses will seem to be more permanent and less likely to yield to treatment.[18,19]

Whether or not one believes in the existence of free will, future advances in the neurosciences may provide new methods of achieving a better understanding of this and relevant concepts.[8,20] For example, neuroimaging research could seek to compare brain activity among individuals who are judged to have decisional capacity on clinical grounds and among a relevant comparison group who lack this capacity. This type of knowledge of brain functioning could create empiric data that are clinically and legally useful as well as philosophically intriguing. The philosopher Patricia Smith Churchland[20] summarizes this potential aptly, "Ultimately, we'd like to have some general understanding of the neural difference between someone who is operating with what we might loosely call free choice and someone who is not. Another way of putting this is that we want to understand the neural difference between someone who, roughly speaking, is *in control* and someone who, also roughly speaking, is *not in control*."

What Role do Emotions have in Moral Decision Making?

fMRI research has also begun to inform another philosophical debate—the role of emotions in moral decision making.[21,22] Briefly, the ancient Greek philosopher Aristotle[23] and others held the view that emotions should and do have an important role in ethical decision making. On the other hand, the eighteenth century German philosopher Immanuel Kant and others argued that human emotions have no legitimate role in ethics or morality, which instead should be based on rational thought and logic.[24] Nevertheless, Kant admitted that divorcing emotions from ethical decision making would be very difficult, and that only a few people could do it.

This philosophical debate has great practical relevance today, especially in the field of bioethics, where some experts defer to the "wisdom of repugnance" as a sort of gut-level guide to judging right and wrong.[25] According to the contemporary bioethicist Leon Kass,[25] "Repugnance is the emotional expression of deep wisdom, beyond reason's power fully to articulate it." This emotion-driven morality has been criticized on several grounds.[26] For example, emotion-based reasoning may not be suitable as a basis for broadly applicable ethics guidelines and public policies, because an individual's emotional responses are influenced by several idiosyncratic factors, including one's personality, life experiences, and cultural background. What is repugnant to one person in a given culture and given time may be entirely benign, or even desirable, to another.

A landmark fMRI study published in 2001 provided a unique, empiric examination of the role of emotions in decision making. Psychologist Joshua D. Greene and colleagues[22] imaged the brains of a small number of male and female undergraduate research participants as they considered three types of dilemmas, some classified as "nonmoral" problems, others as impersonal moral dilemmas (eg, whether or not to keep money found in a wallet or to vote for a policy that may increase death rates), and a third group classified as "personal" moral dilemmas (eg, whether to steal one person's organs to save the lives of five other persons and whether to throw some people off a sinking lifeboat to save others). The researchers reported that as participants contemplated the personal moral dilemmas, there was significantly increased activity in areas of the brain involved in processing emotions (the medial frontal, angular, and anterior cingulate gyri). The patterns of brain activity suggested that emotions influenced decision making and were not merely incidental to the process. Greene and colleagues[22] concluded that moral dilemmas differ in their reliance upon emotional processing, and that these variations in emotional engagement influence ethical judgment.

Such findings suggest that morality is, indeed, to some extent a function of the emotions, at least for the participants who have been studied. By virtue of its empiric nature, this type of research can demonstrate how ethics *is* done, not how it *should* be done. The finding that those studied did use their emotions in ethical decision making would perhaps come as no surprise to Kant, who might nonetheless say that this type of moral thinking is far from ideal.

A promising area for future research might involve testing interventions designed to help individuals make ethical decisions with less emotional engagement. For example, such interventions could theoretically help individuals to become more aware of their emotional reactions to particular dilemmas, and then to consciously set aside emotionally charged aspects of the decisions. Pre- and postintervention neuroimaging could provide some demonstration of whether such interventions might be successful. If not, the results would lend credence to the aristotelian view that ethical decision making is always emotion based. If the interventions did help reduce emotional decision making, the proponents of a kantian view might encourage use of the interventions as an educational aid, at least for physicians, policymakers, and others who are called upon to make ethical choices on behalf of others who may not share their emotional responses.

ETHICAL CONTROVERSIES SURROUNDING NEUROENHANCEMENT

Advances in neuromodulation, psychopharmacology, and genetic manipulation have raised numerous ethical concerns, which are arguably the most prevalent and contentious topics in the field of neuroethics.[2,4,8,12,27,28] These therapies include brain implants to affect mood and behavior, genetic testing or gene therapy to alter the genetic makeup of individuals or prevent the birth of genetically disadvantaged children, and medications to alter mood, personality, wakefulness, memory, focus, attention, and cognition. All of these technologies could (in theory at least) be used for the enhancement of normal range characteristics as well as for the treatment of diagnosable disorders and illnesses.

Interest in mental enhancement as a subject of bioethics study has been fueled by recent reporting of the increasing use of pharmacologic agents among mentally healthy individuals to become "better than well."[29] Selective serotonin reuptake inhibitors may have some usefulness as "personality enhancers" as well as psychiatric treatments.[30] Beta blockers may have benefit as agents to prevent posttraumatic stress disorder by blocking emotion-laden aspects of memory.[31] Psychostimulants and the wakefulness-enhancing drug modafinil are reportedly being used by students and even scientific researchers to improve mental focus and intellectual ability.[27,32–34] Indeed, the journal *Nature*[32] recently published the results of an online readership survey demonstrating that one in five respondents had used medications for nonmedical enhancement purposes to improve memory, concentration, or focus.

The remainder of this article focuses on the complex and interwoven ethical issues surrounding neuroenhancement, organized by six overlapping areas of inquiry—theological, emotional, philosophical, empiric, medical, and social (**Table 1**). We use the terms *neuroenhancement* and *mental enhancement* interchangeably throughout this discussion to refer to any medication, neuromodulation technique, or genetic technology used to improve a "normal" individual's mood, cognition, memory, attention, or focus.

Is Neuroenhancement within the Appropriate Domain of Human Activity?

Theological, emotional, and philosophical lines of inquiry concern the essential characteristics of the technology, aside from any potential it has to bring good or ill. The

Table 1
Modes of inquiry into the ethics of neuroenhancement

Modes of Inquiry	Questions Posed	Examples
Theological	Is neuroenhancement technology within the appropriate realm of human activity?	Some belief systems may identify certain technologies as impinging on the realm of God or "playing God."
Emotional	What is one's emotional reaction to neuroenhancement technology?	Some individuals may find a new technology immoral because they feel repugnance toward it, and because they believe that feeling is a kind of innate moral wisdom.
Philosophical	Is the new technology congruent with essential qualities of humanity, such as authenticity, dignity, and personal identity?	The philosophical debate over neuroenhancement technologies has focused largely upon the concept of authenticity, that is, how enhancement of a person's mood, cognition, or memory could either bolster or detract from the person's authentic self.
Empirical	What are the benefits, risks, and utility of the new technology? How can individual decision making about these risks and benefits be enhanced?	These questions can be partially answered by conceptual/philosophical analysis and extrapolation from historical examples. Full answers may require empiric data through scientific research, such as randomized controlled trials with longitudinal follow-up.
Medical	Should the medical community be responsible for the wise use of the new technology? If so, what are the parameters for appropriate medical care?	These questions may be answered based on an analysis of the risks and benefits of the technology, and the best means of protecting patient (or consumer) autonomy.
Social	How should risks and benefits of the new technology be distributed among members of society? How can social coercion and other negative effects be minimized or eliminated?	Technologies that are seen to be highly beneficial with few risks may be offered to all members of society at low cost or even mandated (such as newborn screening for phenylketonuria). Technologies that have high risks and few benefits may be prohibited or made available only with numerous safeguards, such as physician involvement and informed consent.

dominating question is whether the technology itself is within the appropriate sphere of human activity. For example, certain faith traditions believe that human reproduction is the domain of God, not humanity. Adherents of those faiths may consider enhancement that involves the creation, manipulation, or destruction of human embryos by definition immoral. Further analyses of ethical issues such as utility, justice, and autonomy would not be required to make this determination. Instead, the basis for moral decision making would likely include consideration of theological writings and texts, prayer, or other forms of spiritual guidance.

Emotion-based moral decision making may lead some individuals to assert that certain types of enhancement are immoral because features of the technologies involved are repugnant to them.[25] In this realm of ethical inquiry, the emotional response is itself considered a type of moral wisdom, which may or may not require further rational or empiric study. Pharmacology and genetic testing of blood samples seem less likely to provoke strong negative responses than neuromodulation techniques, some of which involve surgical manipulation of the brain and the implantation of electrodes. These later techniques may be perceived as immoral to some people on the basis of negative, gut-level reactions.

A more purely intellectual, philosophical realm of inquiry has tended to focus upon the impact of enhancement on the concepts of human dignity, personal identity, and authenticity.[10] Some philosophers who are sympathetic to Kant object that the use of neuroenhancements violates the categorical imperative, namely, the duty to act always such that one treats persons as ends in themselves, never merely as means.[24] In short, Kant objects to "using" people, that is, deceiving them to obtain their cooperation, forcing them to cooperate, and so on. For Kant, this action is immoral because people have the capacity for free autonomous action. It is wrong to deprive them of the opportunity to exercise their autonomy (eg, when one lies to another to secure assistance, one denies the other person the opportunity to exercise his or her autonomy in choosing whether or not to assist in the real plan). If I use enhancements, I violate the categorical imperative by treating *myself* as a means to an end, namely, my goal of, say, increased focus and attention. Nevertheless, this view is a bit difficult to grasp because my ends are my own, and I cannot force myself or deceive myself into aiding myself on a quest for enhancement. The kantian objection does not seem to actually violate the categorical imperative unless enhancements are forced upon people through passive or active coercion, which will be described later on.

The notion of authenticity, which embraces the idea of being "true to oneself" in the most profound sense, is perhaps more important to this discussion. Striving for authenticity is considered by some philosophers to be the very reason for living. Exactly what it means to be one's authentic self is debatable. What is the authentic self of a person with longstanding dysthymia or characterologic depression? The self that has been shaped over time by chronic low mood, or the self that might come into existence if the depression were lifted? Similarly, what is the authentic self of the formerly jocular war veteran who is now disabled by severe posttraumatic stress disorder, or of the self-mutilating teenager whose early development was derailed by severe abuse and neglect?

Creativity and Gratitude Perspectives on Enhancement

The contemporary bioethicist Erik Parens[11] has described the philosophical debate over pharmacologic and other types of neuroenhancement as two competing views of what it means to be authentically human—the "creativity" and "gratitude" perspectives. In Parens' terminology, the creativity view posits that the essential, authentic nature of humanity is to strive toward perfection, seeking to improve oneself and one's offspring and possessing innate creativity to learn to do so in ever-changing ways. This viewpoint suggests that personal enhancement can be an authentic expression of one's humanity no matter how it is achieved, whether through traditional means such as education or prayer or new technologies such as medication or gene therapy.

At least one proponent of this viewpoint suggests that the use of enhancement may not just be permissible but necessary to achieving full authenticity as human beings.[28]

On the other hand, the gratitude perspective holds that life is a gift and that being authentically human means accepting the gift of one's flawed self wholeheartedly, suffering with one's shortcomings, learning from them, and not seeking a "quick fix" to escape them through technological enhancement. As psychologist Martha Farah[6] succinctly states, "Most of us would love to go through life cheerful and svelte, focusing like a laser beam at work and enjoying rapturous sex each night. Yet most of us also feel uneasy about the idea of achieving these things through drugs."

Other ethicists would also argue that achieving enhancement without hard work or suffering is a violation of human dignity. This view has been expressed by the philosopher Richard Dees,[10] who notes (borrowing from Aristotle and the nineteenth century British philosopher John Stuart Mill) that achieving happiness seems to require more than just being happy. It requires the effort needed to achieve happiness. Happiness is "a complex state that goes beyond how people feel and what is inside their minds. Happiness, then, requires authenticity." Dees notes that the issue is not quite this simple, and as described earlier, more discussion and exploration of these topics is needed.

Examining Risks and Benefits to Individuals

A fourth domain of inquiry is primarily empiric in nature, requiring the gathering and weighing of facts about the risks, benefits, and utility of enhancement for individuals. This domain is primarily focused on the principles of beneficence and nonmaleficence.

Many ethical concerns about neuroenhancement arise specifically from the lack of data about the risks of use in healthy individuals.[35] For example, although there may be sufficient safety data to permit the use of modafinil for the treatment of narcolepsy, whether or not the drug is safe for use by emergency room clinicians to stay awake and alert during 24-hour shifts is not known. There may be so many unknowns about the risks and benefits of emerging enhancement technologies that sustained research efforts will be necessary to achieve clarity. One of many understudied issues is the likelihood of addiction and abuse. History has clearly demonstrated the abuse potential of some pharmacologic agents originally perceived as safe, effective enhancers of mental phenomena such as cognition and mood (eg, cocaine[36]) and psychological insight (eg, 3,4 methylenedioxymethamphetamine [MDMA] or "ecstasy"[37]).These and other concerns are not absolute objections to the use of neuroenhancement in principle but apply only to specific cases in which safety data are lacking. As Dees[10] notes, "The argument from safety does not show we should never use neuroenhancements"; rather, Dees suggests that we ought to be cautious in such use and that more empiric data are needed.

In general, the acceptable level of risk of an intervention is in balance with its benefits and with the risks associated with the underlying illness and with alternative treatments. For example, most psychiatrists consider the risk of agranulocytosis associated with clozapine to be acceptable for the treatment of refractory schizophrenia but would likely find this same risk unacceptable for the treatment of transient anxiety on the grounds of nonmaleficence. A subtle, temporary increase in mental performance seems to be a benefit too small to offset any but the mildest of risks. It is important to note, however, that cosmetic surgery involves enhancement procedures that carry a small risk of death due to the inherent risks of surgery and anesthesia, and many individuals freely choose to accept that risk to achieve the benefits of the enhancement.

Respect for Persons and the Possibility of Coercion

Yet another class of ethical concerns arises from the possibility that if the use of neuro-enhancements were to become more widespread, some individuals who would not otherwise choose to use them might be actively or passively coerced into doing so. Such coercion could be a violation of the ethical principle of respect for persons, which requires that we facilitate and respect the autonomous choices and plans of others (as well as protect those with diminished autonomy, although that aspect is less relevant here). If people are coerced into choosing enhancements, their decisions to do so will not be free and autonomous, thereby violating respect for persons.

Theoretically at least, certain classes of workers might be required by their employers to use enhancement aids to keep or maintain their jobs. For example, pilots could be mandated to take stimulants or modafinil to sustain mental sharpness during long flights. Such requirements could clearly be beneficial in certain industries and the military, in which enhanced human performance might reduce accidents and save lives; however, at least some workers may find the enhancement aid objectionable on moral or other grounds. The resulting tension between the potential benefits to employers and the threat to workers' autonomy has led to the suggestion that legislation be created to prohibit employers from mandating the use of enhancement drugs.[38]

A less overt form of coercion from social pressure may also occur. If enough people avail themselves of mental enhancements, those who choose not to partake may find themselves at a competitive disadvantage in education, careers, or even romantic relationships. If 90% of medical students use medications that improve their grades, the remaining 10% of students who choose not to use them may fall below the curve. A fictional example of social coercion toward enhancement is depicted in the 1997 film *Gattaca*, which has become something of a cultural touchstone for ethical concerns about human genetics. The film features a society in which the use of in vitro fertilization and pre-implantation genetic diagnosis has become so widespread that couples feel social pressure to "give your child the best possible start" in life by selecting embryos for implantation with the most favorable genetic profiles.

Dees[10] has argued that concerns over social coercion are misplaced "as long as plenty of reasonably equivalent alternatives exist." According to Dees, even if a particular career path requires that workers use enhancements to be competitive, as long as the workers have other options for meaningful employment, they are not coerced. Nevertheless, it is difficult to imagine a wide range of desirable jobs and careers in which mental enhancements would not be helpful. Focus, intelligence, the ability to work long hours, cheerfulness, and attention are fundamental advantages regardless of one's career; therefore, the possibility of coercion remains one of the more troubling objections to enhancement, and one in which neuroenhancement may differ substantively from other types such as cosmetic surgery, because mental enhancements could be greatly advantageous in many endeavors.

Medical Professionalism and the Ethical Provision of Enhancements

The role of the medical profession in providing enhancements is highly controversial, with many experts arguing that enhancement is never a legitimate use of the practice of medicine,[9,10,39,40] just as the provision of futile treatments is also outside the purview of ethical medical practice. Nevertheless, such a distinction between treatment and enhancement is difficult to maintain, because it fails to account for the fact that some enhancements are routinely and ethically offered by physicians in medical settings (eg, cosmetic surgery and cosmetic dermatology).

Furthermore, the distinction between treatment and enhancement also rests on the assumption that there is a clear demarcation between illness, which merits treatment, and normality, which does not. Many psychiatric diagnoses hinge on the patient's level of distress or dysfunction. The line between "disease-level" distress or functional disability and "normal level" is not always clear-cut. When precisely is a mild, chronic, low mood properly diagnosed as dysthymia, and when is it just someone's personality? Consider another example of two children with measured IQs of 69 and 70. Hypothetically, both might benefit if prescribed a cognition-improving medication developed in the future exclusively for the treatment of mental retardation. It would seem unfair and illogical that prescribing the medication to only one of the children would be considered medically legitimate as treatment, merely because of a 1-point difference in IQ, which is likely neither clinically significant nor ethically salient.[40]

Concerns about the Impact of Mental Enhancement upon Society

Finally, we consider the potential for mental enhancement technologies to affect society for good or ill. Although most scholars have tended to focus on the negative effects, some have perceived positive ones. For example, there could be a tremendous social benefit if at least some citizens use interventions to improve their mental abilities. Having smarter, more focused, and more creative scientists, doctors, legislators, teachers, artists, and even parents might advance humankind in ways never before possible. Indeed, in an era in which the world is beset with environmental, economic, and humanitarian crises, one could argue on the grounds of beneficence that national decision makers should avail themselves of any form of intellectual enhancement possible.

On the other hand, many neuroethicists fear that enhancements will be deeply damaging to society, in part, because they will exacerbate inequality. Emerging enhancement technologies may be expensive, and if they are not covered by medical insurance or public assistance, they will be out of the reach of the poor and perhaps even the middle class. The result could be to widen the gap between the school performance and career potentials of the rich and the poor.[6] Some point out that this possibility is not an objection to neuroenhancement, per se, but rather a greater concern about social inequality in general.[10,39] In other words, if we are seriously concerned about social inequality, why do we allow wealthy parents to send their children to private schools, enroll in test preparation courses, and gain similar advantages? Nevertheless, the fact that society allows some inequalities in opportunity does not mean that all inequalities must be tolerated. The inequalities that may result from neuroenhancements might not be very different in kind from those resulting from access to private schools, but the cumulative effect of numerous enhancements might be unjust.

The potential injustice caused by mental enhancement may well be addressable through legislation and policy.[28] For example, policies regarding newborn screening and childhood immunizations demonstrate how low-risk, high-benefit enhancements could (theoretically at least) be made available to all members of society.

It is possible that overvaluation of enhancement technologies may "enable" society to depend on them to solve structural problems that could be addressed more humanely in other ways.[41] Neuroenhancement technologies, especially pharmacologic agents that increase wakefulness, could become a relatively inexpensive means of increasing the productivity of the American workforce and allowing working parents to interact more with their children, facilitating an apparent trend of Americans "multitasking" more and sleeping less.[42] An estimated 70 million Americans suffer from sleep deprivation, chronic sleepiness, or sleep disorders.[43] The apparent acceptability of the use of wakefulness-enhancing drugs among the readers of *Nature*[32] may perhaps say less about the intellectual striving of these individuals and more about the demands of their careers and lifestyle.

To thrive, human beings need adequate time for rest, family life, and recreation as well as work. Long work hours have been associated with a variety of poor health indicators, including poor mental health.[44] As a matter of respect for persons, it would be more ethical to set reasonable limits on expectations of human work performance rather than use technology to sidestep them. For example, consider two possible strategies for reducing the rate of medical errors in American medicine: (1) limiting the number of hours that clinical personnel are required to work per shift versus (2) encouraging their use of wakefulness-enhancing drugs. Of these two options, limiting required work hours is likely to be a more expensive option but is also more humane, reducing errors by acknowledging the human needs of health care workers and perhaps nurturing more compassionate clinicians in the process.

SUMMARY

This review has touched upon some of the major ethical issues surrounding emerging technologies in neuroscience and genetics. Although at first glance these issues may seem somewhat peripheral to the clinical practice of psychiatry, we suggest that they may have unanticipated effects upon the care of patients with mental illness. Certainly, the philosophical issues surrounding free will are of tremendous consequence to persons who commit crimes while suffering severe symptoms of mental illness. In addition, the opening up of a lucrative new "enhancement" market for the sale of new therapies could divert commercial resources away from the development of therapies for mental illness, although it is also possible that some enhancements will have secondary benefits as treatments for disease. Social acceptance of enhancement therapies could have a beneficial, normalizing effect on public attitudes toward those who receive mental health treatment. On the other hand, a moral backlash against enhancements as "quick fixes" that deprive individuals of authenticity could have a secondary effect of increasing the stigma of mental health treatment. For all of these reasons, it has become increasingly important for psychiatrists to be informed about and active participants in the public conversation about neuroethics. Psychiatric patients appear to have much at stake in these ethical debates, and psychiatrists have valuable expertise to offer as professionals with intimate knowledge of the human mind, its limitations, and its potential.

ACKNOWLEDGMENTS

The authors gratefully acknowledge the assistance of Ann Tennier, BS, and Krisy Edenharder, BA, in the preparation of this manuscript.

REFERENCES

1. Kosslyn SM, Andersen RA. Frontiers in cognitive neuroscience. Cambridge (MA): MIT Press; 1992.
2. Merkel R. Intervening in the brain: changing psyche and society. Berlin: Springer; 2007. New York.
3. Insel TR, Lehner T. A new era in psychiatric genetics? Biol Psychiatry 2007;61: 1017–8.

4. Synofzik M, Schlaepfer TE. Stimulating personality: ethical criteria for deep brain stimulation in psychiatric patients and for enhancement purposes. Biotechnol J 2008;3:1511–20.
5. Corrigan PW, Watson AC. At issue: stop the stigma. Call mental illness a brain disease. Schizophr Bull 2004;30:477–9.
6. Farah MJ. Emerging ethical issues in neuroscience. Nat Neurosci 2002;5:1123–9.
7. Illes J, Bird SJ. Neuroethics: a modern context for ethics in neuroscience. Trends Neurosci 2006;29:511–7.
8. Roskies A. Neuroethics for the new millennium. Neuron 2002;35:21–3.
9. Cheshire WP Jr. Drugs for enhancing cognition and their ethical implications: a hot new cup of tea. Expert Rev Neurother 2006;6:263–6.
10. Dees RH. Better brains, better selves? The ethics of neuroenhancements. Kennedy Inst Ethics J 2007;17:371–95.
11. Parens E. Authenticity and ambivalence: toward understanding the enhancement debate. Hastings Cent Rep 2005;35:34–41.
12. Wolpe PR. Treatment, enhancement, and the ethics of neurotherapeutics. Brain Cogn 2002;50:387–95.
13. Uhl GR, Grow RW. The burden of complex genetics in brain disorders. Arch Gen Psychiatry 2004;61:223–9.
14. Faraone S, Tsuang M, Tsuang D. Genetics of mental disorders: a guide for students, clinicians, and researchers. New York: Guilford Press; 1999.
15. Nuffield Council on Bioethics. Genetics and human behavior: the ethical context. Available at: http://www.nuffieldbioethics.org/go/ourwork/behaviouralgenetics/publication_311.html. Accessed January 4, 2008.
16. Bernet W, Vnencak-Jones CL, Farahany N, et al. Bad nature, bad nurture, and testimony regarding MAOA and SLC6A4 genotyping at murder trials. J Forensic Sci 2007;52:1362–71.
17. Attitudes, knowledge and behaviour of general practitioners in relation to HIV infection and AIDS. Commonwealth AIDS Research Grant Committee working party. Med J Aust 1990;153:5–12 [see comments].
18. Phelan JC. Geneticization of deviant behavior and consequences for stigma: the case of mental illness. J Health Soc Behav 2005;46:307–22.
19. Crown S, Lee A, editors. Ethics primer of the American Psychiatric Association. Washington (DC): American Psychiatric Association; 2001.
20. Churchland PS. Brain-wise: studies in neurophilosophy. Cambridge (MA): MIT Press; 2002.
21. Casebeer WD. Natural ethical facts: evolution, connectionism, and moral cognition. Cambridge (MA): MIT Press; 2003.
22. Greene JD, Nystrom LE, Engell AD, et al. The neural bases of cognitive conflict and control in moral judgment. Neuron 2004;44:389–400.
23. Aristotle, Irwin T. Nicomachean ethics. Indianapolis (IN): Hackett Publishing; 1985.
24. Kant I, Ellington JW, Kant I. Uber ein vermeintes Recht aus Menschenliebe zu lügen. [Grounding for the metaphysics of morals with on a supposed right to lie because of philanthropic concerns]. 3rd edition. Indianapolis (IN): Hackett Publishing; 1993.
25. Kass LR. The wisdom of repugnance. New Repub June 2, 1997.
26. Mori M. A moralidade da reprodução assistida e da manipulação genética. Cad Saúde Pública [online] 1999;15. Available at: http://www.scielo.br/scielo.php?script=sci_arttext&pid=S0102 311X1999000500008&lng=en&nr Accessed March 14, 2009.

27. Sahakian B, Morein-Zamir S. Professor's little helper. Nature 2007;450:1157–9.
28. Savulescu J. Justice, fairness, and enhancement. Ann N Y Acad Sci 2006;1093: 321–38.
29. Elliott C. Better than well: American medicine meets the American dream. New York: W.W. Norton; 2004.
30. Kramer PD. Listening to Prozac. New York: Viking; 1993.
31. Larkin M. Can post-traumatic stress disorder be put on hold? Lancet 1999;354: 1008.
32. Maher B. Poll results: look who's doping. Nature 2008;452:674–5.
33. McCabe ER. Clinical genetics: compassion, access, science, and advocacy. Genet Med 2001;3:426–9.
34. Teter CJ, McCabe SE, Boyd CJ, et al. Illicit methylphenidate use in an undergraduate student sample: prevalence and risk factors. Pharmacotherapy 2003;23: 609–17.
35. Glannon W. Psychopharmacological enhancement. Neuroethics 2008;1:45–54.
36. Das G. Cocaine abuse in North America: a milestone in history. J Clin Pharmacol 1993;33:296–310.
37. Parrott AC. The psychotherapeutic potential of MDMA (3,4-methylenedioxyme-thamphetamine): an evidence-based review. Psychopharmacology (Berl) 2007; 191:181–93.
38. Appel JM. When the boss turns pusher: a proposal for employee protections in the age of cosmetic neurology. J Med Ethics 2008;34:616–8.
39. Chatterjee A. Neuroethics: toward broader discussion. Hastings Cent Rep 2004; 34:4 [author reply 4–5].
40. Buchanan AE. From chance to choice: genetics and justice. Cambridge (UK): Cambridge University Press; 2000. New York.
41. Rajczi A. One danger of biomedical enhancements. Bioethics 2008;22:328–36.
42. Warner J. Living the off-label life. NY Times 2008;A25. Available at: http://www. nytimes.com/2008/12/27/opinion/27warner.html?_r=1. Accessed December 27, 2008.
43. Carmona RH. Frontiers of knowledge in sleep and sleep disorders: opportunities for improving health and quality of life. J Clin Sleep Med 2005;1:83–9.
44. Artazcoz L, Cortes I, Escriba-Aguir V, et al. Understanding the relationship of long working hours with health status and health-related behaviours. J Epidemiol Community Health. 2009 Mar 1. [Epub ahead of print].

Index

Note: Page numbers of article titles are in **boldface** type.

A

Abuse reporting, child, 252–253
    elder, 353
Addictions, evolving ethical issues in, 293–294
Adolescents, access to confidential services for, 248
    assessment and diagnosis of, 250–251
    care of, boundary issues in, 251–252
        responsibility for staff members and, 253
    confidentiality and, 248–249
    consent to release of information, 249
    ethical care of, reseach issues in, 253–254
    informed consent and, 248
Advance directives for psychiatric research, 387–388
Alzheimer's disease, decisional capacity in, 398
Alzheimer's disease research, double consent in, 399–400, 403
    proxy consent in, 399–400, 402
    surrogate consent for, 400
Assent, of child, to research participation, 254
        to treatment, 248
Authenticity, neuroenhancement and, 443
Autonomy, and boundaries in community psychiatry, 338
    and informed consent, in geriatric psychiatry, 344–346
    confidentiality and, 388
    dual agency and, 339
    in addiction, 285
    in community psychiatry, 334–336
        balance of, with beneficence and nonmaleficence, 336
        consumer and, allowing to fail, 335
        professional paternalisms and, 334
        recovery and, 334–335
        vs. professional recommendations based on beneficence and
            nonmaleficence, 335
    in substance abuse treatment, 289
    maternal, in perinatal mental health, 261–262, 264, 267
    neuroenhancement and, 443

B

Beneficence, and boundaries in community psychiatry, 338
    confidentiality and, 388
    dual agency and, 339

Psychiatr Clin N Am 32 (2009) 451–463
doi:10.1016/S0193-953X(09)00041-0
0193-953X/09/$ – see front matter © 2009 Elsevier Inc. All rights reserved.

Beneficence (*continued*)
    evidence-based medicine and, 416–417
    in community psychiatry, 335
        competing interests of patient and society, 333
        distributon of resources, 332–333
        weighing of risks and benefits and, 332
    in informed consent, 396
    in perinatal mental health, 260–262
    in research ethics, 383
Best interests, challenges in geriatric psychiatry, 343
    in child and adolescent research, 368
    in psychiatric research, 387
    standard for proxies, 401–405
Bipolar disorder, and decisional capacity of older patient, 398–399
    in perinatal mental health, 260–261
    proxy consent in, 401
Boundaries, in adolescent patient care, 251–252
    in community psychiary, engagement in varied settings and, 337
        ethical principles in, 338
    in military psychiatry, 272, 275–276
        dual roles of psychiatrist and, 272, 275–276
    in psychotherapy, **299–314**
        communicating to patient, 301
        conflicts of interest in therapist-patient relationship, 302
        definitions, examples, characteristics, 304
        nonsexual, 304–306
        recognizing boundary issues, 303–304
        sexual, 305–307
        therapeutic relationship and, 301
        violations of, and ethical principles, 303
    sexual, between patients and psychiatrists, 418–419
        in psychiatric education, 418–419
        in psychotherapy, 305–307
Boundary issues, in adolescent care, 251–252
    in child care, 251–252
    in psychotherapy, recognizing, 303–304
Boundary violations, nonmaleficence and, 333

C

Child abuse reporting, and therapeutic relationship, 253
    conflicts over when and how to, 252
Child and adolescent research, Case A: decision to conduct, 362–366
        conflicts of commitment in, 365
        conflicts of interest in, 364
        difference between research and medical care, 362–363
        financial incentives and, 362–363
        relationship of trust with patients and community, 364, 366
        risk-benefit assessment in, 365
        separation of medical and research records, 366
        staff considerations, 366

Case B: which studies to conduct and communication with patients, 366, 368
 best interests of patient, 368
 communication with patients and families, 368
 contact person for informed consent, 368
 ethical conduct in, 367
 independent review of, 367
 risk–benefit ratio and clinical equipoise, 367
 scientific validity of study, 367
 value of study, scientific, social, clinical, 366
Case C: therapeutic misconception, advising role in, 370
 communication with investigators, 370
 monitoring role in, 370
 motivations for participation, 370
Case D: consent, confidentiality, participant selection, 371–374
 capacity determination in, 373
 child assent in, 371–373
 federal regulations for federally funded research, 371–372
 informed consent in, 371
  of adolescent in, 373
 parental permission in, 371–73
 rule of sevens in, 373
 state laws for consent, 373–374
 therapeutic misconception in, 374
Case E: genetic research and information sharing, 374–376
 clinical usefullness in, 375
 genetic discrimination and, 376
 separation of medical and research records, 376
 value of results in, 375
practical and ethical considerations, **361–380**
Children, assent to treatment by, 248
 assessment and diagnosis of, 250–251
 care of, boundary issues in, 251–252
  challenging situations in, 246–247
  competing world views of child and parents in, 251
  core ethical issues in, 243–244
  professional competence in, 246–247
  psychiatrist responsibility for staff members and, 253
 confidentiality and, 249
 differences from adults, dependence, 245
  individual, 245
  vulnerability, 244–245
 ethical care of, reseach issues in, 253–254
 informed consent and, 247–248
 protecting and child abuse reports, 252–253
 psychopharmacology, ethical aspects of, 247
Children and adolescents, clinical ethics for general psychiatrists, **243–257**
 research in, **361–380**
Clinical equipoise, in child and adolescent research, 367
Coercion, in neuroenhancement, from employer and from social pressure, 445
Cognitive impairment, informed consent and, 344
 voluntarism and, 345–346

Cognitive tests or screens, in assessment of consent capacity, 397
Commitment, conflicts of, in child and adolescent research, 365
Community psychiary, special topics in, boundaries, 337–338
        dual agency, 338–339
        universal application of ethical principles, 339–340
Community psychiatry, **329–332**
    chronic mental illnesses in, treatment of, 330
    ethics in, **329–341**
    Medicaid, choice of physician and system and, 330
    multi-dyadic doctor-patient relationship in, 330
    practice elements in, 329–330
    program development for populations at risk, 331
    traditional medical ethics principles in, autonomy, 334–336
        beneficence, 332–333
        justice, 336–337
        nonmaleficence, 333
    treatment of persons with socioeconomic disadvantage, 330–331
    universal application of principles to other providers, 339–340
Confidentiality, child abuse reports and, 252
    disclosure of requested confidential information, legal, ethical, practical considerations
        in, 309–310
    doctrine of privilege and, 308–309
    electronic records and, 309
    exceptions to, 275
    for children and adolescents, 248–249
        communication with third parties and, 249–250
    HIPAA privacy and, 309
    in military psychiatry, 272–274
    in psychiatric research, 384, 388–389
    in psychotherapy, 308–311
    in substance use disorder treatment, criminal justice system and, 286–287
        public health exceptions to, 285
        regulations for disclosure of information, 284–285
    publication of case material, 310–311
    technology-based comminication, 309–310
    third-party payers and, 309
Conflicts of interest, in child and adolescent research, 364
    in perinatal mental health, 261
    in therapist-patient relationship, 302
    psychiatric education amd, 418–419
    psychiatric research and pharmaceutical industry, 391
    self-interest vs. obligations to patient, 419
Consultation-liaison psychiatry, decision-making approach to, **315–328**
        ethical principles in clinical care, 316–317
        situational diagnosis methodology in, 317
    decision-making methology for, four topics method, 318–319. See also *Four topics
        method of ethical decision making.*
        situational diagnosis methodology in, 317
    ethical issues in, decisional capacity, 317–318
        informed consent, 317–318
Contextual features, in capacity for independent living, 324–325

in case of unclear motivation, 326
in legitimate desire to die, 321
in refusal of evaluation and treatment, 323

D

Decisional capacity, assessment of, bedside cognitive assessment instruments, 345
    instruments for, 346–347
    standarization of, 346–347
  capacities in, 317
  clinical assessment of, 347–348
  for informed consent, 345
    in psychiatric research, 387
  in Alzheimer's disease, 398
  in consultation-liaison psychiatry, 317–318
  in geriatric psychiatry, 344, 346–348
  in substance use disorder treatment, 287–289
    practices to enhance, 291
  of minors, 248
  of suicidal patients, to consent to research, 407
Decision making, by proxy, 399, 401, 405
  emotions in, imaging studies of, 440–441
    interventions to reduce, 441
  in neuroenhancement, emotion-based, 443
Dementia, proxy consent in, 399
Depression, in geriatric psychiatry, decisional capacity and, 398
  in perinatal mental health, 263–264
Dual agency, in community psychiatry, 338–339
  in military psychiatry, 275

E

Evidence-based medicine, conflicts between beneficence and autonomy in, 417
  defined, 416
  strategies of, 416
    beneficence and, 416–417

F

Forensic ethics, **423–425**
  compassion in, 428
  cultural formulation of, 427
  cultural narrative in, 427–428
  of Guantanamo Bay, 429–430
    "exceptionalism" of health care professionals in, 429–430
  robust professionalism in, application of, 432–433
    defining professionalism, 431
    ethical precepts in, 433
    exclusion of historical elements and, 430
    exclusion of recent ethical considerations and, 430–431

Forensic (*continued*)
  integrity in, unitary, 431
  moral grounding in, 431–432
  openness and transparency in, 432
  separate role and view of, 430
  strict role theory in, 430
  striving for objectivity in, 432–433
social justice in, 428–429
Forensic psychiatry, as legal or medical profession, 423–424
  interactions of individuals, institutions, and society in, 424
  primacy of legal ethics in, 424–425
    truth and justice vs. care of individual, 425
  primacy of medical ethics in, 425–426
  robust professionalism in, institutional usefullness of, for disadvantaged patients,
    433–434
  systems approach to, 427
Four topics method of ethical decision making, case examples of, capacity for independent
  living, 323–325
    legitimate desire to die, 320–321
    refusal of evaluation and treatment, 321–323
    unclear motivation, 325–326
  contextual/situational factors in, 319
  medical indications in, 318–319
  patient preferences in, 319
  quality-of-life issues in, 319
Free will, compatibilism and, 439
  emotions and moral decision making and, 440–441
  genetic inheritance and, 439
  neural difference between person *in control* and *not in control* neuroscience, 440
  vs. determinism, 439

G

Genetics, biological basis of illness and, 439
  inheritance and free will and, 439
  in mental illness, 391
  philosophical and ethical issues in, **437–449**
Geriatric psychiatry, **343–359**
  addressing diminished capacity, 350–352
    guardianship, 352
    improvement of capacity in, 350–351
    surrogate decision-maker in, 351–352
  autonomy and informed consent in, 344–346
  capacities in, for driving, 349–350
    for independent living, 348–349
    for management of finance, 349–350
    for sexual activity, 349–350
    for testamentary capacity, 349–350
    for voting, 349–350
  clinical ethics in, **343–359**
  decisional capacity in, 344

assessment of, 346–348
   dementia patient care, 352–354
   dementia patient care in, antipsychotics in, 353
      diagnosis of AD and, 353
      elder abuse and reporting requirements, 353
      genetic testing in, 352
      paliiative care in, 353–354
      social justice and allocation of resources and, 353
   end-of-life issues in, 354
   research ethics in, decisional capacity of older participant, 398–399, 406
Geriatric psychiatry research, advanced research directives for, 400, 406
   decision-making capacity in, 398–399, 406
   double consent to, 399–400
   ethics issues in, **395–411**
   influence on proxies' willingness to enroll relatives, 401
   on depression and suicide, 405, 407
   Prevention of Suicide in Primary Care Elderly study, 405–406
   proxy consent in, 399–402
   schizophrnia, proxy consent in, 401
   suicide, 405–407
   surrogate consent for, 399–406
   surrogate/proxy consent in, 400–401, 406
   with cognitively impaired patients, ethicist positions, 404
      ethics codes, federal regulations, and state laws for, 402–403
      organizational position statements/proposed guidelines, 403–404
Guardianship, in geriatric psychiatry, 352

I

Informed consent, beneficence in, 396
   capacity assessments and, 396
   capacity for, instruments for assessment of, 397
   components in process of, 396
   components of, 317
   decisional capacity in, 396, 398–399
   in child and adolescent research, 368
   in consultation-liaison psychiatry, 317–318
   information, comprehension, voluntariness in, 387
   in geriatric psychiatry, cognitive impairment and, 345
      decisional capacity for, 344–347
      educational interventions in, 399
      factors affecting, 399
      institutionalization and, 345
      mood disorders and, 344–345
      schizophrenia and, 345
   in military psychiatry, 274
   in psychiatric research, 385
      advance directive for psychiatric research, 387–388
      decisional capacity in, 387
      information provided to participants, 387
      surrogate decision-making in, 387

Informed (*continued*)
    in psychotherapy, 301–302
    in substance use disorder research, 288–290
    in substance use disorder treatment, behavioral manifestations and, 288
        cognitive deficits and, 287–288
        free will vs. coercive factors in, 288
        involuntary commitment and protective custody, 288
        mandated treatment and, 289
        responsibility of user in, 288
    justice in, 396
    legal standards for, 396
    of children and adolescents, 247–248
    parents and legal guardians, 248
    respect for persons in, 395–396
    to treatment during pregnancy, 262–263

J

Justice, and boundaries in community psychiatry, 338
    dual agency and, 339
    in community psychiatry, distributive, 336–337
        systems level, 336
    in informed consent, 396
    in perinatal mental health, 261
    in preconception planning consultation with woman with schizophrenia, 264–265
    in psychiatric research, 384
    in reporting mental illness, 266
    in research ethics, 383

M

Maternal mental health screens, justice and report of risk for child maltreatment, 266
    pediatricians' obligations and, 266–267
Medical indications, in ethical decision making, 318–319
        in capacity for independent living, 324
        in case of unclear motivation, 325
        in legitimate desire to die, 320
        in refusal of evaluation and treatment, 322
Military psychiatry, confidentiality in, 272–274
    detainees, ethical considerations related to, 276–277
        professional ethics and primacy of mission in military ethics, 277
    dual agency of psychiatrist in, 275
    ethical issues in, **271–281**
    fitness for deployment, 272, 277–278
    fitness for duty vs. disability, 279–280
    informed consent in, basic elements in, 274
        perception of diminished self-determination in, 274
    maintaining boundaries in, 272, 275–276
    minimum mental health standards for deployment, 277–278
    psychotropic medication use in combat, 278–279
    separation from military, 279–280
    soldier's disposition from military, 272
Morality, emotion-driven, 440–441

N

Narrative ethics, in forensic psychiatry, 427–428
  in medical ethics, 428
Neuroenhancement, creativity perspective on, 444
    ethical controversies in, 441–443
        emotional, 442–443
        empirical, 442, 444
        impact on dignity, identity, authenticity, 443
        medical professionalism, 442, 445–446
        modes of inquiry into, 441–442
        philosophical, 443
        respect for persons and possible coercion, 444–445, 447
        risks and benefits to individuals, 442, 444
        social impact of, 442, 446–447
        theological, 441–442
    gratitude perspective on, 444
Neuroethics, 438
Neuroscience, philosophical and ethical issues in, **437–449**
    philosophical questions in, do human beings have free will, 439–440
        is mind independent from brain? 438–439
Nonmaleficence, and boundaries in community psychiatry, 338
    bias-free approach childbearing by women with psychotic disorders, 265
    boundary violations and, 333
    confidentiality and, 388
    dual agency and, 339
    in community psychiatry, 333, 335
    patient exploitation, 333
    seclusion and restraint and, 333

O

Omission bias, in perinatal mental health, 264

P

Parental notification, confidentiality and, 249
Parents, confidentiality and, 249
Patient preferences, in capacity for independent living, 324
    in case of unclear motivation, 325
    in legitimate desire to die, 320–321
    in refusal of evaluation and treatment, 322
Perinatal mental health, autonomy, beneficence, and relational ethics in, 260–261
    autonomy of mother in, 264
    conflict of interests in, 261
    decisional capacity of mother in, 261
    denial of pregnancy, preventive ethics and, 263
        psychiatric advance directives, 263
        substitute decision maker in, 262–263
    ethical assessment of parenting risks, 264–265
    ethical dilemmas in, 267
    ethical issues in, **259–270**
    ethics in, autonomy in, 260

Perinatal (*continued*)
>   beneficence in, 260
>   relational, 260–261
>   justice and directive counseling in, 261–262
>   major depression in, 263–264
>   maternal autonomy vs. beneficence to fetus, 260–262, 267
>   medication decisions and omission bias in, 263–264
>   omission bias in, 264
>   parenting risks in, assessment of, 264–265
>   preventive ethics in, 265
>   refusal of obstetric care in, 261–262
>   autonomy vs. beneficece to mother and fetus, 261–262
>   justice and directive counseling, 261–262
>   schizoaffective disorder patient, 262–263
>   screening for maternal mental illness, 266–267
>   substitute decision makers and preventive ethics, 262–263
>   surrogate decision-maker in, 261
Personal values, in forensic psychiatry, 434
Privacy, in psychiatric research, 384
Proxy consent, best interests standards for, 401, 405
>   decision-making ability of proxy, 401
>   in geriatric psychiatry research, 399–402
>   in patients with dementia, 400–401
>   substituted judgment standard for, 401, 405
Psychiatric advance directives, 263
Psychiatric education, cultivating Gregory's virtues, 417–420
>   ethical issues in, conflicts of interest, 419–420
>   sexual boundaries, patients and psychiatrists, 418–419
>   suicidal patients, 417–418
>   ethics of, **413–421**
>   John Gregory's ethics of medicine and, four fundamental virtues of, 415
>   interests and needs of patients before self interest, 415
>   lack of intellectual trust in physicians and, 414–415
>   psychiatric educators, teaching standards of intellectual and moral excellence, 416
>   teaching evicence-based medicine, 416–417
Psychiatric research, ethical issues in, **381–394**
>   confidentiality, 384, 388–389
>   conflicts of interest, 390–391
>   current, 389–392
>   ethical expertise of reseach team, 385–386
>   genetic technology, 390–391
>   informed consent, 385, 387–388
>   justice, 384
>   key concepts and safeguards, 385–389
>   National Bioethics Advisory Commission report on, 384
>   practical implications of empirical research, 389–390
>   privacy, 384
>   regulatory oversight in, 389
>   safeguards in, 390
>   stigma of mental illness, 384
>   study design and recruitment in, 385

veterans of Operation Enduring Freedom/Operation of Iraqi Freedom, 391–392
    vulnerable population in, 384, 386
Psychotherapy, boundaries in, nonsexual, 304–306
    sexual, 305–306
    violations of, 300–308
  confidentiality and privacy in, disclosure of information and, 309–310
    electronic records and, 309
    e-mail and, 309–310
    publication of case material, 309–311
  conflict of interest in, 301–302
  ethics in, **299–314**
  informed consent in, 301
  professional and therapeutic ethics in, 300–308

Q

Quality of life, in capacity for independent living, 324
  in case of unclear motivation, 325
  in legitimate desire to die, 321
  in refusal of evaluation and treatment, 323

R

Relational ethics, in perinatal mental health, 264
Research, child participants, capacity to assent and, 254
        vulnerability and need for safeguards in, 253
  clinical research organizations for, 362
  ethical issues in, **381–394**
  in child and adolescent psychiatry, **361–380**
  industry-sponsored studies, 362
  in geriatric psychiatry, **395–411**
  in private-practice offices, 362
  mature minor in, risk-benefit ratio and, 254
    waiver of parental permission for, 254
  need for, 381
  practice-based research networks for, 362
  prevalence of mental illness in U.S., 381
  site management organizations for, 362
Research ethics, general, 382–383
    Belmont Report of key issues with human participants, 383, 387
    federal regulatory framework for protection of human participants in research, 383
    history of abuses in U.S., 382–383
    Nuremberg Code and, 382
  in psychiatry, **381–394**
Respect for persons, in ethics of neuroenhancement, 447
  in forensic psychiatry, 434
  in informed consent, 395–396
  in research ethics, 383
  neuroenhancement and, 444–445
Risk–benefit, assessment in child and adolescent research, 365
  in child and adolescent research, 367

Risk–benefit ratio, for child and adolescent research participants, 254
Roles, in community psychiatry, 338–339
    in military psychiatry, 275
    in treatment of children, 251–252

S

Schizoaffective disorder, in perinatal mental health, 262–263
Schizophrenia, and decisional capacity of older patient, 398
    preconception planning consultation and, 264–265
Schizophrenia research, proxy consent in, 401
Sexual boundary violations, 305
    between patients and psychiatrists, 418–419
    consequences of, 307
    in psychiatric education, 418–419
    prevention of, 307
        Exploitation Index in, 308
        referral of patient elsewhere, 308
        supervision, 308
    understanding and preventing, 305, 307
Social justice, challenges in geriatric psychiatry, 343–344
    in forensic ethics, 428–429
    substance use disorder treatment and, 291–292
Stigma of mental illness, confidentiality and, 384, 388–389
    principle of justice and, 384
    protection of privacy and, 384
Substance use disorders (SUDs), addictions in, ethical issues in, 293–294
    confidentiality in, 284–287
    consequences of, mental health and psychosocial, 283–284
    economic costs of, 283
    ethics in treatment of, **283–297**
    informed consent and decisional capacity in, 287–290
    medical ethics applied to addiction, 284–285
    parity and, 290–293
        criminal justice system and, 292
        education deficit in health profession training, 291
        gap in services for women, 292
    prevalence of, 283
    social justice and, 290–293
Substitute decision-maker, in perinatal mental health, 261, 264
Substituted judgement, 261
    for proxies, 401, 405
    in psychiatric research, 387
Suicidal patients, ethical issues in, beneficence, 417
        emotional responses of caregivers, 417
        prevention and appropriate treatment, 417
        self-effacement and self-sacrifice and, 418
Surrogate decision maker, in geriatric psychiatry, 351–352
    in perinatal treatment, 261
    in psychiatric research, 387

T

Therapeutic misconception, in child and adolescent research, 369–370

V

Voluntarism, and cognitive impairment, 345–346
 and perception of diminished self-dtermination in service member-patient, 274
 in informed consent, 345–346, 388
 in substance use disorder treatment, 287–288, 291
Voluntarism capacity, 317

Related Interest:

Child and Adolescent Psychiatry Clinics of North America
Bipolar Disorder, April 2009
Jeffrey I. Hunt, MD and Daniel P. Dickstein, MD, *Guest Editors*

1. **The Concept of Bipolar Disorder in Children: A History of the Bipolar Controversy**, Gabrielle A. Carlson and Ira Glovinsky

2. **Phenomenology, Longitudinal Course, and Outcome of Children and Adolescents with Bipolar Spectrum Disorders**, Regina Sala, David Axelson, and Boris Birmaher

3. **Comorbidity in Pediatric Bipolar Disorder**, Gagan J. Sini and Timothy Wilens

4. **The Adverse Consequences of Sleep Disturbance in Pediatric Bipolar Disorders: Implications for Intervention**, Allison G. Harvey

5. **Suicidality in Pediatric Bipolar Disorder**, Tina R. Goldstein

6. **The Assessment of Children and Adolescents with Bipolar Disorder**, Eric A. Youngstom, Andrew J. Freeman, and Melissa McKeown Jenkins

7. **Preschool Bipolar Disorder**, Joan L. Luby, Mini Tandon, and Andy Belden

8. **Affect Regulation in Pediatric Bipolar Disorder**, Daniel P. Dickstein, Alison C. Brazel, Lisa D. Goldberg, and Jeffrey I. Hunt

9. **Magnetic Resonance Imaging Studies in Early Onset Bipolar Disorder: An Updated Review**, Janine Terry, Melissa Lopez-Larson, and Jean A. Frazier

10. **Family and Genetic Association Studies of Bipolar Disorder in Children**, Eric Mick and Stephen V. Faraone

11. **Pharmacologic Treatment of Pediatric Bipolar Disorder**, Jayasree J. Nandagopal, Melissa P. DelBello, and Robert Kowatch

12. **Psychosocial Treatments for Childhood and Adolescent Bipolar Disorder**, Amy E. West and Mani N. Pavuluri

13. **Alternative Treatments in Pediatric Bipolar Disorder**, Mona Potter, Alana Moses, and Janet Wozniak

14. **Raising a Bipolar Child: A Family Perspective**, Susan Resko

Moving?

Make sure your subscription moves with you!

To notify us of your new address, find your **Clinics Account Number** (located on your mailing label above your name), and contact customer service at:

E-mail: elspcs@elsevier.com

800-654-2452 (subscribers in the U.S. & Canada)
314-453-7041 (subscribers outside of the U.S. & Canada)

Fax number: 314-523-5170

Elsevier Periodicals Customer Service
11830 Westline Industrial Drive
St. Louis, MO 63146

*To ensure uninterrupted delivery of your subscription, please notify us at least 4 weeks in advance of move.

Printed and bound by CPI Group (UK) Ltd, Croydon, CR0 4YY

03/10/2024

01040452-0006